Estimation and Inferential Statistics

Pradip Kumar Sahu · Santi Ranjan Pal
Ajit Kumar Das

Estimation and Inferential Statistics

Springer

Pradip Kumar Sahu
Department of Agricultural Statistics
Bidhan Chandra Krishi Viswavidyalaya
Mohanpur, Nadia, West Bengal
India

Ajit Kumar Das
Department of Agricultural Statistics
Bidhan Chandra Krishi Viswavidyalaya
Mohanpur, Nadia, West Bengal
India

Santi Ranjan Pal
Department of Agricultural Statistics
Bidhan Chandra Krishi Viswavidyalaya
Mohanpur, Nadia, West Bengal
India

ISBN 978-81-322-3421-0 ISBN 978-81-322-2514-0 (eBook)
DOI 10.1007/978-81-322-2514-0

Springer New Delhi Heidelberg New York Dordrecht London

Softcover re-print of the Hardcover 1st edition 2015

Printed on acid-free paper

Springer (India) Pvt. Ltd. is part of Springer Science+Business Media (www.springer.com)

Preface

Nowadays one can hardly find any field where statistics is not used. With a given sample, one can infer about the population. The role of estimation and inferential statistics remains pivotal in the study of statistics. Statistical inference is concerned with problems of estimation of population parameters and test of hypotheses. In statistical inference, drawing a conclusion about the population takes place on the basis of a portion of the population. This book is written, keeping in mind the need of the users, present availability of literature to cater to these needs, their merits and demerits under a constantly changing scenario. Theories are followed by relevant worked-out examples which help the user grasp not only the theory but also practice them.

This work is a result of the experience of the authors in teaching and research work for more than 20 years. The wider scope and coverage of the book will help not only the students, researchers and professionals in the field of statistics but also several others in various allied disciplines. All efforts are made to present the "estimation and statistical inference", its meaning, intention and usefulness. This book reflects current methodological techniques used in interdisciplinary research, as illustrated with many relevant research examples. Statistical tools have been presented in such a manner, with the help of real-life examples, that the fear factor about the otherwise complicated subject of statistics will vanish. In its seven chapters, theories followed by examples will make the readers to find most suitable applications.

Starting from the meaning of the statistical inference, its development, different parts and types have been discussed eloquently. How someone can use statistical inference in everyday life has remained the main point of discussion in examples. How someone can draw conclusions about the population under varied situations, even without studying each and every unit of the population, has been discussed taking numerous examples. All sorts of inferential problems have been discussed, at one place supported by examples, to help the students not only in meeting their examination need and research requirement, but also in daily life. One can hardly get such a compilation of statistical inference in one place. The step-by-step procedure will immensely help not only the graduate and Ph.D. students but also other researchers and professionals. Graduate and postgraduate students, researchers and the professionals in various fields will be the user of the book. Researchers in medical and social and other disciplines will be greatly benefitted from the book. The book would also help students in various competitive examinations.

Written in a lucid language, the book will be useful to graduate, postgraduate and research students and practitioners in diverse fields including medical, social and other sciences. This book will also cater the need for preparation in different competitive examinations. One can find hardly a single book, in which all topics related to estimation and inference are included. Numerous relevant examples for related theories are added features of this book. An introduction chapter and an annexure are special features of this book which will help readers in getting basic ideas and plugging the loopholes of the readers. Chapter-wise summary of the content of the proposed book is presented below.

Estimation and Inferential Statistics

- Chapter 1: The chapter relates to introduction to the theory of point estimation and inferential statistics. Different criteria for a good estimator are discussed. The chapters also present real-life worked-out problems that help the reader understand the subject. Compared to partial coverage of this topic in most books on statistical inference, this book aims at elaborate coverage about the subject of point estimation.
- Chapter 2: This chapter deals with different methods of estimation like least square method, method of moments, method of minimum χ^2 and method of maximum likelihood estimation. Not all these methods are equally good and applicable in all situations. Merits, demerits and applicability of these methods have been discussed in one place, which otherwise have remained mostly dispersed or scattered in the competing literature.
- Chapter 3: Testing of hypotheses has been discussed in this chapter. This chapter is characterized by typical examples in different forms and spheres including Type A1 testing, which is mostly overlooked in many of the available literature. This has been done in this book.
- Chapter 4: The essence and technique of likelihood ratio test has been discussed in this chapter. Irrespective of the nature of tests for hypotheses (simple and composite), this chapter emphasizes how easily the test could be performed, supported by a good number of examples. Merits and drawbacks have also been discussed. Some typical examples are discussed in this chapter that one can hardly find in any other competing literature.

- Chapter 5: This chapter deals with interval estimation, techniques of interval estimation under different situations, problems and prospects of different approaches of interval estimation has been discussed with numerous examples in one place.
- Chapter 6: This chapter deals with non-parametric methods of testing hypotheses. All types of non-parametric tests have been put together and discussed in detail. In each case, suitable examples are the special feature of this chapter.
- Chapter 7: This chapter is devoted to the discussion of decision theory. This discussion is particularly useful to students and researchers interested in inferential statistics. In this chapter, attempt has been made to present the decision theory in an exhaustive manner, keeping in mind the requirement and the purpose of the reader for whom the book is aimed at. Bayes and mini-max method of estimation have been discussed in the Annexure. Most of the available literature on inferential statistics lack due attention on these important aspects of inference. In this chapter, the importance and utilities of the above methods have been discussed in detail, supported with relevant examples.
- Annexure: The authors feel that the Annexure portion would be an asset to varied types of readers of this book. Related topics, proofs, examples, etc., which could not be provided in the text itself, during the discussion of various chapter for the sake of maintenance of continuity and flow are provided in this section. Besides many useful proofs and derivations, this section includes transformation of statistics, large sample theories, exact tests related to binomial, Poisson population, etc. This added section will be of much help to the readers.

In each chapter, theories are followed by examples from applied fields, which will help the readers of this book to understand the theories and applications of specific tools. Attempts have been made to familiarize the problems with examples on each topic in a lucid manner. During the preparation of this book, a good number of books and articles from different national and international journals have been consulted. Efforts have been made to acknowledge and provide these in the bibliography section. An inquisitive reader may find more material from the literature cited.

The primary purpose of the book is to help students of statistics and allied fields. Sincere efforts have been made to present the material in the simplest and easy-to-understand form. Encouragements, suggestions and help received from our colleagues at the Department of Agricultural Statistics, Bidhan Chandra Krishi Viswavidyalaya are sincerely acknowledged. Their valuable suggestions towards improvement of the content helped a lot and are sincerely acknowledged. The authors thankfully acknowledge the constructive suggestions received from the reviewers towards the improvement of the book. Thanks are also due to Springer for the publication of this book and for continuous monitoring, help and suggestion during this book project. The authors acknowledge the help, cooperation, encouragement received from various corners, which are not mentioned here. The effort will be successful, if this book is well accepted by the students, teachers, researchers and other users to whom this book is aimed at. Every effort has been made to avoid errors. Constructive suggestions from the readers in improving the quality of this book will be highly appreciated.

Mohanpur, Nadia, India

Pradip Kumar Sahu
Santi Ranjan Pal
Ajit Kumar Das

Contents

About the Authors

P.K. Sahu is associate professor and head of the Department of Agricultural Statistics, Bidhan Chnadra Krishi Viswavidyalaya (a state agriculture university), West Bengal. With over 20 years of teaching experience, Dr. Sahu has published over 70 research papers in several international journals of repute and has guided several postgraduate students and research scholars. He has authored four books: *Agriculture and Applied Statistics*, Vol. 1, and *Agriculture and Applied Statistics*, Vol. 2 (both published with Kalyani Publishers), *Gender, Education, Empowerment: Stands of Women* (published with Agrotech Publishing House) and *Research Methodology: A Guide for Researchers In Agricultural Science, Social Science and Other Related Fields* (published by Springer) as well as contributed a chapter to the book *Modelling, Forecasting, Artificial Neural Network and Expert System in Fisheries and Aquaculture*, edited by Ajit Kumar Roy and Niranjan Sarangi (Daya Publishing House). Dr. Sahu has presented his research papers in several international conferences. He also visited the USA, Bangladesh, Sri Lanka, and Vietnam to attend international conferences.

S.R. Pal is former eminent professor at the Department of Agricultural Statistics at R.K. Mission Residential College and Bidhan Chandra Krishi Viswavidyalaya (a state agriculture university). An expert in agricultural statistics, Prof. Pal has over 35 years of teaching experience and has guided several postgraduate students and research scholars. He has several research papers published in statistics and related fields in several international journals of repute. With his vast experience in teaching, research and industrial advisory role, Prof. Pal has tried to incorporate the problems faced by the users, students, and researchers in this field.

A.K. Das is professor at the Department of Agricultural Statistics, Bidhan Chandra Krishi Viswavidyalaya (a state agriculture university). With over 30 years of teaching experience, Prof. Das has a number of good research articles to his credit published in several international journals of repute and has guided several postgraduate students and research scholars. He has coauthored a book, *Agriculture and Applied Statistics*, Vol. 2 (both published with Kalyani Publishers), and contributed a chapter to the book, *Modelling, Forecasting, Artificial Neural Network and Expert System in Fisheries and Aquaculture*, edited by Ajit Kumar Roy and Niranjan Sarangi (Daya Publishing House).

Introduction

In a statistical investigation, it is known that for reasons of time or cost, one may not be able to study each individual element of the population. In such a situation, a random sample should be taken from the population, and the inference can be drawn about the population on the basis of the sample. Hence, statistics deals with the collection of data and their analysis and interpretation. In this book, the problem of data collection is not considered. We shall take the data as given, and we study what they have to tell us. The main objective is to draw a conclusion about the unknown population characteristics on the basis of information on the same characteristics of a suitably selected sample. The observations are now postulated to be the values taken by random variables. Let X be a random variable which describes the population under investigation and F be the distribution function of X. There are two possibilities. Either X has a distribution function of F_θ with a known functional form (except perhaps for the parameter θ, which may be vector), or X has a distribution function F about which we know nothing (except perhaps that F is, say, absolutely continuous). In the former case, let Θ be the set of possible values of unknown parameter θ, then the job of statistician is to decide on the basis of suitably selected samples, which member or members of the family $\{F_\theta, \theta \in \Theta\}$ can represent the distribution function of X. These types of problems are called *problems of parametric statistical inference*. The two principal areas of statistical inference are the "area of estimation of parameters" and the "tests of statistical hypotheses". The problem of estimation of parameters involves both point and interval estimation. Diagrammatically, let us show components and constituents of statistical inference as in chart.

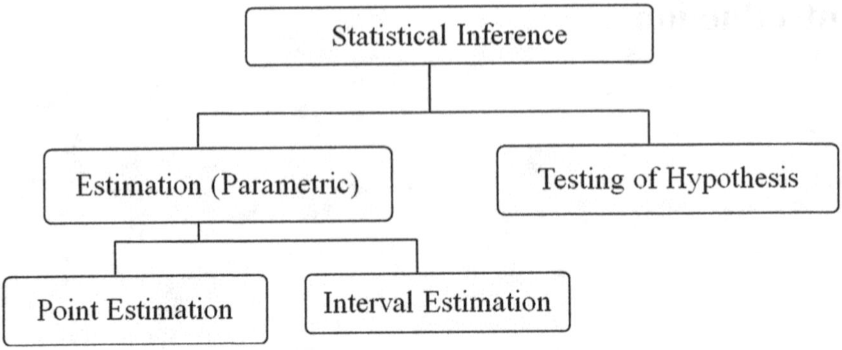

Problem of Point Estimation

The problem of point estimation relates to the estimating formula of a parameter based on random sample of size n from the population. The method basically comprises of finding out an estimating formula of a parameter, which is called the *estimator* of the parameter. The numerical value, which is obtained on the basis of a sample while using the estimating formula, is called *estimate*. Suppose, for an example, that a random variable X is known to have a normal distribution $N(\mu, \sigma^2)$, but we do not know one of the parameters, say μ. Suppose further that a sample $X_1, X_2, \ldots, X_n$ is taken on X. The problem of point estimation is to pick a statistic $T(X_1, X_2, \ldots, X_n)$ that best estimates the parameter μ. The numerical value of T when the realization is $x_1, x_2, \ldots, x_n$ is called an *estimate* of μ, while the statistic T is called an *estimator* of μ. If both μ and σ^2 are unknown, we seek a joint statistic $T = (U, V)$ as an estimate of (μ, σ^2).

Example Let $X_1, X_2, \ldots, X_n$ be a random sample from any distribution F_θ for which the mean exists and is equal to θ. We may want to estimate the mean θ of distribution. For this purpose, we may compute the mean of the observations $x_1, x_2, \ldots, x_n$, i.e., say

$$\bar{x} = \frac{1}{n}\sum_{i=1}^{n} x_i.$$

This $\bar{x}$ can be taken as the point estimate of θ.

Example Let $X_1, X_2, \ldots, X_n$ be a random sample from Poisson's distribution with parameter λ, i.e., $P(\lambda)$, where λ is not known. Then the mean of the observations $x_1, x_2, \ldots, x_n$, i.e.,

$$\bar{x} = \frac{1}{n}\sum_{i=1}^{n} x_i$$

is a point estimate of λ.

Example Let $X_1, X_2, \ldots, X_n$ be a random sample from a normal distribution with parameters μ and σ^2, i.e., $N(\mu, \sigma^2)$, where both μ and σ^2 are unknown. μ and σ^2 are the mean and variance respectively of the normal distribution. In this case, we may take a joint statistics $(\bar{x}, s^2)$ as a point estimate of $N(\mu, \sigma^2)$, where

$$\bar{x} = \frac{1}{n}\sum_{i=1}^{n} x_i = \text{sample mean}$$

and

$$s^2 = \frac{1}{n-1}\sum_{i=1}^{n} (x_1 - \bar{x})^2 = \text{sample mean square.}$$

Problem of Interval Estimation

In many cases, instead of point estimation, we are interested in constructing of a family of sets that contain the true (unknown) parameter value with a specified (high) probability, say $100(1-\alpha)\%$. This set is taken to be an interval, which is known as *confidence interval* with a confidence coefficient $(1-\alpha)$ and the technique of constructing such intervals is known as *interval estimation.*

Let $X_1, X_2, \ldots, X_n$ be a random sample from any distribution F_θ. Let $\underline{\theta}(x)$ and $\bar{\theta}(x)$ be functions of $x_1, x_2, \ldots, x_n$. If $P[\underline{\theta}(x) < \theta < \bar{\theta}(x)] = 1-\alpha$, then $(\underline{\theta}(x), \bar{\theta}(x))$ is called a $100(1-\alpha)\%$ confidence interval for θ, whereas $\underline{\theta}(x)$ and $\bar{\theta}(x)$ are, respectively, called lower and upper limits for θ.

Example Let $X_1, X_2, \ldots, X_n$ be random sample from $N(\mu, \sigma^2)$, whereas both μ and σ^2 are unknown. We can find $100(1-\alpha)\%$ confidence interval of μ. To estimate the population mean μ and population variance σ^2, we may take the observed sample mean

$$\bar{x} = \frac{1}{n}\sum_{i=1}^{n} x_i$$

and the observed sample mean square

$$s^2 = \frac{1}{n-1}\sum_{i=1}^{n} (x_i - \bar{x})^2$$

respectively. $100(1-\alpha)\%$ confidence interval of μ is given by

$$\bar{x} \pm t_{\frac{\alpha}{2},n-1} \frac{s}{\sqrt{n}}$$

where $t_{\frac{\alpha}{2},n-1}$ is the upper $\frac{\alpha}{2}$ point of the t-distribution with $(n-1)$ d.f.

Problem of Testing of Hypothesis

Besides point estimation and interval estimation, we are often required to decide which value among a set of values of a parameter is true for a given population distribution, or we may be interested in finding out the relevant distribution to describe a population. The procedure by which a decision is taken regarding the plausible value of a parameter or the nature of a distribution is known as the *testing of hypotheses*. Some examples of hypothesis, which can be subjected to statistical tests, are as follows:

1. The average length of life μ of electric light bulbs of a certain brand is equal to some specified value μ_0.
2. The average number of bacteria killed by tests drops of germicide is equal to some number.
3. Steel made by method A has a mean hardness greater than steel made by method B.
4. Penicillin is more effective than streptomycin in the treatment of disease X.
5. The growing period of one hybrid of corn is more variable than the growing period for other hybrids.
6. The manufacturer claims that the tires made by a new process have mean life greater than the life of a tire manufactured by an earlier process.
7. Several varieties of wheat are equally important in terms of yields.
8. Several brands of batteries have different lifetimes.
9. The characters in the population are uncorrelated.
10. The proportion of non-defective items produced by machine A is greater than that of machine B.

The examples given are simple in nature, and are well established and have well-accepted decision rules.

Problems of Non-parametric Estimation

So far we have assumed in statistical inference (parametric) that the distribution of the random variable being sampled is known except for some parameters. In practice, the functional form of the distribution is unknown. Here, we are not concerned to the techniques of estimating the parameters directly, but with certain pertinent hypothesis relating to the properties of the population, such as equalities of distribution, tests of randomness of the sample without making any assumption about the nature of the distribution function. Statistical inference under such a setup is called non-parametric.

Bayes Estimator

In case of parametric inference, we consider density function $f(x/\theta)$, where θ is a fixed unknown quantity which can take any value in parametric space Θ. In Bayesian approach, it is assumed that θ itself is a random variable and density $f(x/\theta)$ is the density of x for a given θ. For example, suppose we are interested in estimating P, the fraction of defective items in a consignment. Consider a collection of lots, called superlots. It may happen that the parameter P may differ from lot to lot. In the classical approach, we consider P as a fixed unknown parameter, whereas in Bayesian approach, we say that P varies from lot to lot. It is random variable having a density $f(P)$, say. Bayes method tries to use this additional information about P.

Example Let $X_1, X_2, \ldots X_n$ be a random sample from PDF

$$f(x;a,b) = \frac{1}{\beta(a,b)} x^{a-1}(1-x)^{b-1},\ 0<x<1; a,b>0.$$

Find the estimators of a and b by the method of moments.

Answer
We know

$$E(x) = \mu_1^1 = \frac{a}{a+b} \quad \text{and} \quad E(x^2) = \mu_2^1 = \frac{a(a+1)}{(a+b)(a+b+1)}$$

Hence

$$\frac{a}{a+b} = \overline{x},\ \frac{a(a+1)}{(a+b)(a+b+1)} = \frac{1}{n}\sum_{i=1}^{n} x_i^2$$

Solving, we get

$$\widehat{b} = \frac{(\overline{x}-1)\left(\sum x_i^2 - n\overline{x}\right)}{\left(\sum x_i - \overline{x}\right)^2} \quad \text{and} \quad \widehat{a} = \frac{\overline{x}\widehat{b}}{1-\overline{x}}$$

Example Let $X_1, X_2, \ldots X_n$ be a random sample from PDF

$$f(x;\theta,r) = \frac{1}{\theta^r \sqrt{r}} e^{-x/\theta} x^{r-|1},\ x>0; \theta>0, r>0$$

Find estimator of θ and r by

(i) Method of moments
(ii) Method of maximum likelihood

Answer
Here

$$E(x) = \mu_1^1 = r\theta, E(x^2) = \mu_2^1 = r(r+1)\theta^2 \text{ and } m_1^1 = \bar{x},\ m_2^1 = \frac{1}{n}\sum_{i=1}^{n} x_i^2$$

Hence

$$r\theta = \bar{x}, r(r+1)\theta^2 = \frac{1}{n}\sum_{i=1}^{n} x_i^2$$

Solving, we get

$$\widehat{r} = \frac{n\bar{x}^2}{\sum\limits_{i=1}^{n}(x_i - \bar{x})^2} \quad \text{and} \quad \widehat{\theta} = \frac{\sum\limits_{i=1}^{n}(x_i - \bar{x})^2}{n\bar{x}}$$

(i) $L = \frac{1}{\theta^{nr}(\sqrt{r})^n} e^{-\frac{1}{\theta}\sum\limits_{i=1}^{n} x_i} \prod\limits_{i=1}^{n} x_i^{r-1}$

(ii) $\log L = -nr\log\theta - n\log\sqrt{n} - \frac{1}{\theta}\sum\limits_{i} x_i + (r-1)\sum\limits_{i=1}^{n} wgx_i$

Now,

$$\frac{\partial \log L}{\partial \theta} = -\frac{nr}{\theta} + \frac{n\bar{x}}{\theta^2} = 0 \Rightarrow \widehat{\theta} = \frac{\bar{x}}{r}$$

Or

$$\frac{\partial \log L}{\partial r} = -n\log\theta - n\frac{\partial \log\sqrt{r}}{\partial r} + \sum_{i=1}^{n}\log x_i$$
$$= n\log r - n\frac{\tau(r)}{\sqrt{r}} - n\log\bar{x} + \sum_{i}^{n}\log x_i$$

It is, however, difficult to solve the equation

$$\frac{\partial \log L}{\partial r} = 0$$

and to get the estimate of r. Thus, for this example, estimators of θ and r are more easily obtained by the method of moments than the method of maximum likelihood.

Example Find the estimators of α and β by the method of moments.

Proof We know

$$E(x) = \mu_1^1 = \frac{\alpha+\beta}{2} \quad \text{and} \quad V(x) = \mu_2 \frac{(\beta-\alpha)^2}{12}$$

Hence

$$\frac{\alpha+\beta}{2} = \bar{x} \quad \text{and} \quad \frac{(\beta-\alpha)^2}{12} = \frac{1}{n}\sum_{i=1}^{n}(x_i-\bar{x})^2$$

Solving, we get

$$\widehat{\alpha} = \bar{x} - \sqrt{\frac{3\sum(x_i-\bar{x})^2}{n}} \quad \text{and} \quad \widehat{\beta} = \bar{x} + \sqrt{\frac{3\sum(x_i-\bar{x})^2}{n}}$$

Example If a sample of size one be drawn from the PDF $f(x,\beta) = \frac{2}{\beta^2}(\beta - x),\ 0 < x < \beta$ find $\widehat{\beta}$, the MLE of β and β^* the estimator of β based on method of moments. Show that $\widehat{\beta}$ is biased but β^* is unbiased. Show that the efficiency of $\widehat{\beta}$ with respect to β^* is 2/3.

Solution
Here suppose

$$L = \frac{2}{\beta^2}(\beta - x)$$

Then

$$\text{Log}L = \text{Log}2 - 2\log\beta + \log(\beta - x)$$

Or

$$\frac{\partial \log L}{\partial \beta} = -\frac{2}{\beta^2} + \frac{1}{\beta - x} = 0 \Rightarrow \beta = 2x$$

Now,

$$E(x) = \frac{2}{\beta}\int_0^{\beta}(\beta x - x^2)\,dx = \frac{\beta}{3}$$

Hence

$$\frac{\beta}{3} = x \Rightarrow \beta = 3x$$

Thus the estimator of β based on method of moments is given as $\beta^* = 3x$. Now,

$$E(\widehat{\beta}) = 2 \times \frac{\beta}{3} = \frac{2\beta}{3} \neq \beta$$
$$E(\beta^*) = 3 \times \frac{\beta}{3} = \beta$$

Hence $\widehat{\beta}$ is biased but β^* is unbiased.
Again

$$E(x^2) = \frac{2}{\beta^2} \int_0^\beta (\beta x^2 - x^3)\, dx = \frac{\beta^2}{6}$$

Therefore,

$$V(x) = \frac{\beta^2}{6} - \frac{\beta^2}{9} = \frac{\beta^2}{18}$$

Solving, we get

$$V(\beta^*) = 9V(x) = \frac{\beta^2}{9}$$
$$V(\widehat{\beta}) = 4V(x) = \frac{2}{9}\beta^2$$

Hence

$$M(\widehat{\beta}) = V(\widehat{\beta}) + \left[E(\widehat{\beta}) - \beta\right]^2$$
$$= \frac{2}{9}\beta^2 + \left(\frac{2}{3}\beta - \beta\right)^2$$
$$= \frac{1}{3}\beta^2$$

Thus the efficiency of $\widehat{\beta}$ with respect to β^* is 2/3.

Example Let $(x_1, x_2, \ldots x_n)$ be a given sample of size n. It is to be tested whether the sample comes from some Poisson distribution with unknown mean μ. How do you estimate μ by the method of modified minimum chi-square?

Solution

Let $x_1, x_2, \ldots x_n$ be arranged in K groups such that there are ni observations with $x = i, i = r+1, \ldots, r+k-2$, n_L observations $x \leq r$, and n_u observations with $x \geq r+k-1$, so that the smallest and the largest values of x that are fewer are pooled together and

$$n_L + \sum_{i=r+1}^{r+k-2} n_i + n_u = n$$

Let

$$\pi_i(\mu) = P(x = i) = \frac{e^{-u}\mu^i}{i!}$$

$$\pi_L(\mu) = P(x \leq r) = \sum_{i=0}^{n} \pi_i(\mu)$$

$$\pi_u(\mu) = P(x \geq r+k-1) = \sum_{i=r+k-1}^{\infty} \pi_i(\mu)$$

Now, by using

$$\sum_{i=1}^{k} \frac{n_i}{\pi_i(\theta)} \frac{\partial \pi_i(\theta)}{\partial \theta_j} = 0 j = 1, 2, \ldots .p$$

We have

$$n_L \frac{\sum_{i=0}^{r} \left(\frac{i}{\mu} - 1\right)\pi_i(\mu)}{\sum_{i=0}^{r} \pi_i(\mu)} + \sum_{i=r+1}^{r+k-2} n_i\left(\frac{i}{\mu} - 1\right) + n_u \frac{\sum_{i=r+k-1}^{\infty} \left(\frac{i}{\mu} - 1\right)\pi_i(\mu)}{\sum_{i=r+k-1}^{\infty} \pi_i(\mu)} = 0$$

Since there is only one parameter, i.e., $p = 1$ we get the only above equation. Solving,we get

$$n\hat{\mu} = n_L \frac{\sum_{i=0}^{r} i\pi_i(\mu)}{\sum_{i=0}^{r} \pi_i(\mu)} + \sum_{i=r+1}^{r+k-2} in_i + n_u \frac{\sum_{i=r+k-1}^{\infty} i\pi_i(\mu)}{\sum_{i=r+k-1}^{\infty} \pi_i(\mu)}$$

$$= \text{sum of all } x\text{'s}$$

Hence $\hat{\mu}$ is approximately the sample mean $\bar{x}$

Example In general, we consider n uncorrelated observations $y_1, y_2, \ldots y_n$ such that $E(y_i) = \beta_1 x_{1i} + \beta_2 x_{2i} + \ldots\ldots\ldots\ldots + \beta_k x_{ki}$ and $V(y_i) = \sigma^2, i = 1, 2, \ldots\ldots, n,\ x_{1i} = 1 \forall i$, where $\beta_1, \beta_2 \ldots\ldots\ldots\ldots \beta_k$ and σ^2 are unknown parameters. If Y and β^* stand for column vectors of the variables y_i and parameters β_j and if $X = (x_{ji})$ be an $(n \times k)$ matrix of known coefficients x_{ji} the above equation can be written as

$$E(Y) = X\beta^* \quad \text{and} \quad V(e) = E(ee') = \sigma^2 I$$

Where $e = Y - X\beta^*$ is an $(n \times 1)$ vector of error random variable with $E(e) = 0$ and I is an $(n \times n)$ identity matrix. The least square method requires that β's be calculated such that $\phi = ee' = (Y - X\beta^*)'(Y - X\beta^*)$be the minimum. This is satisfied when

$$\frac{\partial \phi}{\partial \beta^*} = 0 \quad \text{on} \quad 2X'(Y - X\beta^*) = 0$$

The least square estimators β' s is thus given by the vector $\hat{\beta}^* = (X'X)^{-1}X'Y$.

Example Let $y_i = \beta_1 x_{1i} + \beta_2 x_{2i} + \ldots\ldots\ldots\ldots + \beta_k x_{ki},\ i = 1, 2, \ldots\ldots, n$ or $E(y_i) = \beta_1 x_{1i} + \beta_2 x_{2i},\ x_{1i} = 1$ for all i. Find the least square estimates of β_1 and β_2. Prove that the method of maximum likelihood and the method of least square are identical for the case of normal distribution.

Solution

In matrix notation, we have

$$E(Y) = X\beta^* \text{ where } X = \begin{pmatrix} 1 & x_{21} \\ 1 & x_{22} \\ \vdots & \vdots \\ 1 & x_{2n} \end{pmatrix},\ \beta^* = \begin{pmatrix} \beta_1 \\ \beta_2 \end{pmatrix} \quad \text{and} \quad Y = \begin{pmatrix} y_1 \\ y_2 \\ \vdots \\ y_n \end{pmatrix}$$

Now,

$$\hat{\beta}^* = (X'X)^{-1}X'Y$$

Here

$$X'X = \begin{pmatrix} 1 & 1 & \ldots & 1 \\ x_{21} & x_{22} & \ldots & x_{2n} \end{pmatrix} \begin{pmatrix} 1 & x_{21} \\ 1 & x_{22} \\ \vdots & \vdots \\ 1 & x_{2n} \end{pmatrix} = \begin{pmatrix} n & \sum x_{2i} \\ \sum x_{2i} & \sum x_{2i}^2 \end{pmatrix}$$

$$X'Y = \begin{pmatrix} \sum y_i \\ \sum x_{2i} y_i \end{pmatrix}$$

Then

$$\hat{\beta}^* = \frac{1}{n\sum x_{2i}^2 - (\sum x_{2i})^2}\begin{pmatrix} \sum x_{2i}^2 & -\sum x_{2i} \\ -\sum x_{2i} & n \end{pmatrix}\begin{pmatrix} \sum y_i \\ \sum x_{2i}y_i \end{pmatrix}$$

$$= \frac{1}{n\sum x_{2i}^2 - (\sum x_{2i})^2}\begin{pmatrix} \sum x_{2i}^2 \sum y_i - \sum x_{2i} \sum x_{2i}y_i \\ -\sum x_{2i}\sum y_i + n\sum x_{2i}\sum y_i \end{pmatrix}$$

Hence

$$\hat{\beta}_2 = \frac{n\sum x_{2i}\sum y_i - \sum x_{2i}\sum y_i}{n\sum x_{2i}^2 - (\sum x_{2i})^2}$$

$$= \frac{\sum x_{2i}\sum y_i - n\bar{x}_2\bar{y}}{\sum x_{2i}^2 - n\bar{x}_2^2}$$

$$= \frac{\sum (x_{2i} - \bar{x}_2)(y_i - \bar{y})}{\sum (x_{2i} - \bar{x}_2)^2}$$

and

$$\hat{\beta}_1 = \frac{\sum x_{2i}^2 \sum y_i - \sum x_{2i}\sum x_{2i}y_i}{n\sum x_{2i}^2 - (\sum x_{2i})^2}$$

$$= \frac{\bar{y}\sum x_{2i}^2 - \bar{x}_2\sum x_{2i}y_i}{\sum x_{2i}^2 - n\bar{x}^2}$$

$$= \bar{y} + \frac{\bar{y}n\bar{x}_2^2 - \bar{x}_2\sum x_{2i}y_i}{\sum x_{2i}^2 - n\bar{x}_2^2}$$

$$= \bar{y} - \bar{x}_2\hat{\beta}_2$$

Let y_i be an independent $N(\beta_1 + \beta_2 x_i, \sigma^2)$ variate, $i = 1, 2, \ldots\ldots, n$ so that $E(y_i) = \beta_1 + \beta_2 x_{i.}$ The estimators of β_1 and β_2 are obtained by the method of least square on minimizing

$$\phi = \sum_{i=1}^{n} (y_i - \beta_1 - \beta_2 x_i)^2$$

The likelihood estimate is

$$L = \left(\frac{1}{\sqrt{2\pi}\sigma}\right)^n e^{\frac{1}{2\sigma^2}\sum (y_i - \beta_1 - \beta_2 x_i)^2}$$

L is maximum when $\sum_{i=1}^{n} (y_i - \beta_1 - \beta_2 x_i)^2$ is minimum. By the method of maximum likelihood we choose β_1 and β_2 such that $\sum_{i=1}^{n} (y_i - \beta_1 - \beta_2 x_i)^2 = \phi$ is minimum. Hence both the methods of least square and maximum likelihood estimator are identical.

Chapter 1
Theory of Point Estimation

1.1 Introduction

In carrying out any statistical investigation, we start with a suitable probability model for the phenomenon that we seek to describe (The choice of the model is dictated partly by the nature of the phenomenon and partly by the way data on the phenomenon are collected. Mathematical simplicity is also a point that is given some consideration in choosing the model). In general, model takes the form of specification of the joint distribution function of some random variables $X_1, X_2, \ldots X_n$ (all or some of which may as well be multidimensional). According to the model, the distribution function F is supposed to be some (unspecified) member of a more or less general class $\mathbb{F}$ of distribution functions.

Example 1.1 In many situations, we start by assuming that $X_1, X_2, \ldots X_n$ are iid (independently and identically distributed) unidimensional r.v's (random variables) with a common but unspecified distribution function, F_1, say. In other words, the model states that F is some member of the class of all distribution functions of the form

$$F(x_1, x_2, \ldots, x_n) = \prod_{i=1}^{n} F_1(x_i).$$

Example 1.2 In traditional statistical practice, it is frequently assumed that $X_1, X_2 \ldots X_n$ have each the normal distribution (but its mean and/or variance being left unspecified), besides making the assumption that they are iid r.v's.

In carrying out the statistical investigation, we then take as our goal, the task of specifying F more completely than is done by the model. This task is achieved by taking a set of observations on the r.v's $X_1, X_2, \ldots, X_n$. These observations are the raw material of the investigation and we may denote them, respectively, by $x_1, x_2, \ldots, x_n$. These are used to make a guess about the distribution function F, which is partly unknown.

P.K. Sahu et al., *Estimation and Inferential Statistics*,
DOI 10.1007/978-81-322-2514-0_1

The process is called Statistical Inference, being similar to the process of inductive inference as envisaged in classical logic. For here too the problem is to know the general nature of the phenomenon under study (as represented by the distribution of the r.v's) on the basis of the particular set of observations. The only difference that in a statistical investigation induction is achieved within a probabilistic framework. Probabilistic considerations enter into the picture in three ways. Firstly, the model used to represent the field of study is probabilistic. Second, certain probabilistic principles provide the guidelines in making the inference. Third, as we shall see in the sequel, the reliability of the conclusions also is judged in probabilistic terms.

Random Sampling

Consider a statistical experiment that culminate in outcomes x which are the values assumed by a r.v. X. Let F be the distribution function of X. One can also obtain n independent observations on X. This means that the n values observed as $x_1, x_2, \ldots, x_n$ are assumed by the r.v. X [This can be obtained by replicating the experiment under (more or less) identical conditions]. Again each x_i may be regarded as the value assumed by a r.v. X_i, $i = 1\ (1)n$, where $X_1, X_2, \ldots X_n$ are independent random variables with common distribution function F. The set $X_1, X_2, \ldots X_n$ of iid r.v's is known as a random sample from the distribution function F. The set of values $(x_1, x_2, \ldots, x_n)$ is called a realization of the sample $(X_1, X_2, \ldots, X_n)$.

Parameter and Parameter Space

A constant which changes its value from one situation to another is knownparameter. The set of all admissible values of a parameter is often called the parameter space. Parameter is denoted by θ (θ may be a vector). We denote the parameter space by Θ.

Example 1.3

(a) Let $y = 2x + \theta$. Here, θ is a parameter and

$$\Theta = \{\theta, -\propto < \theta < \propto\}.$$

(b) Let $x \sim b(1, \pi)$. Here, π is a parameter and

$$\Theta = \{\pi, 0 < \pi < 1\}.$$

(c) Let $x \sim P(\lambda)$ Here, λ is a parameter and

$$\Theta = \{\lambda, \lambda > 0\}.$$

(d) Let $x \sim N(\mu_0, \sigma^2)$, μ_0 is a known constant.
Here, σ is a parameter and $\Theta = \{\sigma, \sigma > 0\}$.

(e) Let $x \sim N(\mu, \sigma^2)$, both μ and σ are unknown.
Here, $\theta = \begin{pmatrix} \mu \\ \sigma \end{pmatrix}$ is a parameter and $\Theta = \left\{ \binom{\mu}{\sigma}, -\infty < \mu < \infty, \sigma > 0 \right\}$

Family of distributions
Let $X \sim F_\theta$ where $\theta \, \varepsilon \, \Theta$. Then the set of distribution functions $\{F_\theta, \theta \, \varepsilon \, \Theta\}$ is called a family of distribution functions.

Similarly, we define family of p.d.f's and family of p.m.f's.

Remark

(1) If functional form of F_θ is known, then θ can be taken as an index.
(2) In the theory of estimation, we restrict ourselves to the case $\Theta \subseteq R^k$ when k is the number of unknown functionally unrelated parameters.

Statistic
A statistic is a function of observable random variable which must be free from unknown parameter(s), that is a Borel measurable function of sample observations $\underset{\sim}{X} = (x_1, x_2, \ldots, x_n) \in R^n \; f : R^n \to R^k$ is often called a statistic.

Example 1.4 Let $X_1, X_2 \ldots X_n$ be a random sample from $N(\mu, \sigma^2)$. Thus $\sum X_i, \sum X_i^2, (\sum X_i, \sum X_i^2)$ each of these is a statistic.

Estimator and estimate
Any statistic which is used to estimate (or to guess) $\tau(\theta)$, a function of unknown parameter θ, is said to be an estimator of $\tau(\theta)$. The experimentally determined value of an estimator is called an estimate.

Example 1.5 Let $X_1, X_2, \ldots, X_5$ be a random sample from $P(\lambda)$.

An estimator of λ is $\bar{X} = \frac{1}{5}\sum_{i=1}^{5} X_i$.

Suppose the experimentally determined values are $X_1 = 1$, $X_2 = 4$, $X_3 = 2$, $X_4 = 6$ and $X_5 = 0$.

Then the estimate of λ is $\frac{1+4+2+6+0}{5} = 2.6$.

1.2 Sufficient Statistic

In statistics, the job of a statistician is to interpret the data that he has collected and to draw statistically valid conclusion about the population under investigation. But, in many cases the raw data, which are too numerous and too costly to store, are not suitable for this purpose. Therefore, the statistician would like to condense the data by computing some statistics and to base his analysis on these statistics so that there is no loss of relevant information in doing so, that is the statistician would like to choose those statistics which exhaust all information about the parameter, which is contained in the sample. Keeping this idea in mind, we define sufficient statistics as follows:

Definition Let $\underset{\sim}{X} = (X_1, X_2, \ldots, X_n)$ be a random sample from $\{F_\theta, \; \theta \in \Theta\}$. A statistic $T(\underset{\sim}{X})$ is said to be sufficient for θ [or for the family of distribution $\{F_\theta, \; \theta \in \Theta\}$] iff the conditional distribution of $\underset{\sim}{X}$ given T is free from θ.

Illustration 1.1 Suppose we want to study the nature of a coin. To do this, we want to estimate p, the probability of getting head in a single toss. To estimate p, n tosses are performed. Suppose the results are $X_1, X_2, \ldots, X_n$ where

$$X_i = \begin{cases} 0 & \text{if tail appears} \\ 1 & \text{if head appears (in } i\text{th toss).} \end{cases}$$

Intuitively, it sums unnecessary to mention the order of occurrences of head. To estimate p, it is enough to keep the record of the number of heads. So the statistic $T = \Sigma X_i$ should be sufficient for p.

Again, conditional distribution of $X_1 = x_1, X_2 = x_2, \ldots, X_n = x_n$ given $T(\underset{\sim}{X}) = t$ where $t = T\ (X_1 = x_1, X_2 = x_2, \ldots, X_n = x_n)$ is given by

$$\begin{cases} \frac{P(X_1 = x_1, X_2 = x_2, \ldots, X_n = x_n, T = t)}{P(T = t)} & \text{if } T = t \\ 0 & \text{otherwise} \end{cases}$$

$$= \begin{cases} \frac{p^{\sum x_i}(1-p)^{n-\sum x_i}}{\binom{n}{t} p^t (1-p)^{n-t}} & \text{if } \quad T = t \\ 0 & \text{otherwise} \end{cases}$$

$$= \begin{cases} \frac{1}{\binom{n}{t}} & \text{if } \quad T = t \\ 0 & \text{otherwise} \end{cases}$$

which is free from parameter p.

So from definition of sufficient statistics, we observe that Σx_i is a sufficient statistic for p.

Illustration 1.2 Let $X_1, X_2, \ldots, X_n$ be a random samples from $N(\mu, 1)$ where μ is unknown. Consider an orthogonal transformation of the form

$$y_1 = \frac{X_1 + X_2 + \cdots + X_n}{\sqrt{n}}$$

$$\text{and} \quad y_k = \frac{(k-1)X_k - (X_1 + X_2 + \cdots + X_{k-1})}{\sqrt{k(k-1)}}, \quad k = 2(1)n.$$

Clearly, $y_1 \sim N(\sqrt{n}\,\mu, 1)$ and each of $y_k \sim N(0, 1)$.

Again, $y_1, y_{2,\ldots}, y_n$ are independent.

Note that the joint distribution of $y_2, y_3, \ldots, y_n$ does not involve μ, i.e. $y_2, \ldots, y_n$ do not provide any information on μ. So to estimate μ, we use either the observations on $X_1, X_2, \ldots X_n$ or simply the observed value of y_1. So any analysis based on y_1, is just as effective as the analysis that is based on all observed values on $X_1, X_2, \ldots X_n$. Hence, we can suggest that y_1 is a sufficient statistic for μ.

From the above discussion, we see that the conditional distribution of $(y_2, y_3, \ldots, y_n)$ given y_1 is same as the unconditional distribution of $(y_2, y_3, \ldots, y_n)$. Hence, the conditional distribution of $\underset{\sim}{X}$ given y_1 will be free from μ.

Thus according to the definition of sufficient statistics, y_1 will be a sufficient statistic for μ.

However, this approach is not always fruitful. To overcome this, we consider a necessary and sufficient condition for a statistic to be sufficient.

We first consider the Fisher–Neyman criterion for the existence of a sufficient statistic for a parameter.

Let $\underset{\sim}{X} = (X_1, X_2, \ldots, X_n)$ be a random sample from a population with continuous distribution function F_θ, $\theta \in \Theta$. Let $T(\underset{\sim}{X})$ be a statistic whose probability density function is $\{g\{T(\underset{\sim}{x}); \theta\}\}$. Then $T(\underset{\sim}{X})$ is a sufficient statistic for θ iff the joint probability density function $f(\underset{\sim}{x}, \theta)$ of $X_1, X_2, \ldots, X_n$ can be expressed as $f(\underset{\sim}{X}, \theta) = g\{T(\underset{\sim}{x}); \theta\}h(\underset{\sim}{x})$ whose, for every fixed value of $T(\underset{\sim}{x})$, $h(\underset{\sim}{x})$ does not depend upon θ.

Example 1.5 Let $X_1, X_2, \ldots, X_n$ be a random sample from the distribution that has probability mass function

$f(x, \theta) = \theta^x (1-\theta)^{1-x}$, $x = 0, 1; 0 < \theta < 1$. The statistic $T\left(\underset{\sim}{X}\right) = \sum_{i=1}^{n} X_i$ has the probability mass function

$$g(t; \theta) = \frac{n!}{t!(n-t)!}\theta^t (1-\theta)^{n-t}, t = 0, 1, 2, \ldots, n$$

Thus the joint probability mass function of $X_1, X_2, \ldots, X_n$ may be written

$$f\left(\underset{\sim}{x}, \theta\right) = \theta^{x_1 + x_2 + \cdots + x_n} \cdot (1-\theta)^{n-(x_1 + x_2 + \cdots + x_n)}$$

$$= \frac{n!}{t!(n-t)!}\theta^t (1-\theta)^{n-t} \ldots \frac{t!(n-t)!}{n!}$$

By Fisher–Neyman criterion, $T\left(\underset{\sim}{X}\right) = X_1 + X_2 + \cdots + X_n$ is a sufficient statistic for θ. In some cases, it is quite tedious to find the p.d.f or p.m.f of a certain statistic which is or is not a sufficient statistic for θ. This problem can be avoided if we use the following

Fisher–Neymann factorization theorem

Let $\underset{\sim}{X} = (X_1, X_2, \ldots X_n)$ be a random sample from a population with c.d.f. F_θ, $\theta \,\varepsilon\, \Theta$. Furthermore, let all $X_1, X_2, \ldots X_n$ are of discrete type or of continuous type. Then a statistic $T(\underset{\sim}{x})$ will be sufficient for θ or for $\{F_\theta, \theta \varepsilon \Theta\}$ iff the joint p.m.f. or p.d.f. $f(\underset{\sim}{X}, \theta)$, of $X_1, X_2, \ldots X_n$ can be expressed as

$$f(\underset{\sim}{X}, 0) = g\{T(\underset{\sim}{X}), \theta\} \cdot h(\underset{\sim}{x})$$

where the first factor $g\{T(\underset{\sim}{x}), \theta\}$ is a function of θ and x only through $T(\underset{\sim}{x})$ and for fixed $T(\underset{\sim}{x})$ the second factor $h(\underset{\sim}{x})$ is free from θ and is non-negative.

Remark 1.1 When we say that a function is free from θ, we do not only mean that θ does not appear in the **functional form** but also the domain of the function does not involve θ.

e.g. the function

$$f(x) = \begin{cases} 1/2, & \theta - 1 < x < \theta + 1 \\ 0 & \text{otherwise} \end{cases}$$

does depend upon θ.

Corollary 1.1 *Let* $T\left(\underset{\sim}{X}\right)$ *be a sufficient statistic for* θ *and* $T'\left(\underset{\sim}{X}\right) = \psi\left\{T\left(\underset{\sim}{X}\right)\right\}$ *be a one-to-one function of T. Then* $T'\left(\underset{\sim}{X}\right)$ *is also sufficient for the same parameters* θ.

Proof Since T is sufficient for θ, by factorization theorem, we have

$$f(\underset{\sim}{x}, \theta) = g\{T(\underset{\sim}{x}), \theta\} \cdot h(\underset{\sim}{x})$$

Since the function $T'\left(\underset{\sim}{x}\right)$ is one-to-one

$$f(\underset{\sim}{x}, \theta) = g\left[\psi^{-1}\{T'(\underset{\sim}{x})\}, \theta\right] h(\underset{\sim}{x}).$$

□

Clearly, the first factor of R.H.S. depends on θ and $\underset{\sim}{x}$ only through $T'(\underset{\sim}{x})$ and the second factor $h(\underset{\sim}{x})$ is free from θ and is non-negative.

Therefore, according to factorizability criterion, we can say that $T'(\underset{\sim}{x})$ is also sufficient for the same parameter θ.

Example 1.6 Let $X_1, X_2, \ldots X_n$ be a random sample from $b(1, \pi)$. We show that $^1/_n$ ΣX_i is a sufficient statistic for π.

P.m.f. of x is

$$f_\theta(x) = \begin{cases} \theta^X(1 - \theta)^{1-X} & \text{if } x = 0,\ 1 \quad [\theta \equiv \pi] \\ 0 & \text{otherwise} \end{cases}$$

where $0 < \theta < 1$, i.e. the parameter space is $\Theta = (0, 1)$. Writing $f_\theta(x)$ in the form

$$f_\theta(x) = C(x)\theta^x(1 - \theta)^{1-x} \qquad \text{with } C(x) = \begin{cases} 1 & \text{if } x = 0,\ 1 \\ 0 & \text{Otherwise.} \end{cases}$$

We find that joint p.m.f. of $X_1, X_2, \ldots X_n$ is

$$\prod_i f_\theta(x_i) = \theta^{\Sigma \mathrm{Xi}}(1 - \theta)^{n-\Sigma \mathrm{Xi}} \quad \prod_i C(x_i)$$
$$= g_\theta(t)\, h(x_1, x_2, \ldots x_n) \qquad \text{(Say)}$$

where $t = \Sigma x_i$, $g_\theta(t) = \theta^t(1 - \theta)^{n-t}$ and $h(x_1, x_2, \ldots, x_n) = \prod_i C(x_i)$.

Hence, the factorization criterion is met by the joint distribution, implying that $T = \Sigma X_i$ is sufficient for θ. So is T/n, the sample proportion of successes being one-to-one correspondence with T.

Example 1.7 Let $X_1, \ldots, X_n$ be a random sample from $P(\lambda)$. We show that $1/n\ \Sigma X_i$ is a sufficient statistic for λ.

The p.m.f. of the Poisson distribution is

$$f_\theta(x) = \begin{cases} \frac{e^{-\theta}\theta^x}{x!} & \text{if } x = 0, 1, 2 \ldots [\theta \equiv \lambda] \\ 0 & \text{otherwise} \end{cases}$$

where $0 < \theta \propto$, i.e. $\Theta = (0, \propto)$

Let us write the p.m.f. in the form $f_\theta(x) = C(x)e^{-\theta}\theta^X$

$$\text{with } C(x) = \begin{cases} \frac{1}{x!} & \text{if } x = 0, 1, 2, \ldots \\ 0 & \text{otherwise} \end{cases}$$

We may represent the joint p.m.f. of $X_1, X_2, \ldots X_n$ as

$$\prod_i f_\theta(x_i) = e^{-n\theta}\ \theta^{\sum \mathrm{Xi}} \prod_i C(x_i)$$
$$= g_\theta(t)h(x_1, x_2 \ldots x_n), \qquad \text{(Say)}$$

where $t = \sum x_i$, $g_\theta(t) = e^{-n\theta}\theta^t$ and $h(x_1, x_2, \ldots x_n) = \prod_i C(x_i)$.

The factorizability condition is thus observed to hold, so that $T = \Sigma X_i$ is sufficient for θ; so is $T/n = \overline{X}$, the sample mean.

Example 1.8 Let $X_1, X_2, \ldots, X_n$ be a random sample from $N(\mu, \sigma^2)$. Show that (i) if σ is known, ΣX_i is a sufficient statistic for μ, (ii) if μ is known $\Sigma(X_i - \mu)^2$ is a sufficient statistic for σ^2, and (iii) if both μ and σ are unknown $\left(\Sigma X_i, \Sigma X_i^2\right)$ is a sufficient statistic for (μ, σ^2).

Ans. (i) we may take the variance to be σ^2 and the unknown mean to be μ, varying over the space $\Theta = (-\infty, \infty)$. Here, the joint p.d.f. of $X_1, X_2, \ldots, X_n$ is $\prod_i \left\{\frac{1}{\sigma\sqrt{2\pi}} e^{-\frac{1}{2\sigma^2}(x_i-\mu)^2}\right\}$

$$= \frac{1}{\left(\sigma\sqrt{2\pi}\right)^n} e^{-\frac{1}{2\sigma^2}\sum_i (x_i-\mu)^2}$$

$$= e^{\frac{-n(\bar{x}-\mu)^2}{2\sigma^2}} \left\{ e^{\frac{-\sum_i (x_i-\bar{x})^2}{2\sigma^2}} \cdot \frac{1}{\left(\sigma\sqrt{2n}\right)^n} \right\}$$

$$= g_\mu(t) \cdot h(x_1, x_2, \ldots, x_n), \qquad \text{(Say)}$$

where $t = \bar{x}$, $g_\mu(t) = e^{-n(\bar{X}-\mu)^2/2\sigma^2}$

and $h(x_1, x_2, \ldots, x_n) = \frac{1}{\left(\sigma\sqrt{2\pi}\right)^n} e^{-\frac{1}{2\sigma^2}\sum (x_i-\bar{x})^2}$

Thus the factorizability condition holds with respect to $T = \bar{X}$, the sample mean, which is therefore sufficient for μ. So the sum is $\sum_i X_i$

(ii) The unknown variance $\sigma^2 = \theta$, say, is supposed to vary over $\Theta = (0, \infty)$. The joint p.d.f. of $X_1, X_2, \ldots X_n$ may be written as

$$\prod_i \left\{\frac{1}{\sigma\sqrt{2\pi}} e^{-\frac{1}{2\sigma^2}(x_i-\mu)^2}\right\} = \frac{1}{\left(\sigma\sqrt{2\pi}\right)^n} e^{\frac{-1}{2\sigma^2}\sum_i (x_i-\mu)^2} = g_\theta(t)\, h(x_1, x_2 \ldots x_n), \text{ say,}$$

where $t = \sum_i (x_i - \mu)^2, g_\theta(t) = \frac{1}{\left(\sqrt{2\pi\sigma}\right)^n} e^{-\frac{1}{2\sigma^2}\sum (x_i-\mu)^2}$

$\sigma^2 \equiv \theta$ and $h\left(\underset{\sim}{x}\right) = 1$. Hence, $T = \sum (X_i - \mu)^2$ is a sufficient statistic for θ. So is

$S_0^2 = \frac{1}{n}\sum_i (x_i - \mu)^2$, which is in this situation commonly used to estimates σ^2.

(iii) Taking the unknown mean and variance to be θ_1 and θ_2, respectively, we now have for θ a vector $\theta = (\theta_1,\ \theta_2)$ varying over the parameter space (which is a half-plane) $\Theta = \{(\theta_1,\ \theta_2)\,/-\infty < \theta_1 < \infty,\ 0 < \theta_2 < \infty\}$.

The jt. p.d.f. of $X_1,\ X_2,\ \ldots, X_n$ may now be written as

$$\prod_i \left\{ \frac{1}{\sqrt{2\pi\theta_2}} e^{-\frac{1}{2\theta_2}(x_i-\theta_1)^2} \right\} = \frac{1}{(2\pi\theta_2)^{\frac{n}{2}}} e^{-\frac{1}{2\theta_2}[n(\bar{x}-\theta_1)^2 + (n-1)s^2]}$$

$$= g_\theta(t_1,\ t_2)\, h(\underset{\sim}{x}),\ \text{say, where } t_1 = \bar{x},\ t_2 = s^2 = \sum_i (x_i - \bar{x})^2 \Big/ (n-1)$$

$$g_\theta(t_1,\ t_2) = \frac{1}{(2\pi\theta_2)^{\frac{n}{2}}} e^{-\frac{1}{2\theta_2}[n(\bar{x}-\theta_1)^2 + (n-1)s^2]} \text{ and } h\left(\underset{\sim}{x}\right) = 1\ .$$

The factorizability condition is thus observed to hold with regard to the statistics $T_1 = \overline{X}$, the sample mean and $T_2 = s^2$, the sample variance.

Hence, $\overline{X}$ and s^2 are jointly sufficient for θ_1 and θ_2, i.e. $\left(\Sigma X_i, \Sigma X_i^2\right)$ is a joint sufficient statistic for $(\mu,\ \sigma^2)$.

Example 1.9 Let $X_1,\ X_2,\ \ldots, X_n$ be a random sample from $R(0,\ \theta)$.

Show that $X_{(n)} = \max\limits_{1 \le i \le n} X_i$ is a sufficient statistic for θ.

Ans.: The jt. p.d.f. of $x_1,\ x_2, \ldots,\ x_n$ is

$$f\left(\underset{\sim}{x}, \theta\right) = \begin{cases} \frac{1}{\theta^n} & \text{if } 0 < x_i < \theta \quad \forall i \\ 0 & \text{otherwise} \end{cases}$$

$$= \begin{cases} \frac{1}{\theta^n} & \text{if } 0 < x_{(n)} < \theta \\ 0 & \text{otherwise} \end{cases}$$

$$= \frac{1}{\theta^n} I_{(0,\theta)}\left(x_{(n)}\right) \quad \text{where } I_{(\alpha,\beta)}(x) = \begin{cases} 1 & \text{if } \alpha < x < \beta \\ 0 & \text{otherwise} \end{cases}$$

$$= g\{x_{(n)}, \theta\} \cdot h(\underset{\sim}{x}),\ \text{say}$$

where $g\{x_{(n)}, \theta\} = \frac{1}{\theta^n} I_{(0,\theta)}\{x_{(n)}\}$ & $h(\underset{\sim}{x}) = 1$.

Note that $g\{x_{(n)},\ \theta\}$ is a function of θ and $\underset{\sim}{x}$ only through $x_{(n)}$ whereas for fixed $x_{(n)}$, $h(\underset{\sim}{x})$ is free from θ.

Hence, $x_{(n)}$ is a sufficient statistic for θ.

Example 1.10 Let $X_1,\ X_2, \ldots, X_n$ be a random sample from $R(\theta_1,\ \theta_2)$. Show that $\{X_{(1)}, X_{(n)}\}$ is a sufficient statistic for $\theta = (\theta_1,\ \theta_2)$ where $X_{(1)} = \min\limits_{1 \le i \le n} X_i$, $X(n) = \max\limits_{1 \le i \le n} X_i$.

Solution Joint p.d.f. of $X_1, X_2, \ldots, X_n$ is

$$f\left(\underset{\sim}{x},\theta\right) = \begin{cases} \frac{1}{(\theta_2-\theta_1)^n} & \text{if } \theta_1 < x_i < \theta_2 \quad \forall i \\ 0 & \text{otherwise} \end{cases}$$

$$= \begin{cases} \frac{1}{(\theta_2-\theta_1)^n} & \text{if } \theta_1 < x_{(1)} < x_{(n)} < \theta_2 \\ 0 & \text{otherwise} \end{cases}$$

$$= \frac{1}{(\theta_2-\theta_1)^n} I_{1(\theta_1,\infty)}\{x_{(1)}\} I_{2(-\infty,\theta_2)}\{x_{(n)}\}$$

where

$$I_{1(\theta_1,\infty)}\{x_{(1)}\} = \begin{cases} 1 & \text{if } \theta_1 < x_{(1)} < \propto \\ 0 & \text{otherwise} \end{cases}$$

and $I_2(-\propto, \theta_2)\{x_{(n)}\} = \begin{cases} 1 & \text{if } -\propto < x_n < \theta_2 \\ 0 & \text{otherwise} \end{cases}$, i.e. $f(\underset{\sim}{x},\ \theta) = g[\{x_{(1)},\ x_{(n)}\},$ $(\theta_1, \theta_2)]h\left(\underset{\sim}{x}\right)$ where $g[\{x_{(1)},\ x_{(n)}\},\ (\theta_1, \theta_2)] = \frac{1}{(\theta_2-\theta_1)^n} I_{1(0_1,\propto)}\{x(1)\} I_{2(-\infty,\theta_2)}$ $\{x_{(n)}\}$ and $h\left(\underset{\sim}{x}\right) = 1.$

Note that g is a function of $(\theta_1,\ \theta_2)$ and $\underset{\sim}{x}$ only through $\{x_{(1)},\ x_{(n)}\}$ where as for fixed $\{x_{(1)},\ x_{(n)}\}$, $h\left(\underset{\sim}{x}\right)$ is free from θ.

Hence, $\{x_{(1)},\ x_{(n)}\}$ is a sufficient statistic for $(\theta_1,\ \theta_2)$.

Example 1.11 Let $X_1,\ X_2,\ \ldots,\ X_n$ be a random sample from a population having p.d.f.

$$f(x,\theta) = \begin{cases} e^{-(x-\theta)}, & x > \theta \\ 0 & \text{otherwise} \end{cases}$$

Show that $X_{(1)} = \min\limits_{1 \le i \le n} X_i$ is a sufficient statistic for θ.

Solution The p.d.f. can equivalently be written as

$$f(x,\theta) = \begin{cases} e^{-(X-\theta)}, & x_{(1)} > \theta \\ 0 & \text{otherwise} \end{cases}$$

Now, the joint p.d.f. of $X_1,\ X_2,\ \ldots, X_n$ is

$$f(\underset{\sim}{x},\theta) = \begin{cases} e^{-\sum_i (x_i-\theta)}, & x_{(1)} > \theta \\ 0 & \text{otherwise} \end{cases}$$

$$f(\underset{\sim}{x},\theta) = e^{-\sum_i (x_i-\theta)} I_{(\theta,\propto)}\{x_{(1)}\} \quad \text{where } I_{(\theta,\propto)}\{x_{(1)}\} = \begin{cases} 1 & \text{if } x_{(1)} > \theta \\ 0 & \text{otherwise} \end{cases}$$

$$= g\ \{x_{(1)},\theta\}\ .\ h\left(\underset{\sim}{x}\right), \quad \text{say}$$

where $g\{x_{(1)},\theta\} = e^{-\sum_i (x_i-\theta)} I_{(\theta,\propto)}\{x_{(1)}\}$ and $h\left(\underset{\sim}{x}\right) = 1$.

Note that $g\{x_{(i)},\ \theta\}$ is a function of θ and $\underset{\sim}{x}$ only through $x_{(1)}$ and for fixed $x_{(1)}$, $h(x)$ is free from θ. Hence, according to factorizability criterion, $x_{(1)}$ is a sufficient statistic for θ.

Note In the above three problems the domain of the probability density depends upon the parameter θ. In this situation, we should aware to apply Fisher–Neyman factorization theorem and we should give proper consideration to the domain of the function $h\left(\underset{\sim}{x}\right)$ for every fixed value of $T\left(\underset{\sim}{X}\right)$. In these situations, it is better to use Fisher–Neyman criterion. Let us solve Example 1.10 by using Fisher–Neyman criterion:

$$f(x) = \frac{1}{\theta_2-\theta_1}, \theta_1 < x < \theta_2$$

Let $X_{(1)} = \min\limits_{1\le i\le n} X_i = y_1,\ X_{(n)} = \max\limits_{1\le i\le n} X_i = y_2$

The joint p.d.f. of y_1, y_2 is

$$g(y_1,y_2;\theta_1,\theta_2) = \frac{n(n-1)}{(\theta_2-\theta_1)^n}(y_2-y_1)^{n-2}, \theta_1 < y_1 < y_2 < \theta_2$$

The joint p.d.f. of $X_1, X_2, \ldots, X_n$ is

$$f\left(\underset{\sim}{x};\theta_1,\theta_2\right) = \frac{1}{(\theta_2-\theta_1)^n}$$

$$= \frac{n(n-1)}{(\theta_2-\theta_1)^n}\left(x_{(n)}-x_{(1)}\right)^{n-2} \frac{1}{n(n-1)\left(x_{(n)}-x_{(1)}\right)^{n-2}}$$

$$= g\left(x_{(n)},x_{(1)};\theta_1,\theta_2\right) h\left(\underset{\sim}{x}\right)$$

By the Fisher–Neyman criterion, $\{x_{(1)}, x_{(n)}\}$ is a sufficient statistic for $\theta = (\theta_1, \theta_2)$

Example 1.12 Let $X \sim N(0, \sigma^2)$, show that $|X|$ is sufficient for σ.

Solution

$$\begin{aligned} f(x, \sigma) &= \frac{1}{\sqrt{2\lambda}\sigma} e^{-\frac{x^2}{2\sigma^2}}, \qquad \sigma > 0 \\ &= \frac{1}{\sqrt{2\lambda}\sigma} e^{-\frac{|x|^2}{2\sigma^2}} \cdot 1 \\ &= g(t, \sigma)\, h(x), \qquad h(x) = 1 \end{aligned}$$

where $g(t, \sigma)$ is a function of σ and x only through $t = |x|$ and for fixed t, $h(x) = 1$ is free from σ.

Hence, by Fisher–Neymam factorization theorem, $|X|$ is sufficient for σ.

Example 1.13 Let $X_1, X_2, \ldots X_n$ be a random sample from a double-exponential distribution whose p.d.f. may be taken as $f_\theta(X) = \frac{1}{2}\exp\left(-|x_i - \theta|\right)$, and the unknown parameter θ varies over the space $\Theta = (-\infty, \infty)$.

In this case, the joint p.d.f. is $\prod_i f_\theta(x_i) = \frac{1}{2^n}\exp\left(-\sum_i |x_i - \theta|\right)$.

For no single statistic T, it is now not possible to express the joint p.d.f. in the form $g_\theta(t)\, h(x_1, x_2, \ldots x_n)$.

Hence, there exists no statistic T which taken alone is sufficient for θ. The whole set $X_1, X_2, \ldots, X_n$, or the set $X_{(1)}, X_{(2)}, \ldots X_{(n)}$, is of course sufficient.

Remarks 1.2 A single sufficient statistic does not always exist.

e.g. Let $X_1, X_2, \ldots, X_n$ be a random sample from a population having p.d.f.

$$f(x,\theta) = \begin{cases} \frac{1}{\theta}, & k\,\theta < x < (k+1)\,\theta, \quad k > 0 \\ 0 & \text{otherwise} \end{cases}$$

Here, no single sufficient statistic for θ exists. In fact, $\{x_{(1)}, x_{n)}\}$ is sufficient for θ.

Remark 1.3 Not all functions for sufficient statistic are sufficient. For example, in random sampling from $N(\mu, \sigma^2)$, σ^2 being known, $\overline{X}^2$ is not sufficient for μ. (Is $\overline{X}$ sufficient for μ^2 ?)

Remark 1.4 Not all statistic are sufficient.

Let X_1, X_2 be a random sample from $P(\lambda)$. Then $X_1 + 2X_2$ is not sufficient for λ, because in particular, say

$$P\{X_1 = 0, X_2 = 1 | \; X_1 + 2X_2 = 2\} = \frac{P\{X_1 = 0, X_2 = 1 \;\; X_1 + 2X_2 = 2\}}{P\{X_1 + 2X_2 = 2\}}$$

$$= \frac{P\{X_1 = 0, \quad X_2 = 1\}}{P\{X_1 = 0, \quad X_2 = 1\} + P\{X_1 = 2, \quad X_2 = 0\}}$$

$$= \frac{e^{-\lambda} \cdot e^{-\lambda} \cdot \lambda}{e^{-\lambda} \cdot e^{-\lambda} \cdot \lambda + e^{-\lambda} \cdot e^{-\lambda} \cdot \frac{\lambda^2}{2!}}$$

$= \frac{2}{\lambda+2}$ which depends upon λ.

Remarks 1.5 Let $\underline{\theta} = (\theta_1, \theta_2, \ldots, \theta_k)$ and $\underset{\sim}{T} = (T_1, T_2, \ldots T_m)$. Further, let $\underset{\sim}{T}$ be a sufficient statistic for $\underset{\sim}{\theta}$. Then we cannot put any restriction on m, i.e. $m \geq k$, the number of parameters involved in the distribution. Even if $m = k$, then we cannot say that T_i of $\underset{\sim}{T}$ is sufficient for θ_i of $\underset{\sim}{\theta}$. It is better to say that $(T_1, T_2, \ldots T_m)$ are jointly sufficient for $(\theta_1, \theta_2, \ldots \theta_k)$.

Let $X_1, X_2, \ldots, X_n$ be a random sample from $N(\mu, \sigma^2)$. Here, ΣX_i and ΣX_i^2 are jointly sufficient for μ and σ^2.

Remarks 1.6 The whole set of observations $\underset{\sim}{X} = (X_1, X_2, \ldots, X_n)$ is always sufficient for $\underset{\sim}{\theta}$. But we do not consider this to be real sufficient statistic when another sufficient statistic exists. There are a few situations where the whole set of observations is a sufficient statistic. [As shown in the example of double-exponential distribution].

Remarks 1.7 The set of all order statistics $T\{X_{(1)}, X_{(2)}, \ldots, X_{(n)}\}$, $X_{(1)} < X_{(2)}, \ldots, < X_{(n)}$, is sufficient for the family.

Conditional distribution of $(\underset{\sim}{X}/T = t) = \frac{1}{n!}$ because for each $T = t$, we have n-tuples of the form $(x_1, x_2, \ldots x_n)$.

Remarks 1.8: Distribution admitting sufficient statistic Let $X_1, X_2, \ldots, X_n$ be a random sample from $f\left(\underset{\sim}{x}, \theta\right)$ and $T\left(\underset{\sim}{X}\right)$ be a sufficient statistic for θ (θ is a scalar). According to factorization theorem,

$$\sum_i \log f(x_i, \theta) = \log\, g(T, \theta) + \log\, h(\underset{\sim}{x})$$

Differentiating w.r.t. θ, we have

$$\sum_i \frac{\partial \log f(x_i, \theta)}{\partial \theta} = \frac{\partial \log g(T, \theta)}{\partial \theta} = G(T, \theta), \quad \text{(say)} \tag{1.1}$$

Put a particular value of θ in (1.1).

$$\text{Then we have } \sum_{i=1}^{n} u(x_i) = G(T) \tag{1.2}$$

Now differentiating (1.1) and (1.2) w.r.t. x_i, we have

$$\frac{\partial^2 \log f(x_i,\ \theta)}{\partial\theta\partial x_i} = \frac{\partial G(T,\ \theta)}{\partial T} \cdot \frac{\partial T}{\partial x_i} \tag{1.3}$$

$$\frac{\partial u(x_i)}{\partial x_i} = \frac{\partial G(T)}{\partial T} \cdot \frac{\partial T}{\partial x_i} \tag{1.4}$$

(1.3) and (1.4) give us

$$\frac{\partial^2 \log f(x_i, \theta)}{\partial\theta\ \partial x_i} \Big/ \frac{\partial u(x_i)}{\partial x_i} = \frac{\partial G(T, \theta)/\partial T}{\partial G(T)/\partial T} \forall i \tag{1.5}$$

Since the R.H.S. of (1.5) is free from x_i, we can write

$$\begin{aligned}
&\frac{\partial G(T,\theta)}{\partial T} = \frac{\partial\ G(T)}{\partial\ T}\lambda_1(\theta)\\
\Rightarrow\quad & G(T,\theta) = G(T)\lambda_1(\theta) + \lambda_2(\theta)\\
\Rightarrow\quad & \frac{\partial \sum_i \log f(x_i,\theta)}{\partial\theta} = G(T)\lambda_1(\theta) + \lambda_2(\theta)\\
\Rightarrow\quad & \sum_i \log f(x_i,\theta) = G(T)\int \lambda_1(\theta)d\theta + \int \lambda_2(\theta)d\theta + c\left(\underset{\sim}{x}\right)\\
\Rightarrow\quad & \prod_i f(x_i,\theta) = A\left(\underset{\sim}{x}\right)e^{\theta_1 G(T) + \theta_2}
\end{aligned}$$

where $A\left(\underset{\sim}{x}\right) = a$ function of $\underset{\sim}{x}$

θ_1 = a function of θ, and
θ_2 = another function of θ.

Thus if a distribution is to have a sufficient statistic for its parameter, it must be of the form

$$f(x,\theta) = e^{B_1(\theta)u(x) + B_2(\theta) + R(x)}. \tag{1.6}$$

(1.6) is known as Koopman form.

Example Show, by expressing a Poisson p.m.f. in Koopman form, that Poisson distribution possesses a sufficient statistic for itsparameter λ.

Here, $f(x, \lambda) = \frac{e^{-\lambda}\lambda^x}{x!} = e^{-\lambda + x \log \lambda - \log x!}$
which is of the form $e^{B_1(\theta)u(x) + B_2(\theta) + R(x)}$.
Hence, there exists a sufficient statistic for λ.
Completeness A family of distributions is said to be complete

$$\begin{aligned} &\text{if } E\left[g(X)\right] = 0 && \forall\, \theta \in \Theta \\ &\Rightarrow P\{g(x) = 0\} = 1 && \forall\, \theta \in \Theta \end{aligned}$$

A statistic T is said to be complete if family of distributions of T is complete.

Examples 1.14 (a) Let $X_1, X_2, \ldots, X_n$ be a random sample from $b(1, \pi)$, $0 < \pi < 1$. Then $T = \sum_{i=1}^{n} X_i$ is a complete statistic.

$$\begin{aligned} &\text{As } E[g(T)] = 0 && \forall\, \pi \in (0,1) \\ &\Rightarrow \sum_{t=0}^{n} g(t)\binom{n}{t}\pi^t(1-\pi)^{n-t} = 0 \\ &\Rightarrow (1-\pi)^n \sum_{t=0}^{n} g(t)\binom{n}{t}\left(\frac{\pi}{1-\pi}\right)^t = 0 && \forall\, \pi \in (0,1) \\ &\Rightarrow g(t) = 0 \quad \text{for } t = 0, 1, 2 \ldots n && \forall\, \pi \in (0,1) \\ &\Rightarrow P\left\{g(t) = 0\right\} = 1 && \forall\, \pi \end{aligned}$$

(b) Let $X \sim N(0, \sigma^2)$. Then X is not complete

$$\text{as,} \quad E(X) = 0 \not\Rightarrow P(X = 0) = 1 \qquad \forall\, \sigma^2$$

(c) If $X \sim U(0, \theta)$, then X is a complete statistic [or $R(0, \theta)$].

A statistic is said to be complete sufficient statistic if it is complete as well as sufficient.

If $(X_1, X_2, \ldots, X_n)$ is a random sample from b $(1, \pi)$, $0 < \pi < 1$, then $T = \sum X_i$ is also sufficient. So T is a complete sufficient statistic where $T = \sum X_i$.

Minimal Sufficient Statistic

A statistic T is said to be minimal sufficient if it is a function of every other sufficient statistics.

The sufficiency principle

A sufficient statistic for a parameter θ is a statistic that, in a certain sense, captures all the information about θ contained in the sample. Any additional information in the sample, besides the value of sufficient statistic, does not contain any more information about θ. These considerations lead to the data reduction technique known as sufficiency principle.

If $T\left(\underset{\sim}{X}\right)$ is a sufficient statistic for θ, then any inference about θ should depend on the sample $\underset{\sim}{X}$ only through the value $T\left(\underset{\sim}{X}\right)$, that is, if $\underset{\sim}{x}$ and $\underset{\sim}{y}$ are two sample points such that $T\left(\underset{\sim}{x}\right) = T\left(\underset{\sim}{y}\right)$, then the inference about θ should be the same whether $\underset{\sim}{X} = \underset{\sim}{x}$ or $\underset{\sim}{X} = \underset{\sim}{y}$ is observed.

Definition (*Sufficient statistic*) A statistic $T\left(\underset{\sim}{X}\right)$ is a sufficient statistic for θ if the conditional distribution of the sample $\underset{\sim}{X}$ given the value of $T\left(\underset{\sim}{X}\right)$ does not depend on θ.

Factorization theorem: Let $f\left(\underset{\sim}{x}|\theta\right)$ denote the joint pdf/pmf of a sample $\underset{\sim}{X}$. A statistic $T\left(\underset{\sim}{X}\right)$ is a sufficient statistic for θ iff $\exists$ functions $g(t|\theta)$ and $h\left(\underset{\sim}{x}\right)$ such that for all sample points $\underset{\sim}{X}$ and all parameter values θ,

$$f\left(\underset{\sim}{x}|\theta\right) = g(t|\theta)h\left(\underset{\sim}{x}\right)$$

Result: If $T\left(\underset{\sim}{X}\right)$ is a function of $T'\left(\underset{\sim}{X}\right)$, then $T'\left(\underset{\sim}{X}\right)$ is sufficient which implies that $T\left(\underset{\sim}{X}\right)$ is sufficient.

$\left[\text{i.e. sufficiency of } T'\left(\underset{\sim}{X}\right) \Rightarrow \text{sufficiency of } T\left(\underset{\sim}{X}\right), \text{a function of } T'\left(\underset{\sim}{X}\right)\right]$

Proof Let $\{B_{t'}|t' \in \tau'\}$ and $\{A_t|t \in \tau\}$ be the partitions induced by $T'\left(\underset{\sim}{X}\right)$ and $T\left(\underset{\sim}{X}\right)$, respectively. □

Since $T\left(\underset{\sim}{X}\right)$ is a function of $T'\left(\underset{\sim}{X}\right)$, for $t' \in \tau'$ $\therefore$ $B_{t'} \subseteq A_t$, for some $\forall t \in \tau$.

Thus Sufficiency of $T'\left(\underset{\sim}{X}\right)$

$\Leftrightarrow$ Conditional distribution of $\underset{\sim}{X} = \underset{\sim}{x}$ given $T'\left(\underset{\sim}{X}\right) = t'$ is independent of θ, $\forall t' \in \tau'$

$\Leftrightarrow$ Conditional distribution of $\underset{\sim}{X} = \underset{\sim}{x}$ given $\underset{\sim}{X} \in B_{t'}$ is independent of θ, $\forall t' \in \tau'$

$\Rightarrow$ Conditional distribution of $\underset{\sim}{X} = \underset{\sim}{x}$ given $\underset{\sim}{X} \in A_t$ (for some $\forall t \in \tau$) is independent of θ, $\forall t \in \tau$

$\Leftrightarrow$ Conditional distribution of $\underset{\sim}{X} = \underset{\sim}{x}$ given $T\left(\underset{\sim}{X}\right) = t$ is independent of θ, $\forall t \in \tau$.

$\Leftrightarrow$ Sufficiency of $T\left(\underset{\sim}{X}\right)$.

Sufficient statistic for an Exponential family of distributions:

Let $X_1, X_2, \ldots, X_n$ be i.i.d. observations from a pdf/pmf $f\left(x|\underline{\theta}\right)$ that belongs to an exponential family given by

$$f\left(x|\underline{\theta}\right) = h(x)c\left(\underline{\theta}\right)\exp\left(\sum_{i=1}^{k}\omega_i\left(\underline{\theta}\right)t_i(x)\right)$$

where $\underset{\sim}{\theta} = (\theta_1, \theta_2, \ldots \theta_d)$, $d \leq k$. Then

$$T\left(\underset{\sim}{X}\right) = \left(\sum_{j=1}^{n} t_1(X_j), \ldots, \sum_{j=1}^{n} t_k(X_j)\right)$$

is a (complete) sufficient statistic for $\underset{\sim}{\theta}$.

Minimal sufficient statistic

When we introduced the concept of sufficiency, we said that our objective was to condense the data without losing any information about the parameter. In any problem, there are, in fact, many sufficient statistics. In general, we have to consider the choice between alternative sets of sufficient statistics. In a sample of n observations, we always have a set of n sufficient statistics [viz., the observations $\underset{\sim}{X} = (X_1, X_2, \ldots, X_n)$ themselves or the order statistics $\left(X_{(1)}, X_{(2)}, \ldots, X_{(n)}\right)$] for the $k(\geq 1)$ parameters of the distributions. For example, in sampling from $N(\mu, \sigma^2)$ distribution with both μ and σ^2 unknown, there are, in fact, three sets of jointly sufficient statistic: the observations $\underset{\sim}{X} = (X_1, X_2, \ldots, X_n)$, the order statistics $\left(X_{(1)}, X_{(2)}, \ldots, X_{(n)}\right)$ and $(\bar{X}, s^2)$. We naturally prefer the jointly sufficient statistic $(\bar{X}, s^2)$ since they condense the data more than either of the other two. Sometimes, though not always, there will be a set of $s(<n)$ statistics sufficient for the parameters. Often $s = k$ but s may be $<k$ also.

The question that we might ask is as follows: Does $\exists$ a set of sufficient statistic that condenses the data more than $(\bar{X}, s^2)$? The answer is there does not. The notion that we are alluding to is of minimum set of sufficient statistics, which we label minimal sufficient statistic. In other words, we have to ask: what is the smallest number s of statistics that constitute a sufficient set in any problem? It may be said in general that a sufficient statistic T may expected to be minimal sufficient if it has the same dimensions (i.e. the same number of components) as θ.

Statistics and partition

It may be noted that every statistic induces a partition of $\mathscr{X}$. The same is true for a set of statistics; a set of statistics induces a partition of $\mathscr{X}$. Loosely speaking, the condensation of data that a statistic or a set of statistics exhibits can be measured by the number of subsets in the partition induced by the statistic or a set of statistics. If a set of statistics has fewer subsets (co-sets) in its induced partition than the induced partition of another set of statistics, then we say that the first statistic condenses the data more than the later. Still loosely speaking, a minimal sufficient set of statistics is then a sufficient set of statistics that has fewer subsets (co-sets) in its partition than the induced partition of any other set of sufficient statistics. So a set of sufficient statistic is minimal if no other set of sufficient statistics condenses the data more without losing sufficiency.

Thus T is minimal sufficient if any further reduction of data is not possible without losing sufficiency, i.e. T is minimal sufficient if there does not exist a function $U = \psi(T)$ such that U is sufficient.

Definition (*Minimal sufficient statistic*) A sufficient statistic $T(\underset{\sim}{X})$ is called minimal sufficient if, for every other sufficient statistic $T'(\underset{\sim}{X})$, $T(\underset{\sim}{X})$ is a function of $T'(\underset{\sim}{X})$.

To say that $T(\underset{\sim}{X})$ is a function of $T'(\underset{\sim}{X})$ simply means that if $T'(\underset{\sim}{x}) = T'(\underset{\sim}{y})$, then $T(\underset{\sim}{x}) = T(\underset{\sim}{y})$. In terms of the partition sets, if $B_{t'}|t' \in \tau'$ are the partition sets for $T'(\underset{\sim}{X})$ and $A_t|t \in T$ are the partition sets for $T(\underset{\sim}{X})$, then the above definition of minimal sufficient statistic states that every $B_{t'}$ is a subset of some A_t. Thus, the partition associated with a minimal sufficient statistic is coarsest possible partition for a sufficient statistic, and a minimal sufficient statistic achieves the greatest possible data reduction for a sufficient statistic.

Example Let $X_i(i = I, 2, \ldots, n) \sim$ independent $P(\theta)$ distribution. Then $T = \sum_{i=1}^{n} X_i$ is sufficient for θ and, in fact, it is minimal sufficient.

Since $T = \sum_{i=1}^{n} X_i$ is minimal sufficient; therefore, any further reduction of the data is not possible without losing sufficiency, i.e. there does not exist a function $U = \psi(T)$ such that U is sufficient. Suppose that T is sufficient and if possible, $\exists$ a function

$$U = \psi(t) \ni \psi(t_1) = \cdots = \psi(t_k) = u.$$

Then

$$P_\theta[T = t|U = u] = \begin{cases} \dfrac{\frac{(n\theta)^{t_i}}{t_i!}}{\sum\limits_{i=1}^{k} \frac{(n\theta)^{t_i}}{t_i!}} & \text{if } t = t_i (i = 1, 2, \ldots, k) \\ 0 & \text{otherwise} \end{cases}$$

$\rightarrow$ depends on θ ,

so that U is not sufficient retaining sufficiency. Hence, $T = \sum_{i=1}^{n} X_i$ is minimal sufficient statistic.

Remark 1 Since minimal sufficient statistic is a function of sufficient statistic, therefore, a minimal sufficient statistic is also sufficient.

Remark 2 Minimal sufficient statistic is not unique since any one-to-one function of minimal sufficient statistic is also a minimal sufficient statistic.

Definition of minimal sufficient statistic does not help us to find a minimal sufficient statistic except for verifying whether a given statistic is minimal sufficient statistic. Fortunately, the following result of Lehman and Scheffe (1950) gives an easier way to find a minimal sufficient statistic.

Theorem *Let $f\left(\underset{\sim}{x}|\theta\right)$ be the pmf/pdf of a sample $\underset{\sim}{X}$. Suppose $\exists$ a function $T\left(\underset{\sim}{X}\right) \ni$ for every two sample points $\underset{\sim}{x}$ and $\underset{\sim}{y}$, and the ratio of $f\left(\underset{\sim}{x}|\theta\right)\Big/f\left(\underset{\sim}{y}|\theta\right)$ is constant as a function of θ (i.e. independent of θ) iff $T\left(\underset{\sim}{x}\right) = T\left(\underset{\sim}{y}\right)$. Then $T\left(\underset{\sim}{X}\right)$ is minimal sufficient statistic.*

Proof Let us assume $f\left(\underset{\sim}{x}|\theta\right) > 0$, $\underset{\sim}{x} \in \mathscr{X}$ and θ. First, we show that $T\left(\underset{\sim}{X}\right)$ is a sufficient statistic. Let $\tau = \left\{t/t = T(\underset{\sim}{x}), x \in \mathscr{X}\right\}$ be the image of $\mathscr{X}$ under $T(\underset{\sim}{x})$. Define the partition sets induced by $T(\underset{\sim}{X})$ as $A_t = \left\{\underset{\sim}{x}|T\left(\underset{\sim}{x}\right) = t\right\}$. For each A_t, choose and fix one element $\underset{\sim t}{x} \in A_t$. For any $\underset{\sim}{x} \in \mathscr{X}$, $\underset{\sim T(\underset{\sim}{x})}{x}$ is the fixed element that is in the same set A_t, as $\underset{\sim}{x}$. Since $\underset{\sim}{x}$ and $\underset{\sim T\left(\underset{\sim}{x}\right)}{x}$ are in the same set A_t, $T\left(\underset{\sim}{x}\right) = T\left(\underset{\sim T\left(\underset{\sim}{x}\right)}{x}\right)$ and, hence, $f\left(\underset{\sim}{x}|\theta\right)\Big/f\left(\underset{\sim T\left(\underset{\sim}{x}\right)}{x}|\theta\right)$ is constant as a function of θ. Thus, we can define a function on $\mathscr{X}$ by $h\left(\underset{\sim}{x}\right) = \dfrac{f\left(\underset{\sim}{x}|\theta\right)}{f\left(\underset{\sim T\left(\underset{\sim}{x}\right)}{x}|\theta\right)}$ and h does not depend on θ. □

Define a function on τ by $g(t|\theta) = f\left(\underset{\sim t}{x}|\theta\right)$. Then

$$f(\underset{\sim}{x}|\theta) = \frac{f\left(\underset{\sim T(\underset{\sim}{x})}{x}|\theta\right)f\left(\underset{\sim}{x}|\theta\right)}{f\left(\underset{\sim T(\underset{\sim}{x})}{x}|\theta\right)} = g(t|\theta)h(\underset{\sim}{x})$$ and by factorization theorem, $T(\underset{\sim}{X})$ is sufficient for θ. Now to show that $T(\underset{\sim}{X})$ is minimal, let $T'(\underset{\sim}{X})$ be any other sufficient statistic. By factorization theorem, $\exists$ functions g' and h' such that

$$f(\underset{\sim}{x}|\theta) = g'\left(T'(\underset{\sim}{x})|\theta\right)h'(\underset{\sim}{x})$$

Let $\underset{\sim}{x}$ and $\underset{\sim}{y}$ be any two sample points with $T'(\underset{\sim}{x}) = T'(\underset{\sim}{y})$. Then

$$\frac{f(\underset{\sim}{x}|\theta)}{f(\underset{\sim}{y}|\theta)} = \frac{g'(T'\ \underset{\sim}{x}|\theta)\,h'(\underset{\sim}{x})}{g'(T'\ \underset{\sim}{y}|\theta)h'\ \underset{\sim}{y}} = \frac{h'\left(\underset{\sim}{x}\right)}{h'\left(\underset{\sim}{y}\right)}.$$

Since this ratio does not depend on θ, the assumptions of the theorem imply $T(\underset{\sim}{x}) = T(\underset{\sim}{y})$. Thus $T(\underset{\sim}{x})$ is a function of $T'(\underset{\sim}{x})$ and $T(\underset{\sim}{x})$ is minimal.

Example (Normal minimal sufficient statistic) Let $X_1, X_2, \ldots X_n$ be iid $N(\mu, \sigma^2)$, both μ and σ^2 unknown. Let $\underset{\sim}{x}$ and $\underset{\sim}{y}$ denote two sample points, and let $(\bar{x}, s^2_{\underset{\sim}{x}})$ and $(\bar{y}, s^2_{\underset{\sim}{y}})$ be the sample means and variances corresponding to the $\underset{\sim}{x}$ and $\underset{\sim}{y}$ samples, respectively. Then we must have

$$\frac{f\left(\underset{\sim}{x}|\mu,\sigma^2\right)}{f\left(\underset{\sim}{y}|\mu,\sigma^2\right)} = \frac{(2\pi\sigma^2)^{-n/2}\exp\left(-\left[n(\bar{x}-\mu)^2+(n-1)s^2_{\underset{\sim}{x}}\right]\Big/(2\sigma^2)\right)}{(2\pi\sigma^2)^{-n/2}\exp\left(-\left[n(\bar{y}-\mu)^2+(n-1)s^2_{\underset{\sim}{y}}\right]\Big/(2\sigma^2)\right)}$$

$$= \exp\left(\left[-n(\bar{x}^2-\bar{y}^2)+2n\mu(\bar{x}-\bar{y})-(n-1)\left(s^2_{\underset{\sim}{x}}-s^2_{\underset{\sim}{y}}\right)\right]\Big/2\sigma^2\right)$$

This ratio will be constant as a function of μ and σ^2 iff $\bar{x} = \bar{y}$ and $s^2_{\underset{\sim}{x}} = s^2_{\underset{\sim}{y}}$, i.e. $(\bar{x}, s^2_{\underset{\sim}{x}}) \equiv (\bar{y}, s^2_{\underset{\sim}{y}})$. Then, by the above theorem, $(\bar{X}, s^2)$ is a minimal sufficient statistic for (μ, σ^2).

Remark Although minimal sufficiency $\Rightarrow$ sufficiency, the converse is not necessarily true. For a random sample $X_1, X_2, \ldots X_n$ from $N(\mu, \mu)$ distribution, $\left(\sum_{i=1}^n X_i, \sum_{i=1}^n X_i^2\right)$ is sufficient but not minimal sufficient statistic. In fact,

$\sum_{i=1}^{n} X_i$ and $\sum_{i=1}^{n} X_i^2$ are each singly sufficient for μ, $\sum_{i=1}^{n} X_i^2$ being minimal. (This particular example also establishes the fact that single sufficiency does not imply minimal sufficiency.)

1.3 Unbiased Estimator and Minimum-Variance Unbiased Estimator

Let X be a random variable having c.d.f. F_θ, $\theta \in \Theta$. The functional form of F_θ is known, but the parameter θ is unknown. Here, we wish to find the true value of θ on the basis of the experimentally determined values $x_1, x_2, \ldots, x_n$, corresponding to a random sample $X_1, X_2, \ldots, X_n$ from F_θ. Sine the observed values $x_1, x_2, \ldots, x_n$ change from one case to another, leading to different estimates in different cases, we cannot expect that the estimate in each case will be good in the sense of having small deviation from the true value of the parameter. So, we first choose an estimator T of θ such that the following condition holds:

$$P\{|T - \theta| < c\} \geq P\{|T' - \theta| < c\} \;\; \forall\, \theta \in \Theta \text{ and } \forall\, c \tag{1.7}$$

where T' is any rival estimator.

Surely, (1.7) is an ideal condition, but the mathematical handling of (1.7) is very difficult. So we require some simpler condition. Such a condition is based on mean square error (m.s.e.). In this case, an estimator will be best if its m.s.e. is least. In other words, an estimator T will be best in the sense of m.s.e. if

$$E(T - \theta)^2 \leq E(T' - \theta)^2 \;\forall\, \theta \text{ and for any rival estimator } T' \tag{1.8}$$

It can readily be shown that there exists no T for which (1.8) holds. [e.g. Let θ_0 be a value of θ and consider $T' = \theta_0$. Note that m.s.e. of T' at $\theta = \theta_0$ is '0', but m.s. e. of T' for other values of θ may be quite large.]

To sidetrack this, we introduce the concept of unbiasedness.

Actually, we choose an estimator on the basis of a set of criteria. Such a set of criteria must depend on the purpose for which we want to choose an estimator. Usually, a set consists of the following criteria: (i) unbiasedness; (ii) minimum-variance unbiased estimator; (iii) consistency, and (iv) efficiency.

Unbiasedness

An estimator T is said to be an unbiased estimator (u.e.) of θ [or $\gamma(\theta)$] iff $E(T) = \theta$ [or $\gamma(\theta)$] $\forall \theta \in \Theta$.

Otherwise, it will be called a biased estimator. The quantity $b(\theta, T) = E_\theta(T) - \theta$ is called the bias. A function $\gamma(\theta)$ is estimable if it has an unbiased estimator.

Let $X_1, X_2, \ldots, X_n$ be a random sample from a population with mean μ and variance σ^2. Then $\bar{X}$ and $s^2 = \frac{1}{n-1}\sum_{i=1}^{n}(X_i - \bar{X})^2$ are u.e's of μ and σ^2, respectively.

Note

(i) Every individual observation is an unbiased estimator of population mean.
(ii) Every partial mean is an unbiased estimator of population mean.
(iii) Every partial sample variance [e.g. $\frac{1}{k-1}\sum_1^k (X_i - \bar{X}_k)^2$, $\bar{X}_k = \frac{1}{k}\sum_1^k X_i$ and $k < n$] is an unbiased estimator of σ^2.

Example 1.15 Let $X_1, X_2, \ldots, X_n$ be a random sample from $N(\mu, \sigma^2)$. Then $\bar{X}$ and $s^2 = \frac{1}{n-1}\sum_1^n (X_i - \bar{X})^2$ are u.e's for μ and σ^2, respectively. But estimator $s = \sqrt{\frac{1}{n-1}\sum_1^n (X_i - \bar{X})^2}$ is a biased estimator of σ.

The bias $b(s, \sigma) = \sigma\left[\sqrt{\frac{2}{n-1}}\Gamma(n/2)\left\{\Gamma\left(\frac{n-1}{2}\right)\right\}^{-1} - 1\right]$.

Remark 1.9 An unbiased estimator may not exist.

Example (a) Let $X \sim b\,(1, \pi), \quad 0 < \pi < 1$.
Then there is no estimator $T(X)$ for which $E\{T(X)\} = \pi^2 \quad \forall \quad \pi \in (0, 1)$ i.e. π^2 is not estimable. Similarly, $\frac{1}{\pi}$ has no unbiased estimator.

(b) For
$$f(x, \theta) = \frac{\binom{m}{x}\binom{\theta-m}{n-x}}{\binom{\theta}{n}}, \quad x = 0, 1, 2 \ldots n$$
$$\theta = m, m+1, \ldots$$
then there is no unbiased estimator for θ.

Remark 1.10 Usually, unbiased estimator is not unique. Starting from two unbiased estimators, we can construct an infinite number of unbiased estimators.

Example Let $X_1, X_2, \ldots, X_n$ be a random sample from $P(\lambda)$. Then both $\bar{X}$ and $s^2 = \frac{1}{n-1}\sum_1^n (X_i - \bar{X})^2$ are unbiased estimators of λ as mean = variance = λ for $P(\lambda)$.

Let $T_\alpha = \alpha\bar{X} + (1-\alpha)s^2$; $0 \le \alpha \le 1$. Here, T_α is an unbiased estimator of λ.

Remark 1.11 An unbiased estimator may be absurd.

Example Let $X \sim P(\lambda)$. Then $T(X) = (-2)^X$ is an unbiased estimator of $e^{-3\lambda}$ since

$$E\{T(X)\} = \sum_x \frac{e^{-\lambda}\lambda^x}{x!}(-2)^x$$
$$= e^{-\lambda}\sum_x \frac{(-2\lambda)^x}{x!} = e^{-\lambda}\cdot e^{-2\lambda} = e^{-3\lambda}.$$

$$\text{Note that } T(X) > 0 \text{ for even } X$$
$$< 0 \text{ for odd } X.$$

$\therefore$ T(X) which is an estimator of a positive quantity $\left(e^{-3\lambda} > 0\right)$ may occasionally be negative.

Example Let $X \sim P(\lambda)$. Construct an unbiased estimator of $e^{-\lambda}$.

Ans Let $T(x) = \begin{cases} 1 \text{ if } x = 0 \\ 0, \text{ otherwise} \end{cases}$

$$\therefore E\{T(X)\} = 1 \cdot P(X = 0) + O \cdot P(X \neq 0) = e^{-\lambda} \quad \forall \lambda.$$

$\therefore$ T(X) is an unbiased estimator of $e^{-\lambda}$.

Remark 1.12 Mean square error of an unbiased estimator (i.e. variance of unbiased estimator) may be greater than that of a biased estimator and then we prefer the biased estimator.

$$\begin{aligned} E(T-\theta)^2 &= E[T - E(T) + \{E(T) - \theta\}]^2 \\ &= V(T) + b^2(T,\theta) \qquad \text{where } b(T,\theta) = E(T) - \theta. \end{aligned}$$

Let T_1 be a biased estimator and T_2 an unbiased estimator, i.e. $E(T_1) \neq \theta$ but $E(T_2) = \theta$.

$$\begin{aligned} \therefore \text{MSE}(T_1) &= V(T_1) + b^2(T_1,\theta) \\ \text{MSE}(T_2) &= V(T_2) \\ \text{if } V(T_2) &> V(T_1) + b^2(T_1,\theta), \text{ then we prefer } T_1. \end{aligned}$$

e.g. Let $X_1, X_2, \ldots, X_n$ be a random sample from $N(\mu, \sigma^2)$. Then $s^2 = \frac{1}{n-1}\sum_i (X_i - \bar{X})^2$ is an unbiased estimator of σ^2. Clearly, $\frac{1}{n+1}\sum_i (X_i - \bar{X})^2 = \frac{n-1}{n+1}s^2$ is a biased estimator of σ^2.

$$\text{As} \frac{(n-1)S^2}{\sigma^2} \sim \chi^2_{n-1} \quad \therefore V\left[\frac{(n-1)S^2}{\sigma^2}\right] = 2(n-1)$$

$$\therefore V\left(s^2\right) = \frac{2}{n-1}\sigma^4 = \text{MSE of } s^2.$$

On the other hand, MSE of $\frac{n-1}{n+1}s^2 = V\left(\frac{n-1}{n+1}s^2\right) + \left(\frac{n-1}{n+1}\sigma^2 - \sigma^2\right)^2$

$$= \left(\frac{n-1}{n+1}\right)^2 \frac{2}{n-1}\sigma^4 + \frac{4\sigma^4}{(n+1)^2} = \frac{2\sigma^4}{(n+1)^2}(n-1+2) = \frac{2\sigma^4}{n+1} < \frac{2\sigma^4}{n-1}$$

$\Rightarrow$ MSE of s^2 > MSE of $\frac{n-1}{n+1}s^2$, i.e. MSE (Unbiased estimator) > MSE (biased estimator).

Remark 1.13: Pooling of information Let T_i be an unbiased estimator of θ obtained from the ith source, $i = 1, 2 \ldots, k$. Suppose T_i's are independent and $V(T_i) = \sigma_i^2 < \sigma^2$ $\forall i$. Then $\bar{T}_k = \frac{1}{k} = (T_1 + T_2 + \cdots + T_k)$ is also an unbiased estimator of θ with $V(\overline{T}_k) = \frac{1}{k^2}\sum_1^k \sigma_i^2 < \frac{\sigma^2}{k} \to 0$ as $k \to \propto$.

The implication of this statement is that $\overline{T}_k$ gets closer and closer to the true value of the parameter as $k \to \propto$ (k becomes larger and larger).

On the other hand if T_i's are biased estimator with common bias β, then $\overline{T}_k$ approaches to the wrong value $\theta + \beta$ instead of the true value θ even if $k \to \propto$.

Problem 1.1 Let $X_1, X_2, \ldots, X_n$ be a random sample from $b(1, \overline{\wedge})$.

Show that

(i) $\frac{X(X-1)}{n(n-1)}$ is an unbiased estimator of $\overline{\wedge}^2$

(ii) $\frac{X(n-X)}{n(n-1)}$ is an unbiased estimator of $\overline{\wedge}(1-\overline{\wedge})$

where X = number of success in n tosses = $\sum_{i=1}^n X_i$.

Minimum-VarianceUnbiased Estimator (MVUE)

Let U be the set of all u.e's (T) of θ with $E(T^2) < \propto \forall\theta \in \Theta$, and then an estimator $T_0 \in U$ will be called a minimum-variance unbiased estimator (MVUE) of θ\{or $\gamma(\theta)$\} if $V(T_0) \leq V(T)$ $\forall\theta$ and for every $T \in U$.

Result 1.1 Let U be the set of all u.e's (T) of θ with $E(T^2) < \propto$, $\forall\theta \in \Theta$. Furthermore, let U_0 be the class of all u.e's (v) of '0' {Zero} with $E(v^2) < \propto \forall\theta$, i.e. $U_0 = \{v: E(v) = 0\ \forall\theta$ and $E(v^2) < \propto]$.

Then an estimator $T_0 \in U$ will be an MVUE of θ iff

$$\text{Cov}(T_0, v) = E(T_0 v) = 0\ \forall\,\theta, \forall v \in U_0.$$

Proof **Only if part** Given that T_0 is an MVUE of θ, we have to prove that

$$E(T_0 v) = 0\ \forall\theta,\ \forall v \in U_0 \tag{1.9}$$

Suppose the statement (1.9) is wrong.

$\therefore E(T_0 v) \neq 0$ for some θ_0 and for some $v_0 \in U_0$. □

Note that for every real λ, $T_0 + \lambda v_0$ is an u.e. of θ.
Again, $T_0 + \lambda v_0 \in U$, as $E(T_0 + \lambda v_0)^2 < \infty$
Now $V_{00}(T_0 + \lambda v_o) = V_{00}(T_0) + \lambda^2 E_{00}(V_0^2) + 2\lambda E(v_0 T_0)$.
Choose a particular setting $\lambda = -\frac{E_{00}(T_0 v_0)}{E_{00}\left(V_0^2\right)}$ assuming $E_{00}(v_0^2) > 0$
(If $E_{00}(v_0^2) = 0$ then $P_{00}(v_0 = 0) = 1$, and hence $E_{00}(T_0 v_0) = 0$)
We have $V_{00}(T_0 + \lambda v_0) = V_{00}(T_0) - \frac{E_{00}^2(T_o v_o)}{E_o(V_o^2)} < V_{00}(T_0)$ which contradicts the fact that T_0 is a minimum-variance unbiased estimator of θ.

(if part) It is given that $\text{Cov}(T_0 v) = 0\ \forall\ \theta, \forall\ v \in U_0$. We have to prove that T_0 is an MVUE of θ. Let T be an estimator belonging to U, then $(T_0 - T) \in U_0$.
$\therefore$ From the given condition, $\text{Cov}(T_0, T_0 - T) = 0$

$$\Rightarrow V(T_0) - \text{Cov}(T_0, T) = 0 \quad \Rightarrow \text{Cov}\left(T_0, T\right) = V(T_0) \tag{1.10}$$

Now, $V(T_0 - T) \geq 0$

$$\begin{aligned} &\Rightarrow V(T_0) + V(T) - 2\ \text{Cov}(T_0, T) \geq 0 \\ &\Rightarrow V(T_0) + V(T) - 2\ V(T_0) \geq 0 \qquad \text{(by (1.10))} \\ &\Rightarrow V(T) \geq V(T_0) \qquad \forall \theta \in \Theta. \end{aligned}$$

Since T is an arbitrary member of U so that result.

Result 1.2 Minimum-variance unbiased estimator is unique.

Proof Suppose T_1 and T_2 are MVUE's of θ.
Then

$$\begin{aligned} &E\left\{T_1(T_1 - T_2)\right\} = 0 \qquad \text{(from Result 1.1)} \\ &\Rightarrow E\left(T_1^2\right) = E(T_1 T_2) \qquad \Rightarrow \rho_{T_1 T_2} = 1 \end{aligned}$$

as $V(T_1) = V(T_2)\ \forall \theta \Rightarrow T_1 = \beta T_2 + \alpha$ with probability 1.
Now $V(T_1) = \beta^2 V(T_2)\ \forall \theta \quad \Rightarrow \beta^2 = 1 \Rightarrow \beta = 1$ (as $\rho_{T_1 T_2} = 1$).
Again $E(T_1) = \beta E(T_2) + \alpha \quad \forall \theta \quad \Rightarrow \alpha = 0$
as $E(T_1) = E(T_2) = \theta$ and $\beta = 1 \quad \therefore P(T_1 = T_2) = 1$ □

Remark Correlation coefficient between T_1 and T_2 (where T_1 is an MVUE of θ and T_2 is any unbiased estimator of θ) is always non-negative.

$$\begin{aligned} &E\left\{T_1\ (T_1 - T_2)\right\} = 0 \quad \ldots \text{(from Result 1.1)} \\ &\Rightarrow \text{Cov}\ (T_1, T_2) = V(T_1) \geq 0. \end{aligned}$$

Result 1.3 Let T_1 be an MVUE of $\gamma_1(\theta)$ and T_2 be an MVUE of $\gamma_2(\theta)$. Then $\alpha T_1 + \beta T_2$ will be an MVUE of $\alpha\gamma_1(\theta) + \beta\gamma_2(\theta)$.

Proof Let v be an u.e. of zero.

Then

$$E(T_1 v) = 0 = E(T_2 v)$$

Now

$$E\{(\alpha T_1 + \beta T_2)v\} = \alpha E(T_1 v) + \beta E(T_2 v) = 0$$
$$\Rightarrow (\alpha T_1 + \beta T_2) \text{ is an MVUE of } \alpha\gamma_1(\theta) + \beta\gamma_2(\theta).$$

□

Result 1.4: (Rao–Cramer inequality) Let $X_1, X_2, \ldots, X_n$ be a random sample from a population having p.d.f. $f(x, \theta), \theta \in \Theta$. Assume that θ is a non-degenerate open interval on the real line. Let T be an unbiased estimator of $\gamma(\theta)$. Again assume that the joint p.d.f. $f(\underset{\sim}{x}, \theta)\left[= \prod_{i=1}^{n} f(x_i, \theta)\right]$ of $\underset{\sim}{X} = (X_1, X_2, \ldots, X_n)$ satisfies the following regularity conditions:

(a) $\frac{\partial f(\underset{\sim}{x}, \theta)}{\partial \theta}$ exists

(b) $\frac{\partial}{\partial \theta} \int f(\underset{\sim}{x}, \theta) d\underset{\sim}{x} = \int \frac{\partial f(\underset{\sim}{x}, \theta)}{\partial \theta} d\underset{\sim}{x}$

(c) $\frac{\partial}{\partial \theta} \int T(\underset{\sim}{x}) f(\underset{\sim}{x}, \theta) d\underset{\sim}{x} = \int T(\underset{\sim}{x}) \frac{\partial f(\underset{\sim}{x}, \theta)}{\partial \theta} d\underset{\sim}{x}$

and

(d) $0 < I(\theta) < \alpha$

where $I(\theta) = E\left[\frac{\partial \log f(\underset{\sim}{X}, \theta)}{\partial \theta}\right]^2$, information on θ supplied by the sample of size n.

Then

$$V(T) \geq \frac{(\gamma'(\theta))^2}{I(\theta)} \qquad \forall \theta.$$

Proof Since $1 = \int_{R^n} f(\underset{\sim}{x}, \theta) d\underset{\sim}{x}$

∴ We have from the condition (b)

$$O = \int_{R^n} \frac{\partial f(\underset{\sim}{x}, \theta)}{\partial \theta} d\underset{\sim}{x} = \int_{R^n} \frac{\partial \log f(\underset{\sim}{x}, \theta)}{\partial \theta} f(\underset{\sim}{x}, \theta) d\underset{\sim}{x} \qquad (1.11)$$

□

Again, since $T\left(\underset{\sim}{X}\right)$ is an u.e. of $\gamma(\theta)$, we have from condition (c)

$$\gamma'(\theta) = \int_{R^n} T(\underset{\sim}{x}) \frac{\partial \log f(\underset{\sim}{x}, \theta)}{\partial \theta} f(\underset{\sim}{x}, \theta) d\underset{\sim}{x} \tag{1.12}$$

Now, (1.12)–(1.11). $\gamma(\theta)$ gives us

$$\begin{aligned} \gamma'(\theta) &= \int_{R^n} [T(\underset{\sim}{x}) - \gamma(\theta)] \frac{\partial \log f(\underset{\sim}{x}, \theta)}{\partial \theta} f(\underset{\sim}{x}, \theta) d\underset{\sim}{x} \\ &= \text{Cov}\left\{T(\underset{\sim}{X}), \frac{\partial \log f(\underset{\sim}{X}, \theta)}{\partial \theta}\right\}. \end{aligned}$$

From the result, $[\text{Cov}(X, Y)]^2 \leq V(X)\,V(Y)$, we have

$$\{\gamma'(\theta)\}^2 = \left[\text{Cov}\left\{T(\underset{\sim}{X}), \frac{\partial \log f(\underset{\sim}{X}, \theta)}{\partial \theta}\right\}\right]^2$$

$$\leq V\{T(\underset{\sim}{X})\} \cdot V\left\{\frac{\partial \log f(\underset{\sim}{X}, \theta)}{\partial \theta}\right\}$$

$$= V\left\{T(\underset{\sim}{X})\right\} \cdot E\left(\frac{\partial \log f(\underset{\sim}{X}, \theta)}{\partial \theta}\right)^2 \qquad \left(\text{as from (1.11) } E\frac{\partial \log f(\underset{\sim}{X}, \theta)}{\partial \theta} = 0\right)$$

$$= V\,\{T(X)\} \cdot I(\theta)$$

$$\Rightarrow V\,(T) \geq \frac{\{\gamma'(\theta)\}^2}{I(\theta)}, \quad \forall\, \theta.$$

□

Remark 1 If the variables are of discrete type, the underlying condition and the proof of the Cramer–Rao inequality will also be similar, only the multiple integrals being replaced by multiple sum.

Remark 2 For any set of estimators T, having expectation $\gamma(\theta)$,

$$\text{MSE} = E(T-\theta)^2 = V(T) + B^2(T,\theta) \geq \frac{\{\gamma'(\theta)\}^2}{I(\theta)} + B^2(T,\theta) =$$

$$\frac{[1+B'(T,\theta)]^2}{I(\theta)} + B^2(T,\theta) \quad [\text{where } \gamma(\theta) = \theta + B(T,\theta)].$$

Remark 3 Assuming that $f\left(\underset{\sim}{x},\ \theta\right)$ is differentiable not only once but also twice, we have

$$0 = \int\limits_{R^n} \frac{\partial^2 \log f(\underset{\sim}{x},\theta)}{\partial\theta^2} f(\underset{\sim}{x},\theta)d\underset{\sim}{x} + \int\limits_{R^n} \left\{\frac{\partial \log f(\underset{\sim}{x},\theta)}{\partial\theta}\right\}^2 f(\underset{\sim}{x},\theta)d\underset{\sim}{x}$$

$$\Rightarrow \quad I(\theta) = -E\left\{\frac{\partial^2 \log f(\underset{\sim}{x},\theta)}{\partial\theta^2}\right\}.$$

Remark 4 Since $X_1, X_2, \ldots, X_n$ are iid random variables,

$$I(\theta) = -n\, E\left\{\frac{\partial^2 \log f(\underset{\sim}{x},\theta)}{\partial\theta^2}\right\}.$$

Remark 5 An estimator T for which the Cramer–Rao lower bound is attained is often called a minimum-variance bound estimator (MVBE). In this case, we have

$$\frac{\partial \log f(\underset{\sim}{x},\theta)}{\partial\theta} = \lambda(\theta)\{T - \gamma(\theta)\}.$$

Note that every MVBE is an MVUE, but the converse may not be true.

Remark 6 Distributions admitting an MVUE

A distribution having an MVUE of $\lambda(\theta)$ must satisfy $\frac{\partial \log f(x,\theta)}{\partial\theta} = \lambda(\theta)\{T - \gamma(\theta)\}$. It is a differential equation. So

$$\log f(x,\theta) = T\int \lambda(\theta)\, d\theta - \int \lambda(\theta)\, \gamma(\theta)d\theta + c(x)$$

$$\Rightarrow f(x,\theta) = \mathrm{A}e^{T\theta_1 + \theta_2}$$

where $\theta_i, i = 1,2$ are functions of θ and $A = e^{c(x)}$

Note If T be a sufficient statistic for θ, then

$$L = g(T,\ \theta)\, h(x_1,\ x_2,\ldots, x_n)$$

$$\text{or,}\quad \frac{\partial \log\ L}{\partial\theta} = \frac{\partial \log\ g(T,\theta)}{\partial\theta} \tag{1.13}$$

which is a function of T and θ.

Now the condition that T be an MVB unbiased estimator of θ is that $\phi = \frac{\partial \log\ L}{\partial\theta} = B(T-\theta)$ which is a linear function of T and θ and $V(T) = 1/B$. Thus if there exists an MVB unbiased estimator of θ it is also sufficient. The converse is not necessarily true. Equation (1.13) may be a non-linear functions of T and θ in which case T is not an MVB unbiased estimator of θ. Thus the existence of MVB unbiased estimator implies the existence of a sufficient estimator, but the existence of sufficient statistic does not necessarily imply the existence of an MVB unbiased estimator. It also follows that the distribution possessing an MVB unbiased estimator for its parameter can be expressed in Koopman form. Thus, when $L = e^{A'T + B(\theta) + R(x_1, x_2, \ldots x_n)}$, T is an MVB unbiased estimator of θ with variance $1/(\frac{\partial A'}{\partial \theta})$, which is also MVB.

Example $x_1, x_2, \ldots, x_n$ is a random sample from $N(\mu, 1)$

Here, $L = \left(\frac{1}{\sqrt{2\pi}}\right)^n e^{-\frac{1}{2}\sum_{i=1}^{n}(x_i-\mu)^2} = e^{-\frac{1}{2}\left\{\sum_{i=1}^{n}(x_i-\bar{x})^2 + n\bar{x} + n\mu^2 - 2n\mu\bar{x}\right\} - \frac{n}{2}\log 2\pi}$

Take $A'T = n\mu\bar{x}$ where $T = \bar{x}$. MVB $= 1/(\frac{\partial(n\mu)}{\partial\mu}) = \frac{1}{n}$.

Example $x_1, x_2, \ldots, x_n$ is a random sample from $b(1, \pi)$ distribution.

Here, $L = \pi^{\sum_i x_i}(1-\pi)^{n-\sum_i x_i} = e^{\left(\sum_{i=1}^{n} x_i\right)\log\pi + (n-\sum_i x_i)\log(1-\pi)} = e^{n\bar{x}\log\frac{\pi}{1-\pi} + n\log(1-\pi)}$.

Take $= A'T = n\log\frac{\pi}{1-\pi}\bar{x}$ where $T = \bar{x} = \frac{k}{n}$, k = number of successes in n trials.

$$\text{MVB} = 1\Bigg/\left(\frac{\partial n\log\frac{\pi}{1-\pi}}{\partial\pi}\right) = \frac{\pi(1-\pi)}{n}.$$

Remark 7 A necessary condition for satisfying the regularity conditions is that the domain of positive p.d.f. must be free from θ.

Example 1.16 Let $X \sim U[0, \theta]$, let us compute $nE\left(\frac{\partial \log f(x,\theta)}{\partial\theta}\right)^2$ which is $\frac{n}{\theta^2}$. So Cramer–Rao lower bound, in this case, for the variance of an unbiased estimator of θ is $\frac{\theta^2}{n}$ (apparant).

Now, we consider an estimator. $T = \frac{n+1}{n}X_{(n)}, X_{(n)} = \max(X_1, X_2, \ldots, X_n)$. P.d.f. of $X_{(n)}$ is $f_{X_{(n)}}(x) = n\left(\frac{x}{\theta}\right)^{n-1} \cdot \frac{1}{\theta}, 0 \le x \le \theta$.

$$\therefore E\left(X_{(n)}\right) = \frac{n}{\theta^n}\int_0^\theta x^n \mathrm{d}x = \frac{n}{\theta^n}\cdot\left.\frac{x^{n+1}}{n+1}\right]_0^\theta = \frac{n}{n+1}\theta.$$

$\Rightarrow T = \frac{n+1}{n}X_{(n)}$ is an unbiased estimator of θ. It can be shown that $V(T) = \frac{\theta^2}{n(n+2)} < \frac{\theta^2}{n}$.

This is not surprising because the regularity conditions do not hold here. Actually, here $\frac{\partial f(x,\theta)}{\partial \theta}$ exists for $\theta \neq x$ but not for $\theta = x$ since

$$f(x,\theta) = \frac{1}{\theta} \quad \text{if } \theta \geq x$$
$$= 0 \quad \text{if } \theta < x.$$

Result 1.5: Rao–Blackwell Theorem Let $\{F_\theta, \theta \in \Theta\}$ be a family of distribution functions and h be any estimator of $\gamma(\theta)$ in U which is the class of unbiased estimators (h) with $E_\theta(h^2) < \infty\ \forall\theta$.. Let T be a sufficient statistic for the family $\{F_\theta, \theta \in \Theta\}$. Then $E(h/T)$ is free from θ and will be an unbiased estimator of $\gamma(\theta)$. Moreover, $V\{E(h/T)\} \leq V(h) \quad \forall\theta, \theta \in \Theta$.

The equality sign holds iff $h = E(h/T)$ with probability '1'.

Proof Since T is a sufficient for the family $\{F_\theta, \theta \in \Theta\}$, conditional distribution of h given T must be independent of θ.

$\therefore E(h/T)$ will be free from θ.

$$\text{Now, } \gamma(\theta) = E(h) = E_T\left[E_{h/T}(h/T)\right] \quad \forall\, \theta$$
$$\text{i.e. } \gamma(\theta) = E\{E(h/T)\} \quad \forall\, \theta$$

$\Rightarrow E(h/T)$ is an unbiased estimator of $\gamma(\theta)$.

Again we know that $V(h) = V\{E(h|T)\} + E\{V(h|T)\}$

$$\Rightarrow V(h) \geq V\{E(h|T)\} \quad (\text{since } V(h|T) \geq 0)$$

'=' holds iff $V(h|T) = 0.$, i.e. iff $h = E(h|T)$ with probability '1'

$$\left[V(h|T) = E_{h/T}\{h - E(h|T)\}^2\right]$$

□

Result 1.6: Lehmann–Scheffe Theorem If T be a complete sufficientstatistic for θ and if h be an unbiased estimator of $\gamma(\theta)$, then $E(h|T)$ will be an MVUE of $\gamma(\theta)$.

Proof Let both $h_1, h_2 \in U = [h\ :\ E(h) = \gamma(\theta), E(h^2) < \infty]$.

Then $E\{E(h_1|T)\} = \gamma(\theta) = E\{E(h_2|T)\}$ (from Result 1.5).

Hence, $E\{E(h_1|T) - E(h_2|T)\} = 0 \ldots \forall\theta$

$$\Rightarrow P\{E(h_1|T) = E(h_2|T)\} = 1 \quad (\because T \text{ is complete}).$$

$\therefore E(h|T)$ is unique for any $h \in U$.

Again, applying Result 1.5, we have $V\{E(h|T)\} \leq V(h) \forall\, h \in U$. Now since $E(h|T)$ is unique, it will be an MVUE of $\gamma(\theta)$. □

Remark 1.14 The implication of Result 1.5 is that if we are given an unbiased estimator h, then we can improve upon h by forming the new estimator$E(h|T)$

based on h and the sufficient statistic T. This process of finding an improved estimator starting from an unbiased estimator has been called Blackwellization.

Problem 1.2 Let $X_1, X_2, \ldots, X_n$ be a random sample from $N(\mu, \sigma^2)$, σ^2 known. Let $\gamma(\mu) = \mu^2$.

(a) Show that the variance of any unbiased estimator of μ^2 cannot be less than $\frac{4\mu^2\sigma^2}{n}$

(b) Show that $T = \overline{X}^2 - \frac{\sigma^2}{n}$ is an MVUE of μ^2 with variance $\frac{4\mu^2\sigma^2}{n} + \frac{2\sigma^4}{n}$.

Example 1.17 Let $X \sim P(\lambda)$, then show that $\delta(x) = \begin{cases} 1 & \text{if } X = 0 \\ 0 & \text{otherwise} \end{cases}$ is the only unbiased estimator of $\gamma(\lambda) = e^{-\lambda}$. Is it an MVUE of $e^{-\lambda}$?

Answer

Let $h(x)$ be an unbiased estimator of $e^{-\lambda} = \theta$, say.

Then $E\{h(x)\} = \theta \quad \forall\theta$

$$\Rightarrow \sum_{x=0}^{\infty} h(x) \frac{\theta\left(\log_e \frac{1}{\theta}\right)^x}{x!} = \theta \quad \forall\theta$$

$$\Rightarrow h(x) = \begin{cases} 1 \text{ if } x = 0 \\ 0 \text{ if } x \neq 0 \end{cases}$$

$\Rightarrow h(x)$, i.e., $\delta(x)$ is the only unbiased estimator of $e^{-\lambda}$.

Here, unbiased estimator of $e^{-\lambda}$ is unique and its variance exists. Therefore, $\delta(x)$ will be an MVUE of $\gamma(\lambda) = e^{-\lambda}$.

$$\left[E\{h(x)\}^2 = 1.P(x=0) + 0.\sum_{i=1}^{\infty} P(x=i) = e^{-\lambda} < \infty \right]$$

Remark 1.15 MVUE may not be very sensible.

Example Let $X_1, X_2, \ldots, X_n$ be a random sample from $N(\mu, 1)$, and then $T = \overline{X}^2 - \frac{1}{n}$ is an MVUE of μ^2. Note that $\left(\overline{X}^2 - \frac{1}{n}\right)$ may occasionally be negative, so that an MVUE of μ^2 is not very sensible in this case.

Remark 1.16 An MVUE may not exist even though an unbiased estimator does exist.

Example Let

$P\{X = -1\} = \theta$ and $P\{X = n\} = (1-\theta)^2\theta^n$, $n = 0, 1, 2, \ldots, 0 < \theta < 1$.

No MVUE of θ exists even though an unbiased estimator of θ exists.

$$\text{e.g.} \quad T(X) = \begin{cases} 1 & \text{if } X = -1 \\ 0 & \text{otherwise} \end{cases}$$

Bhattacharya system of Lower Bounds (Sankhya A (1946))
(Generalization of Cramer–Rao lower bound)
Regularity conditions

A family of distribution $P = \{f_\theta(x), \theta \in \Omega\}$ is said to satisfy Bhattacharya regularity conditions if

1. θ lies in an open interval Ω of real line R. Ω may be infinite;
2. $\frac{\partial^i}{\partial\theta^i} f_\theta(x)$ exists for almost all x and $\forall\theta$, $i = 1, 2, \ldots k$;
3. $$\frac{\partial^i}{\partial\theta^i} \int f_\theta(x)\mathrm{d}x = \int \frac{\partial^i}{\partial\theta^i} f_\theta(x)\mathrm{d}x \quad \forall\theta, \quad i = 1, 2 \ldots k; \text{ and}$$
4. $V^{k\times k}(\theta) = \{v_{ij}(\theta)\}, \quad \begin{matrix} i = 1, 2, \ldots k \\ j = 1, 2, \ldots k \end{matrix}$
   exists and is positive definite $\forall\theta$ where

$$v_{ij}(\theta) = E_\theta\left[\frac{1}{f_\theta(x)} \frac{\partial^i}{\partial\theta^i} f_\theta(x) \frac{\partial^j}{\partial\theta^j} f_\theta(x)\right].$$

For $i = 1$, Bhattacharya regularity conditions $\equiv$ Cramer–Rao regularity conditions.

Theorem 1.1 *Let $P = \{f_\theta(x), \theta \in \Omega\}$ be a family of distributions satisfying above-mentioned regularity conditions and $g(\theta)$ be a real valued, estimable, and k times differentiable function of θ. Let T be an unbiased estimator of $g(\theta)$ satisfying*

5. $\frac{\partial}{\partial\theta^i} \int t(x) f_\theta(x)\mathrm{d}x = \int t(x) \frac{\partial}{\partial\theta^i} f_\theta(x)\mathrm{d}x$

Then

$$\mathrm{Var}_\theta(T) \geq g' V^{-1} g \quad \forall\theta$$

where

$$g' = \left\{g^{(1)}(\theta), g^{(2)}(\theta), \ldots, g^{(k)}(\theta)\right\}; g^{(i)}(\theta) = \frac{\partial^i}{\partial\theta^i} g(\theta)$$

Proof

$$\text{Define } \beta_i(x,\theta) = \frac{1}{f_\theta(x)}\frac{\partial^i}{\partial\theta^i}f_\theta(x)$$
$$E[\beta_i(x,\theta)] = \int \frac{1}{f_\theta(x)}\frac{\partial^i}{\partial\theta^i}f_\theta(x)\cdot f_\theta(x)\mathrm{d}x = 0$$
$$V[\beta_i(x,\theta)] = E[\beta_i(x,\theta)]^2 = E\left[\frac{1}{f_\theta(x)}\frac{\partial^i}{\partial\theta^i}f_\theta(x)\right]^2 = v_{ii}(\theta)$$
$$\mathrm{Cov}(\beta_i,\beta_j) = v_{ij}(\theta)$$

$$\mathrm{Cov}(T,\beta_i) = \int t(x)\frac{1}{f_\theta(x)}\frac{\partial^i}{\partial\theta^i}f_\theta(x)\,.\,f_\theta(x)\mathrm{d}x = \frac{\partial^i}{\partial\theta^i}\int t(x)f_\theta(x)\mathrm{d}x = g^{(i)}(\theta)$$

$$\text{Let } \Sigma^{(k+1)x(k+1)} = \text{Disp}\begin{pmatrix} T \\ \beta_1 \\ \beta_2 \\ \cdot \\ \cdot \\ \cdot \\ \beta_k \end{pmatrix}$$

$$= \left\{\begin{matrix} V_\theta(T) & g^{(1)}(\theta) & g^{(2)}(\theta) & \ldots & g^{(k)}(\theta) \\ g^{(1)}(\theta) & v_{11} & v_{12} & \ldots & v_{1k} \\ g^{(2)}(\theta) & v_{21} & v_{22} & \ldots & v_{21} \\ \cdot & \cdot & \cdot & \ldots & \ldots \\ \cdot & \cdot & \cdot & \ldots & \ldots \\ g^{(k)}(\theta) & v_{k1} & v_{k2} & \ldots & v_{kk} \end{matrix}\right\} = \begin{pmatrix} V_\theta(T) & g' \\ g & V \end{pmatrix}$$

$$|\Sigma| = |V|\{V_\theta(T) - g'V^{-1}g\}$$
$$\text{as } |\Sigma| \geq 0, \quad |V| \geq 0$$
$$\Rightarrow V_\theta(T) - g'V^{-1}g \geq 0 \quad \text{i.e. } V_\theta(T) \geq g'V^{-1}g \ \ \forall\theta.$$

Cor: For $k = 1$ $\quad V_\theta(T) \geq \frac{\{g'(\theta)\}^2}{v_{11}(\theta)} = \frac{\{g'(\theta)\}^2}{I(\theta)}$ = Cramer–Rao lower bound. □

Case of equality holds when $|\sum| = 0$

$$\therefore R\left(\sum\right) < k+1 \text{ or } R\left(\sum\right) \leq k,\ R(V) = k \quad \left[R\left(\sum\right) = \text{rank of } \sum\right]$$
$$R\left(\sum\right) \geq R(V) \Rightarrow R\left(\sum\right) = k.$$

Lemma 1.1 Let $X = (x_1, x_2, \ldots, x_p)'$, $D(X) = \sum^{p\times p}$

$\sum$ is of rank $r(\leq p)$ iff $x_1, x_2, \ldots, x_p$ satisfies $(p - r)$ linear restrictions of the form

$$a_{11}\{x_1 - E(x_1)\} + a_{12}\{x_2 - E(x_2)\} + \cdots + a_{1p}\{x_p - E(x_p)\} = 0$$
$$a_{21}\{x_1 - E(x_1)\} + a_{22}\{x_2 - E(x_2)\} + \cdots + a_{2p}\{x_p - E(x_p)\} = 0$$
$$\cdot$$
$$\cdot$$
$$a_{\overline{p-r},1}\{x_1 - E(x_1)\} + a_{\overline{p-r},2}\{x_2 - E(x_2)\} + \cdots + a_{\overline{p-r},p}\{x_p - E(x_p)\} = 0$$

with probability 1.

Put $p = k + 1$, $r = k$; $x_1 = T$, $x_2 = \beta_1, \ldots, x_p = \beta_k$.

Then $R(\Sigma) = k$ iff $T, \beta_1, \beta_2, \ldots, \beta_k$ satisfy one restriction with probability '1' of the form

$$a_1\{T - E(T)\} + a_2\{\beta_1 - E(\beta_1)\} + \cdots + a_{k+1}\{\beta_k - E(\beta_k)\} = 0$$
$$\Rightarrow a_1\{T - g(\theta)\} + a_2\beta_1 + \cdots + a_{k+1}\beta_k = 0$$
$$\Rightarrow T - g(\theta) = b_1\beta_1 + b_2\beta_2 + \cdots + b_k\beta_k = \underset{\sim}{b}'\underset{\sim}{\beta}$$

where $\underset{\sim}{b}' = (b_1, b_2, \ldots, b_k)$ and $\underset{\sim}{\beta} = (\beta_1, \beta_2, \ldots, \beta_k,)'$.

Result

$T - g(\theta) = b'\beta$ with probability '1' $\Rightarrow T - g(\theta) = g'V^{-1}\beta$ with probability '1'.

Proof

$$T - g(\theta) = b'\beta \Rightarrow V_\theta(T) = g'V^{-1}g$$

Consider $V_\theta(b'\beta - g'V^{-1}\beta) = V_\theta(T - g'V^{-1}\beta)$

$$= V_\theta(T) + g'V^{-1}V(\beta)V^{-1}g - 2g'V^{-1}\mathrm{Cov}(T, \beta)$$

$= g'V^{-1}g + g'V^{-1}g - 2g'V^{-1}g = 0 \Rightarrow b'\beta = g'V^{-1}\beta$ with probability '1'. □

A series of lower bounds: $g'V^{-1}g = \{g^{(1)}, g^{(2)}, \ldots, g^{(k)}\}V^{-1}\begin{pmatrix} g^{(1)} \\ g^{(2)} \\ \cdot \\ \cdot \\ g^{(k)} \end{pmatrix}$ gives

nth lower bound $= {g_{(n)}}'{V_n}^{-1}g_{(n)} = \Delta_n, n = 1, 2, .., k$

Theorem 1.2 *The sequence* $\{\Delta_n\}$ *is a non-decreasing sequences, i.e.* $\Delta_{n+1} \geq \Delta_n \forall n$

Proof The $(n+1)$th lower bound $\Delta_{n+1} = g'_{n+1}\, V_{n+1}{}^{-1} g_{n+1}$ where $g'_{n+1} = \left\{g^{(1)}{}_{(\theta)}, g^{(2)}{}_{(\theta)}, \ldots, g^{(n)}{}_{(\theta)}, g^{(n+1)}{}_{(\theta)}\right\} = \{g^1_n, g^{n+1}\}$

$$V_{n+1} = \begin{pmatrix} v_{11} & v_{12} & v_{1n} & v_{1,\overline{n+1}} \\ v_{21} & v_{22} & v_{2n} & v_{2,\overline{n+1}} \\ \cdot & \cdot & \cdot & \cdot \\ \cdot & \cdot & \cdot & \cdot \\ v_{n1} & v_{n2}\cdot\cdot & v_{nn} & v_{n,\overline{n+1}} \\ v_{\overline{n+1},1} & v_{\overline{n+1},2}\cdot\cdot & v_{\overline{n+1},n} & v_{\overline{n+1},\overline{n+1}} \end{pmatrix} = \begin{pmatrix} V_n & v_n \\ v'_n & v_{\overline{n+1},\overline{n+1}} \end{pmatrix}$$

where $v'_n = \left(v_{\overline{n+1},1}\ v_{\overline{n+1},2}\cdots v_{\overline{n+1},n}\right)$.

$$\begin{aligned} \text{Now } \Delta_{n+1} &= g'_{n+1} V^{-1}_{n+1} g_{n+1} \\ &= g'_{n+1} C'(C')^{-1} V^{-1}_{n+1} C^{-1} C g_{n+1} \quad \text{for any non symmetric matrix } C^{\overline{n+1}x\overline{n+1}} \\ &= (Cg_{n+1})'(CV_{n+1}C')^{-1}(Cg_{n+1}) \end{aligned}$$

$$\text{Choose } C = \begin{pmatrix} I_n & \underset{\sim}{o} \\ -v'_n V_n^{-1} & 1 \end{pmatrix}$$

$$\therefore Cg_{n+1} = \begin{pmatrix} I_n & \underset{\sim}{o} \\ -v'_n V_n^{-1} & 1 \end{pmatrix} \begin{pmatrix} g_n \\ g^{n+1} \end{pmatrix} = \begin{pmatrix} g_n \\ g^{n+1} - v'_n V_n^{-1} g_n \end{pmatrix}$$

$$CV_{n+1}C' = \begin{pmatrix} I_n & \underset{\sim}{o} \\ -v'_n V_n^{-1} & 1 \end{pmatrix} \begin{pmatrix} V_n & v_n \\ v'_n & v_{\overline{n+1},\overline{n+1},} \end{pmatrix} \begin{pmatrix} I_n & -V_n^{-1} v_n \\ \underset{\sim}{o} & 1 \end{pmatrix}$$

$$= \begin{pmatrix} I_n & \underset{\sim}{o} \\ -v'_n V_n^{-1} & 1 \end{pmatrix} \begin{pmatrix} V_n & \underset{\sim}{o} \\ v'_n & v_{\overline{n+1},\overline{n+1}} - v'_n V_n^{-1} v_n \end{pmatrix} = \begin{pmatrix} V_n & \underset{\sim}{o} \\ \underset{\sim}{o} & E_{\overline{n+1},\overline{n+1}} \end{pmatrix}$$

Since V_{n+1} is positive definite, $CV_{n+1}C'$ is also +ve definite □

$$E_{\overline{n+1},\overline{n+1},} > 0, \quad (CV_{n+1}C')^{-1} = \begin{pmatrix} V_n^{-1} & \underset{\sim}{o} \\ \underset{\sim}{o} & E^{-1}_{\overline{n+1},\overline{n+1}} \end{pmatrix}$$

Then

$$\Delta_{n+1} = \{g_n, g^{n+1} - v_n' V_n^{-1} g_n\} \begin{pmatrix} V_n^{-1} & \underset{\sim}{o} \\ \underset{\sim}{o} & E^{-1}_{\overline{n+1,n+1}} \end{pmatrix} \begin{pmatrix} g_n' \\ g^{n+1} - v_n' V_n^{-1} g_n \end{pmatrix}$$

$$= \left\{g_n V_n^{-1}, (g^{n+1} - v_n' V_n^{-1} g_n) E^{-1}_{\overline{n+1,n+1}}\right\} \begin{pmatrix} g_n' \\ g^{n+1} - v_n' V_n^{-1} g_n \end{pmatrix}$$

$$= g_n' V_n^{-1} g_n + \frac{\left(g^{n+1} - v_n' V_n^{-1} g_n\right)^2}{E^{-1}_{\overline{n+1,n+1}}} \geq g_n' V_n^{-1} g_n = \Delta_n$$

i.e. $\Delta_{n+1} \geq \Delta_n$.

If there exists no unbiased estimator T of $g(\theta)$ for which $V(T)$ attains the nth Bhattacharya's Lower Bound (BLB), then one can try to find a sharper lower bound by considering the $(n + 1)$th BLB. In case the lower bound is attained at nth stage, then $\Delta_{n+1} = \Delta_n$. However, $\Delta_{n+1} = \Delta_n$ does not imply that the lower bound is attained at the nth stage.

Example 1.18 $X_1, X_2, \ldots, X_n$ is a random sample from iid $N(\theta, 1)$

$$f_\theta(x) = \text{Const. } e^{-\frac{1}{2}\sum (x_i-\theta)^2}, \; g(\theta) = \theta^2$$

$$\overline{X} \sim N\left(\theta, \frac{1}{n}\right) \text{i.e. } E(\overline{X}) = \theta, \;\; V(\overline{X}) = \frac{1}{n}$$

$$\therefore E(\overline{X}^2) - E^2(\overline{X}) = \frac{1}{n} \Rightarrow E(\overline{X}^2) = \theta^2 + \frac{1}{n}$$

$$\therefore E\left(\overline{X}^2 - \frac{1}{n}\right) = \theta^2, \;\; T = \overline{X}^2 - \frac{1}{n}.$$

$$\frac{\partial}{\partial \theta} f_\theta(x) = \text{Const. } e^{-\frac{1}{2}\sum (x_i-\theta)^2} \cdot \sum (x_i - \theta)$$

$$\beta_1 = \frac{1}{f_\theta(x)} \frac{\partial}{\partial \theta} f_\theta(x) = \sum (x_i - \theta)$$

$$\beta_2 = \frac{1}{f_\theta(x)} \frac{\partial^2}{\partial \theta^2} f_\theta(x) = \left\{\sum (x_i - \theta)\right\}^2 - n$$

$$E(\beta_1) = 0, \; E(\beta_2) = 0, \; E(\beta_1^2) = n,$$

$$E(\beta_1 \beta_2) = E\left\{\sum (x_i - \theta)\right\}^3 - nE\left\{\sum (x_i - \theta)\right\} = 0$$

$$E(\beta_2^2) = E\left\{\sum (x_i - \theta)\right\}^4 + n^2 - 2nE\left\{\sum (x_i - \theta)\right\}^2$$

$$= 3n^2 + n^2 - 2n \cdot n = 2n^2$$

$$V = \begin{pmatrix} n & 0 \\ 0 & 2n^2 \end{pmatrix} \Rightarrow V^{-1} = \begin{pmatrix} \frac{1}{n} & 0 \\ 0 & \frac{1}{2n^2} \end{pmatrix}$$

$$g(\theta) = \theta^2, g^{(1)}(\theta) = 2\theta, g^{(2)}(\theta) = 2 \therefore g' = (2\theta, 2)$$

$$\begin{aligned} \Delta_2 = g'V^{-1}g = (2\theta, 2)\begin{pmatrix} \frac{1}{n} & 0 \\ 0 & \frac{1}{2n^2} \end{pmatrix}\begin{pmatrix} 2\theta \\ 2 \end{pmatrix} &= (2\theta, 2)\begin{pmatrix} 2\theta/n \\ 1/n^2 \end{pmatrix} \\ &= \frac{4\theta^2}{n} + \frac{2}{n^2}. \end{aligned}$$

$$\left[n\bar{X}^2 \sim \chi^2_{1,\lambda}, \lambda = n\theta^2; V\left(n\bar{X}^2\right) = 2 + 4n\theta^2; V\left(\bar{X}^2\right) = \frac{2}{n^2} + \frac{4\theta^2}{n}\right]$$

Lower bound is attained if $b'\beta = T - g(\theta) = g'V^{-1}\beta$.

$$\begin{aligned} T - g(\theta) &= (2\theta, 2)\begin{pmatrix} \frac{1}{n} & 0 \\ 0 & \frac{1}{2n^2} \end{pmatrix}\begin{Bmatrix} \sum(x_i - \theta) \\ [\sum(x_i - \theta)]^2 - n \end{Bmatrix} \\ &= (2\theta, 2)\begin{Bmatrix} \bar{x} - \theta \\ \frac{1}{2}(\bar{x} - \theta)^2 - \frac{1}{2n} \end{Bmatrix} = 2\theta(\bar{x} - \theta) + (\bar{x} - \theta)^2 - \frac{1}{n} \\ &= (\bar{x} - \theta)(2\theta + \bar{x} - \theta) - \frac{1}{n} = \bar{x}^2 - \theta^2 - \frac{1}{n}. \end{aligned}$$

Theorem 1.3 *Let $f_\theta(x)$ is of the exponential, i.e.*

$$f_\theta(x) = h(x)e^{k_1(\theta)t(x) + k_2(\theta)} \text{ such that } k_1'(\theta) \neq 0. \tag{1.14}$$

Then the variance of an unbiased estimator of $g(\theta)$, say $\widehat{g}(x)$, attains the kth *lower bound but not* $(k-1)$th *if $\widehat{g}(x)$ is a polynomial of degree k in $t(x)$.*

Proof If $f_\theta(x)$ is of form (1.14), then

$$\begin{aligned} &\frac{\partial}{\partial\theta}f_\theta(x) = f_\theta(x)\left[k_1'(\theta)t(x) + k_2'(\theta)\right] \\ &\beta_1 = \frac{1}{f_\theta(x)}\frac{\partial}{\partial\theta}f_\theta(x) = k_1'(\theta)t(x) + k_2'(\theta) \\ &\frac{\partial^2}{\partial\theta^2}f_\theta(x) = f_\theta(x)\left[\left\{k_1'(\theta)t(x) + k_2'(\theta)\right\}^2 + \left\{k_1''(\theta)t(x) + k_2''(\theta)\right\}\right] \\ &\beta_2 = \frac{1}{f_\theta(x)}\frac{\partial^2}{\partial\theta^2}f_\theta(x) = \left\{k_1'(\theta)t(x) + k_2'(\theta)\right\}^2 + \left\{k_1''(\theta)t(x) + k_2''(\theta)\right\} \end{aligned}$$

Generally, $\beta_i = \frac{1}{f_\theta(x)}\frac{\partial^i}{\partial\theta^i}f_\theta(x) = \left\{k_1'(\theta)t(x) + k_2'(\theta)\right\}^i + P_{i-1}\{t(x), \theta\}$ where $P_{i-1}\{t(x), \theta\}$ = a polynomial in $t(x)$ of degree at most $(i-1)$. □

Let $P_{i-1}\{t(x),\theta\} = \sum_{j=0}^{i-1} Q_{ij}(\theta).t^j(x)$

Then

$$\begin{aligned}\beta_i &= \{k_1'(\theta)t(x) + k_2'(\theta)\}^i + \sum_{j=0}^{i-1} Q_{ij}(\theta).t^j(x) \\ &= \sum_{j=0}^{i-1}\binom{i}{j}\{k_1'(\theta)\}^j.t^j(x)\cdot\{k_2'(\theta)\}^{i-j} + \sum_{j=0}^{i-1} Q_{ij}(\theta).t^j(x) \\ &= a \text{ polynomial in } t(x) \text{ of degree } i \text{ since } k_1'(\theta) \neq 0\end{aligned} \quad (1.15)$$

Condition of equality in BLB
Variance of $\widehat{g}(x)$ attains the kth BLB but not the $(k-1)$th BLB iff

$$\widehat{g}(x) = a_0(\theta) + \sum_{i=1}^{k} a_i(\theta)\beta_i \quad (1.16)$$

with $a_k(\theta) \neq 0$.

Proof **Only if part** Given that $\widehat{g}(x)$ is of the form (1.16), we have to show that $\hat{g}(x)$ is a polynomial of degree k in $t(x)$. From (1.15), β_i is a polynomial of degree i in $t(x)$. So by putting the value of β_i in (1.16), we get $\hat{g}(x)$ as a polynomial of degree k in $t(x)$ since $\alpha_k = 0$.

if part Given that □

$$\begin{aligned}\hat{g}(x) &= \sum_{j=0}^{k} C_j \cdot t^j(x) \\ [C_k \neq 0] &= a \text{ polynomial of degree } k \text{ in } t(x)\end{aligned} \quad (1.17)$$

It is sufficient to show that we can write $\hat{g}(x)$ in the form of (1.16)

$$\begin{aligned}a_0(\theta) + \sum_{i=0}^{k} a_i(\theta)\beta_i = a_0(\theta) &+ \sum_{i=0}^{k} a_i(\theta)\sum_{j=0}^{i-1} Q_{ij}(\theta)\cdot t^j(x) \\ &+ \sum_{i=1}^{k} a_i(\theta)\sum_{j=0}^{i}\binom{i}{j}\{k_1'(\theta)\}^j t^j(x)\{k_2'(\theta)\}^{i-j}\end{aligned}$$

from (1.15)

$$= \sum_{j=0}^{k} t^j(x)\{k_1'(\theta)\}^j \sum_{i=j}^{k} a_i(\theta)\binom{i}{j}\{k_2'(\theta)\}^{i-j} + \sum_{j=0}^{k-1} t^j(x) \sum_{i=j+1}^{k} a_i(\theta)Q_{ij}$$

$$= t^k(x)\{k_1'(\theta)\}^k a_k(\theta) + \sum_{j=0}^{i-1} t^j(x)\{k_1'(\theta)\}^j \sum_{i=j}^{k} a_i(\theta)\binom{i}{j}\{k_2'(\theta)\}^{i-j} + \sum_{j=0}^{k-1} t^j(x) \sum_{i=j+1}^{k} a_i(\theta)Q_{ij}(\theta)$$

$$= t^k(x)\{k_1'(\theta)\}^k a_k(\theta) + \sum_{j=0}^{i-1} t^j(x)\left[\{k_1'(\theta)\}^j a_j(\theta) + \sum_{i=j+1}^{k} a_i(\theta)\left(\binom{i}{j}\{k_1'(\theta)\}^j \cdot \{k_2'(\theta)\}^{i-j} + Q_{ij}(\theta)\right)\right] \tag{1.18}$$

Equating coefficients of t^j from (1.17) and (1.18), we get

$$C_k = a_k(\theta)\{k_1'(\theta)\}^k$$

$$\Rightarrow a_k(\theta) = \frac{C_k}{\{k_1'(\theta)\}^k} \neq 0 \quad \text{and}$$

$$a_j(\theta) = \frac{C_j - \sum_{i=j+1}^{k} a_i(\theta)\left(\binom{i}{j}\{k_1'(\theta)\}^j \cdot \{k_2'(\theta)\}^{i-j} + Q_{ij}(\theta)\right)}{\{k'(\theta)\}^j}$$

for $j = 0, 1, \ldots, k-1$

As such a choice of $a_j(\theta)$ exists with $a_k(\theta) \neq 0$, the result follows.

Result 1 If there exists an unbiased estimator of $g(\theta)$ say $\hat{g}(x)$ such that $\hat{g}(x)$ is a polynomial of degree k in $t(x)$, then

$\Delta_k = k$th BLB to the variance of an unbiased estimator of $g(\theta) = Var\{g(x)\}$.

Result 2 If there does not exist any polynomial in $t(x)$ which is an unbiased estimator of $g(\theta)$, then it is not possible to find any unbiased estimator of $g(\theta)$ where variance attains BLB for some k.

1.4 Consistent Estimator

An estimation procedure should be such that the accuracy of an estimate increases with the sample size. Keeping this idea in mind, we define consistency as follows.

Definition An estimator T_n is said to be (weakly) consistent for $\gamma(\theta)$ if for any two positive numbers $\in$ and δ there exists an n_0 (depending upon $\in$, δ) such that

$\Pr\{|T_n - \gamma(\theta)| \leq \in\} > 1 - \delta$ whenever $n \geq n_0$ and for all $\theta \in \Theta$, i.e. if $T_n \xrightarrow{\Pr} \gamma(\theta)$ as $n \to \infty$

Result 1.7 (Sufficient condition for consistency):

An estimator T_n will be consistent for $\gamma(\theta)$ if $E(T_n) \to \gamma(\theta)$ and $V(T_n) \to 0$ as $n \to \infty$.

Proof By Chebysheff's inequality, for any $\in' > 0$

$$\Pr\{|T_n - E(T_n)| \leq \in'\} > 1 - \frac{V(T_n)}{\in'^2}.$$

$$\text{Now } |T_n - \gamma(\theta)| \leq |T_n - E(T_n)| + |E(T_n) - \gamma(\theta)|$$

$$|T_n - E(T_n)| \leq \in' \Rightarrow |T_n - \gamma(\theta)| \leq \in' + |E(T_n) - \gamma(\theta)|$$

Hence, □

$$\Pr\{|T_n - \gamma(\theta)| \leq \in' + |E(T_n) - \gamma(\theta)|\} \geq \Pr\{|T_n - E(T_n)| \leq \in'\} > 1 - \frac{V(T_n)}{\in'^2}. \tag{1.19}$$

Since $E(T_n) \to \gamma(\theta)$ and $V(T_n) \to 0$ as $n \to \infty$, for any pair of two positive numbers $(\in'', \delta)$, we can find an n_0 (depending on $(\in'', \delta)$) such that

$$|E(T_n) \to \gamma(\theta)| \leq \in'' \tag{1.20}$$

and

$$V(T_n) \leq \in'^2 \delta \tag{1.21}$$

whenever $n \geq n_0$. For such n_0

$$|T_n - \gamma(\theta)| \leq \in' + |E(T_n) - \gamma(\theta)| \Rightarrow |T_n - \gamma(\theta)| \leq \in' + \in''$$
$$\text{and } 1 - \frac{V(T_n)}{\in'^2} \geq 1 - \delta \tag{1.22}$$

Now from (1.19) and (1.22), we have $\Pr\{|T_n - \gamma(\theta)| \leq \in' + \in''\}$

$$\geq \Pr\{|T_n - \gamma(\theta)| \leq \in' + |E(T_n) - \gamma(\theta)|\} > 1 - \delta.$$

Taking $\in = \in' + \in''$

$\therefore \Pr\{|T_n - \gamma(\theta)| \leq \in\} > 1 - \delta$ whenever $n \geq n_0$

Since, $\in'$ $\in''$ and δ are arbitrary positive numbers, the proof is complete.

(It should be remembered that consistency is a large sample criterion)

Example 1.19 Let $X_1, X_2, \ldots, X_n$ be a random sample from a population mean μ and standard deviation σ. Then $\overline{X}_n = \frac{1}{n}\sum_i X_i$ is a consistent estimator of μ.

Proof $E(\overline{X}_n) = \mu$, $V(\overline{X}_n) = \frac{\sigma^2}{n} \to 0$ as $n \to \infty$. Sufficient condition of consistency holds. $\therefore \overline{X}_n$ will be consistent for μ. □

Alt

By Chebysheff's inequality, for any $\in$

$$\Pr\{|\overline{X}_n - \mu| \leq \in\} > 1 - \frac{\sigma^2}{n \in^2}$$

Now for any δ, we can find an n_0 so that
$\Pr\{|\overline{X}_n - \mu| \leq \in\} > 1 - \delta$ whenever $n \geq n_0$ (here $\delta = \frac{\sigma^2}{n \in^2}$)

Example 1.20 Show that in random sampling from a normal population, the sample mean is a consistent estimator of population mean.

Proof For any $\in (>0)$, $\Pr\{|\overline{X}_n - \mu| \leq \in\} = \Pr\left\{|Z| \leq \frac{\in\sqrt{n}}{\sigma}\right\}$

$$= \int_{\frac{-\in\sqrt{n}}{\sigma}}^{\frac{\in\sqrt{n}}{\sigma}} \frac{1}{\sqrt{2\pi}} e^{-\frac{1}{2}t^2} dt \qquad \text{where } Z = \frac{\overline{X}_n - \mu}{\sigma}\sqrt{n} \sim N(0,1)$$

□

Hence, we can choose an n_0 depending on any two positive numbers $\in$ and δ such that

$\Pr\{|\bar{X}_n - \mu| \leq \in\} > 1 - \delta$ whenever $n \geq n_0$

$\therefore \bar{X}_n \xrightarrow{\Pr} \mu$ as $n \to \infty$ $\therefore \bar{X}_n$ is consistent for μ.

Example 1.21 Show that for random sampling from the Cauchy population with density function

$f(x,\mu) = \frac{1}{\pi}\frac{1}{1+(x-\mu)^2}, -\infty < x < \infty$, the sample mean is not a consistent estimator of μ but the sample median is a consistent estimator of μ.

Answer

Let $X_1, X_2, \ldots, X_n$ be a random sample from $f(x,\ \mu) = \frac{1}{\pi}\frac{1}{1+(x-\mu)^2}$. It can be shown that the sample mean $\bar{X}$ is distributed as x.

$$\therefore \Pr\{|\overline{X}_n - \mu| \leq \in\} = \frac{1}{\pi}\int_{-\in}^{\in} \frac{1}{1+Z^2} dZ = \frac{2}{\pi}\tan^{-1} \in \qquad (\text{taking } Z = \overline{X} - \mu)$$

which is free from *n*.

Since this probability does not involve *n*, $\Pr\{|\overline{X}_n - \mu| \leq \in\}$ cannot always be greater than $1 - \delta$, and however large n may be.

It can be shown that for the sample median $\tilde{X}_n$,

$$E(\tilde{X}_n) = \mu + 0\left(\frac{1}{n}\right), \quad V(\tilde{X}_n) = 0\left(\frac{1}{n}\right) + \frac{\pi^2}{4n}$$

$\therefore$ Since $E(\tilde{X}_n) \to \mu$ and $V(\tilde{X}_n) \to 0$ as $n \to \infty$, sufficient condition for consistent estimator holds. $\therefore \tilde{X}_n$, is consistent for μ.

Remark 1.17 Consistency is essentially a large sample criterion.

Remark 1.18 Let T_n be a consistent estimator of $\gamma(\theta)$ and $\psi\{y\}$ be a continuous function. Then $\psi\{T_n\}$ will be a consistent estimator of $\psi\{\gamma(\theta)\}$.

Proof Since T_n is a consistent estimator of $\gamma(\theta)$, for any two +ve numbers $\in_1$ and δ, we can find an n_0 such that □

$\Pr\{|T_n - \gamma(\theta)| \leq \in_1\} > 1 - \delta$ whenever $n \geq n_0$.

Now $\psi\{T_n\}$ is a continuous function of T_n. Therefore, for any $\in$, we can choose an $\in_1$ such that

$$|T_n - \gamma(\theta)| \leq \in_1 \Rightarrow |\psi\{T_n\} - \psi\{\gamma(\theta)\}| \leq \in .$$

$\therefore \Pr\{|\psi\{T_n\} - \psi\{\gamma(\theta)\}| \leq \in\} \geq \Pr\{|T_n - \gamma(\theta)| \leq \in_1\} > 1 - \delta$ whenever $n \geq n_0$

i.e. $\Pr\{|\psi\{T_n\} - \psi\{\gamma(\theta)\}| \leq \in\} > 1 - \delta$ whenever $n \geq n_0$.

Remark 1.19 A consistent estimator is not unique

For example, if T_n is a consistent estimator of θ, then for any fixed a and b $T_n' = \frac{n-a}{n-b} T_n$ is also consistent for θ.

Remark 1.20 A consistent estimator is not necessarily unbiased, e.g. $U : f(x, \theta) = \frac{1}{\theta}, 0 < x < \theta$, consistent estimator of θ is $X_{(n)} = \max_{1 \leq i \leq n} X_i$. But it is not unbiased.

Remark 1.21 An unbiased estimator is not necessarily consistent, e.g. $f(x) = \frac{1}{2} e^{-|x-\theta|}, -\infty < x < \infty$.

An unbiased estimator of θ is $\frac{X_{(1)} + X_{(n)}}{2}$, but it is not consistent.

Remark 1.22 A consistent estimator may be meaningless,

$$\text{e.g. Let } T_n' = \begin{cases} 0 & \text{if} \quad n \leq 10^{10} \\ T_n & \text{if} \quad n \geq 10^{10} \end{cases}$$

If T_n is consistent, then T_n' is also consistent, but T_n' is meaningless for any practical purpose.

Remark 1.23 If T_1 and T_2 are consistent estimators of $\gamma_1(\theta)$ and $\gamma_2(\theta)$, then $(i)(T_1 + T_2)$ is consistent for $\gamma_1(\theta) + \gamma_2(\theta)$ and

$(ii) T_1 T_2$ is consistent for $\gamma_1(\theta)\gamma_2(\theta)$.

Proof (i) Since T_1 and T_2 are consistent for $\gamma_1(\theta)$ and $\gamma_2(\theta)$, we can always choose an n_0 much that

$$\Pr\{|T_1 - \gamma_1(\theta)| \le \in_1\} > 1 - \delta_1$$

and

$$\Pr\{|T_2 - \gamma_2(\theta)| \le \in_2\} > 1 - \delta_2$$

whenever $n \ge n_0$

$\in_1, \in_2, \delta_1, \delta_2$ are arbitrary positive numbers.

$$\text{Now } |T_1 + T_2 - \gamma_1(\theta) - \gamma_2(\theta)| \le |T_1 - \gamma_1(\theta)| + |T_2 - \gamma_2(\theta)|$$

$$\le \in_1 + \in_2 = \in, \text{ (say)}$$

$$\therefore \Pr\{|T_1 + T_2 - \gamma_1(\theta) - \gamma_2(\theta)| \le \in\} \ge \Pr\{|T_1 - \gamma_1(\theta)| \le \in_1, |T_2 - \gamma_2(\theta)| \le \in_2\}$$
$$\ge \Pr\{|T_1 - \gamma_1(\theta)| \le \in_1\} + \Pr\{|T_2 - \gamma_2(\theta)| \le \in_2\} - 1$$

$$[\because P(AB) \ge P(A) + P(B) - 1]$$

$$\ge 1 - \delta_1 + 1 - \delta_2 - 1 = 1 - (\delta_1 + \delta_2) = 1 - \delta \text{ for } n \ge n_0$$

$$\therefore \Pr\{|T_1 + T_2 - \gamma_1(\theta) - \gamma_2(\theta)| \le \in\} > 1 - \delta \text{ for } n \ge n_0$$

Hence, $T_1 + T_2$ is consistent estimator of $\gamma_1(\theta) + \gamma_2(\theta)$.

(ii) Again $|T_1 - \gamma_1(\theta)| \le \in_1$ and $|T_2 - \gamma_2(\theta)| \le \in_2$

$$\Rightarrow |T_1T_2 - \gamma_1(\theta)\gamma_2(\theta)| = |\{T_1 - \gamma_1(\theta)\}\{T_2 - \gamma_2(\theta)\} + T_2\gamma_1(\theta) + T_1\gamma_2(\theta) - 2\gamma_1(\theta)\gamma_2(\theta)|$$
$$\le |\{T_1 - \gamma_1(\theta)\}\{T_2 - \gamma_2(\theta)\}| + |\gamma_1(\theta)||T_2 - \gamma_2(\theta)| + |\gamma_2(\theta)||T_1 - \gamma_1(\theta)|$$
$$\le \in_1\in_2 + |\gamma_1(\theta)| \in_2 + |\gamma_2(\theta)| \in_1 = \in \quad \text{(say)}$$

$$\therefore \Pr\{|T_1T_2 - \gamma_1(\theta)\gamma_2(\theta)| \le \in\} \ge \Pr\{|T_1 - \gamma_1(\theta)| \le \in_1, |T_2 - \gamma_2(\theta)| \le \in_2\}$$
$$\ge \Pr\{|T_1 - \gamma_1(\theta)| \le \in_1\} + \Pr\{|T_2 - \gamma_2(\theta)| \le \in_2\} - 1$$
$$\ge 1 - \delta_1 + 1 - \delta_2 - 1 = 1 - (\delta_1 + \delta_2) = 1 - \delta \text{ whenever } n \ge n_0$$

$\therefore T_1T_2$ is consistent for $\gamma_1(\theta)\gamma_2(\theta)$. □

Example 1.22 Let $X_1, X_2, \ldots, X_n$ be a random sample from the distribution of X for which the moments of order $2r$ (μ'_{2r}) exist. Then show that

(a) $m'_r = \frac{1}{n}\sum_1^n X_i^r$ is a consistent estimator of μ'_r, and

(b) $m_r = \frac{1}{n}\sum (X_i - \bar{X})^r$ is a consistent estimator of μ_r. These can be proved using the following results.

$$\text{As } E\left(m_r'\right) = \mu_r' \text{ and } V\left(m_r'\right) = \frac{\mu_{2r}' - \mu_r'^2}{n}$$

$\therefore V\left(m_r'\right) \to 0$ as $n \to \infty$ $\therefore m_r'$ is consistent for μ_r' and $E(m_r) = \mu_r + 0\left(\frac{1}{n}\right)$

$$V(m_r) = \frac{1}{n}\left[\mu_{2r} - \mu_r^2 - 2r\mu_{r-1}\mu_{r+1} + r^2\mu_{r-1}^2\mu_2\right] + 0\left(\frac{1}{n^2}\right) \to 0 \text{ as } n \to \infty$$

$\therefore m_r$ is consistent for μ_r.

(c) Also it can be shown that b_1 and b_2 are consistent estimators of $\beta_1 = \frac{\mu_3^2}{\mu_2^3}$ and $\beta_2 = \frac{\mu_4}{\mu_2^2}$.

1.5 Efficient Estimator

Suppose the regularity conditions hold for the family of distribution $\{f(x, \theta); \theta \in \Theta\}$. Let an unbiased estimator of $\gamma(\theta)$ be T. Then the efficiency of T is given by

$$\frac{\{\gamma'(\theta)\}^2 / I(\theta)}{V(T)}$$

It is denoted by eff. (*T*)/or *e*(*T*). Clearly, $0 \le e(T) \le 1$.

An estimator *T* will be called (most) efficient if eff(*T*) = 1. An estimator *T* of $\gamma(\theta)$ is said to be asymptotically efficient if $E(T) \to \gamma(\theta)$ and eff (T) $\to 1$ as $n \to \infty$.

Let T_1 and T_2 be two unbiased estimators of $\gamma(\theta)$. Then the efficiency of T_1 relative to T_2 is given by eff.$\left(T_1/T_2\right) = \frac{V(T_2)}{V(T_1)}$.

Remark 1.24 An MVBE will be efficient.

Remark 1.25 In many cases, MVBE does not exist even though the family satisfies the regularity conditions. Again in many cases, the regularity conditions do not hold. In such cases, the above definition fails. If MVUE exists, we take it as an efficient estimator.

Remark 1.26 The efficiency measure has an appealing property of determining the relative sample sizes needed to attain the same precision of estimation as measured by variance.

e.g.: Suppose an estimator T_1 is 80 % efficient and $V(T_1) = \frac{c}{n}$, where c depends upon θ. Then, $V(T_0) = 0.8\frac{c}{n}$. Thus the estimator based on a sample of size 80 will be just as good as an estimator T_1 based on a sample of size 100.

Example 1.23 Let T_1 and T_2 be two unbiased estimators of θ with efficiency e_1 and e_2, respectively. If ρ denotes the correlation coefficient between T_1 and T_2, then

$$\sqrt{e_1e_2} - \sqrt{(1-e_1)(1-e_2)} \le \rho \le \sqrt{e_1e_2} + \sqrt{(1-e_1)(1-e_2)}$$

Proof For any real 'a', $T = aT_1 + (1-a)T_2$ will also be an unbiased estimator of θ. Now

$$V(T) = a^2V(T_1) + (1-a)^2V(T_2) + 2a(1-a)\rho\sqrt{V(T_1)V(T_2)}.$$

Suppose T_0 be an MVUE of θ with variance V_0. Then $V(T) \ge V_0$

$$\Rightarrow a^2\frac{V_0}{e_1} + (1-a)^2\frac{V_0}{e_2} + 2a(1-a)\rho\frac{V_0}{\sqrt{e_1e_2}} \ge V_0$$

$$\Rightarrow a^2\left(\frac{1}{e_1} + \frac{1}{e_2} - \frac{2\rho}{\sqrt{e_1e_2}}\right) - 2a\left(\frac{1}{e_2} - \frac{\rho}{\sqrt{e_1e_2}}\right) + \left(\frac{1}{e_2} - 1\right) \ge 0$$

$$\Rightarrow \left(a - \frac{\frac{1}{e_2} - \frac{\rho}{\sqrt{e_1e_2}}}{\frac{1}{e_1} + \frac{1}{e_2} - \frac{2\rho}{\sqrt{e_1e_2}}}\right)^2 + \frac{\frac{1}{e_2} - 1}{\frac{1}{e_1} + \frac{1}{e_2} - \frac{2\rho}{\sqrt{e_1e_2}}} - \left(\frac{\frac{1}{e_2} - \frac{\rho}{\sqrt{e_1e_2}}}{\frac{1}{e_1} + \frac{1}{e_2} - \frac{2\rho}{\sqrt{e_1e_2}}}\right)^2 \ge 0$$

Taking $a = \frac{\frac{1}{e_2} - \frac{\rho}{\sqrt{e_1e_2}}}{\frac{1}{e_1} + \frac{1}{e_2} - \frac{2\rho}{\sqrt{e_1e_2}}}$, we get

$$\left(\frac{1}{e_2} - 1\right)\left(\frac{1}{e_1} + \frac{1}{e_2} - \frac{2\rho}{\sqrt{e_1e_2}}\right) - \left(\frac{1}{e_2} - \frac{\rho}{\sqrt{e_1e_2}}\right)^2 \ge 0$$

$$\Rightarrow -\rho^2 + 2\rho\sqrt{e_1e_2} - \frac{e_1}{e_2} + (1-e_2)\left(1 + \frac{e_1}{e_2}\right) \ge 0$$

$$\Rightarrow \rho^2 - 2\rho\sqrt{e_1e_2} - 1 + e_1 + e_2 \le 0$$

$$\Rightarrow (\rho - \sqrt{e_1e_2})^2 - (1-e_1)(1-e_2) \le 0$$

$\Rightarrow \left|\rho - \sqrt{e_1e_2}\right| \le \sqrt{(1-e_1)(1-e_2)}$ Hence, the result. □

Remark 1.27 The correlation coefficient between T and the most efficient estimator is $\sqrt{e}$ where e is the efficiency of the unbiased estimator T. Put $e_2 = e$ and $e_1 = 1$ in the above inequality; $\left|\rho - \sqrt{e_1e_2}\right| \le \sqrt{(1-e_1)(1-e_2)}$ and easily we get the result.

Chapter 2
Methods of Estimation

2.1 Introduction

In chapter one, we have discussed different optimum properties of good point estimators viz. unbiasedness, minimum variance, consistency and efficiency which are the desirable properties of a good estimator. In this chapter, we shall discuss different methods of estimating parameters which are expected to provide estimators having some of these important properties. Commonly used methods are:

1. Method of moments
2. Method of maximum likelihood
3. Method of minimum χ^2
4. Method of least squares

In general, depending on the situation and the purpose of our study we apply any one of the methods that may be suitable among the above-mentioned methods of point estimation.

2.2 Method of Moments

The method of moments, introduced by K. Pearson is one of the oldest methods of estimation. Let $(X_1, X_2,\ldots X_n)$ be a random sample from a population having p.d.f. (or p.m.f) $f(x,\theta)$, $\theta = (\theta_1, \theta_2,\ldots, \theta_k)$. Further, let the first k population moments about zero exist as explicit function of θ, i.e. $\mu'_r = \mu'_r(\theta_1, \theta_2, \ldots, \theta_k)$, $r = 1, 2,\ldots,k$. In the method of moments, we equate k sample moments with the corresponding population moments. Generally, the first k moments are taken because the errors due to sampling increase with the order of the moment. Thus, we get k equations $\mu'_r(\theta_1, \theta_2, \ldots, \theta_k), = m'_r$, $r = 1, 2,\ldots, k$. Solving these equations we get the method of moment estimators (or estimates) as $m'_r = \frac{1}{n}\sum_{i=1}^{n} X_i^r$ (or $m'_r = \frac{1}{n}\sum_{i=1}^{n} x_i^r$).

P.K. Sahu et al., *Estimation and Inferential Statistics*,
DOI 10.1007/978-81-322-2514-0_2

If the correspondence between μ'_r and θ is one-to-one and the inverse function is $\theta_i = f_i(\mu'_1, \mu'_2, \ldots, \mu'_k)$, $i = 1, 2,.., k$ then, the method of moment estimate becomes $\hat{\theta}_i = f_i(m'_1, m'_2, \ldots, m'_k)$. Now, if the function $f_i()$ is continuous, then by the weak law of large numbers, the method of moment estimators will be consistent. This method gives maximum likelihood estimators when $f(x, \theta) = \exp(b_0 + b_1x + b_2x^2 + \ldots.)$ and so, in this case it gives efficient estimator. But the estimators obtained by this method are not generally efficient. This is one of the simplest methods. Therefore, these estimates can be used as a first approximation to get a better estimate. This method is not applicable when the theoretical moments do not exist as in the case of Cauchy distribution.

Example 2.1 Let $X_1, X_2, \ldots X_n$ be a random sample from p.d.f. $f(x; a, b) = \frac{1}{\beta(a,b)} x^{a-1}(1-x)^{b-1}, 0 < x < 1; a, b > 0$. Find the estimators of a and b by the method of moments.

Solution

We know $E(x) = \mu_1^1 = \frac{a}{a+b}$ and $E(x^2) = \mu_2^1 = \frac{a(a+1)}{(a+b)(a+b+1)}$.

Hence, $\frac{a}{a+b} = \bar{x}, \frac{a(a+1)}{(a+b)(a+b+1)} = \frac{1}{n}\sum_{i=1}^{n} x_i^2$

By solving, we get $\hat{b} = \frac{(\bar{x}-1)\left(\sum x_i^2 - n\bar{x}\right)}{\sum (x_i - \bar{x})^2}$ and $\hat{a} = \frac{\bar{x}\hat{b}}{1-\bar{x}}$.

2.3 Method of Maximum Likelihood

This method of estimation is due to R.A. Fisher. It is the most important general method of estimation. Let $\underset{\sim}{X} = (X_1, X_2, \ldots, X_n)$ denote a random sample with joint p.d.f or p.m.f. $f\left(\underset{\sim}{x}, \theta\right), \theta \in \Theta$ (θ may be a vector). The function $f\left(\underset{\sim}{x}, \theta\right)$, considered as a function of θ, is called the likelihood function. In this case, it is denoted by $L(\theta)$. The principle of maximum likelihood consists of choosing an estimate, say $\hat{\theta}$, within the admissible range of θ, that maximizes the likelihood. $\hat{\theta}$ is called the maximum likelihood estimate (MLE) of θ. In other words, $\hat{\theta}$ will be an MLE of θ if

$$L\left(\hat{\theta}\right) \geq L(\theta) \forall\, \theta \in \Theta.$$

In practice, it is convenient to work with logarithm. Since log-function is a monotone function, $\hat{\theta}$ satisfies

$$\log L\left(\hat{\theta}\right) \geq \log L(\theta) \forall\ \theta \in \Theta.$$

Again, if $\log L(\theta)$ is differentiable within Θ and $\hat{\theta}$ is an interior point, then $\hat{\theta}$ will be the solution of

$$\frac{\partial \log \mathrm{L}(\theta)}{\partial \theta_i} = \mathrm{o},\ i = 1,\ 2, \ldots, k;\ \underset{\sim}{\theta}^{k \times 1} = (\theta_1, \theta_2, \ldots, \theta_k)'.$$

These equations are known as likelihood equations.

Problem 2.1 Let $(X_1, X_2, \ldots, X_n)$ be a random sample from $b(m, \pi)$, (m known). Show that $\hat{\pi} = \frac{1}{mn}\sum_{i=1}^{n} X_i$ is an MLE of π.

Problem 2.2 Let $(X_1, X_2, \ldots, X_n)$ be a random sample from $P(\lambda)$. Show that $\hat{\lambda} = \frac{1}{n}\sum_{i=1}^{n} X_i$ is an MLE of λ.

Problem 2.3 Let $(X_1, X_2, \ldots, X_n)$ be a random sample from $N(\mu, \sigma^2)$. Show that $\left(\bar{X}, s^2\right)$ is an MLE of (μ, σ^2), where $\bar{X} = \frac{1}{n}\sum_{i=1}^{n} X_i$ and $s^2 = \frac{1}{n}\sum_{i=1}^{n} (X_i - \bar{X})^2$.

Example 2.2 Let $(X_1, X_2, \ldots, X_n)$ be a random sample from a population having p.d.f $f(x, \theta) = \frac{1}{2}e^{-|x-\theta|}, \quad -\infty < x < \infty$.

Show that the sample median $\tilde{X}$ is an MLE of θ.

Answer

$$L(\theta) = \text{ Const. } e^{-\sum_{i=1}^{n} |x_i - \theta|}$$

Maximization of $L(\theta)$ is equivalent to the minimization of $\sum_{i=1}^{n} |x_i - \theta|$. Now, $\sum_{i=1}^{n} |x_i - \theta|$ will be least when $\theta = \tilde{X}$, the sample median as the mean deviation about the median is least. $\tilde{X}$ will be an MLE of θ.

Properties of MLE

(a) If a sufficient statistic exists, then the MLE will be a function of the sufficient statistic.

Proof Let T be a sufficient statistic for the family $\left\{f\left(\underset{\sim}{X}, \theta\right), \theta \in \Theta\right\}$

By the factorisation theorem, we have $\prod_{i=1}^{n} f(x_i, \theta) = g\left\{T\left(\underset{\sim}{X}\right), \theta\right\} h\left(\underset{\sim}{X}\right)$.

To find MLE, we maximize $g\left\{T\left(\underset{\sim}{x}\right), \theta\right\}$ with respect to θ. Since $g\left\{T\left(\underset{\sim}{X}\right), \theta\right\}$ is a function of θ and $\underset{\sim}{x}$ only through $T\left(\underset{\sim}{X}\right)$, the conclusion follows immediately.□

Remark 2.1 Property (a) does not imply that an MLE is itself a sufficient statistic.

Example 2.3 Let $X_1, X_2, \ldots, X_n$ be a random sample from a population having p.d.f. $f\left(\underset{\sim}{X},\theta\right) = \begin{cases} 1 & \forall\, \theta \le x \le \theta+1 \\ 0 & \text{Otherwise} \end{cases}$.

Then, $L(\theta) = \begin{cases} 1 & \text{if } \theta \le \text{Min}X_i \le \text{Max}X_i \le \theta+1 \\ 0 & \text{Otherwise} \end{cases}$.

Any value of θ satisfying $\text{Max}X_i - 1 \le \theta \le \text{Min}X_i$ will be an MLE of θ. In particular, Min X_i is an MLE of θ, but it is not sufficient for θ. In fact, here $(\text{Min}X_i, \text{Max}X_i)$ is a sufficient statistic.

(b) If T is the MVBE, then the likelihood equation will have a solution T.

Proof Since T is an MVBE, $\dfrac{\partial \log f\left(\underset{\sim}{X},\theta\right)}{\partial\theta} = (T-\theta)\lambda(\theta)$

Now, $\dfrac{\partial \log f\left(\underset{\sim}{X},\theta\right)}{\partial\theta} = 0$

$$\Rightarrow \theta = T[\because \lambda(\theta) \neq 0].$$

(c) Let T be an MLE of θ and $\delta = \psi(\theta)$ be a one-to-one function of θ. Then, $d = \psi(T)$ will be an MLE of δ. □

Proof Since T is an MLE of θ, $L\left\{T\left(\underset{\sim}{X}\right)\right\} \ge L(\theta)\forall\theta$,

Since the correspondence between θ and δ is one-to-one, inverse function must exist. Suppose the inverse function is $\theta = \psi^{-1}(\delta)$.

Thus, $L(\theta) = L\{\psi^{-1}(\delta)\} = L_1(\delta)$ (say)

Now,

$$L_1(d) = L\{\psi^{-1}(d)\} = L\left[\psi^{-1}\left\{\psi\left(T\left(\underset{\sim}{X}\right)\right)\right\}\right] = L\left\{T\left(\underset{\sim}{X}\right)\right\} \ge L(\theta) = L_1(\delta).$$

Therefore, 'd' is an MLE of δ.

(d) Suppose the p.d.f. (or p.m.f.) $f(x, \theta)$ satisfies the following regularity conditions:

(i) For almost all x, $\dfrac{\partial f(x,\theta)}{\partial\theta}, \dfrac{\partial^2 f(x,\theta)}{\partial\theta^2}, \dfrac{\partial^3 f(x,\theta)}{\partial\theta^3}$ exists $\forall\, \theta \in \Theta$.

(ii) $\left|\dfrac{\partial f(x,\theta)}{\partial\theta}\right| < A_1(x)$, $\left|\dfrac{\partial^2 f(x,\theta)}{\partial\theta^2}\right| < A_2(x)$ and $\left|\dfrac{\partial^3 f(x,\theta)}{\partial\theta^3}\right| < B(x)$,
where $A_1(x)$ and $A_2(x)$ are integrable functions of x and
$\int_{-\infty}^{\infty} B(x)f(x,\theta)dx < M$, a finite quantity

iii) $\int_{-\infty}^{\infty} \left(\dfrac{\partial \log f(x,\theta)}{\partial\theta}\right)^2 f(x,\theta)dx$ is a finite and positive quantity.

If $\hat{\theta}_n$ is an MLE of θ on the basis of a sample of size n, from a population having p.d.f. (or p.m.f.) $f(x,\theta)$ which satisfies the above regularity conditions, then

$\sqrt{n}\left(\hat{\theta}_n - \theta\right)$ is asymptotically normal with mean '0' and variance $\left[\int\limits_{-\infty}^{\infty} \left(\frac{\partial \log f(x,\theta)}{\partial \theta}\right)^2 f(x,\theta)\mathrm{d}x\right]^{-1}$. Also, $\hat{\theta}_n$ is asymptotically efficient and consistent.

(e) An MLE may not be unique. □

Example 2.4 Let $f(x,\theta) = \begin{cases} 1 & \text{if } \theta \le x \le \theta + 1 \\ 0 & \text{Otherwise} \end{cases}$.

$$\text{Then, } L(\theta) = \begin{cases} 1 & \text{if } \theta \le \min\ x_i \le \max\ x_i \le \theta + 1 \\ 0 & \text{Otherwise} \end{cases}$$

$$\text{i.e. } L(\theta) = \begin{cases} 1 & \text{if } \max\ x_i - 1 \le \theta \le \min\ x_i \\ 0 & \text{Otherwise} \end{cases}$$

Clearly, for any value of θ, say $T_\alpha = \alpha(\text{Max}x_i - 1) + (1 - \alpha)\text{Min}x_i,\ 0 \le \alpha \le 1$, $L(\theta)$ will be maximized. For fixed α, T_α will be an MLE. Thus, we observe that an infinite number of MLE exist in this case.

(f) An MLE may not be unbiased.

Example 2.5

$$f(x,\theta) = \begin{cases} \frac{1}{\theta} & \text{if } 0 \le x \le \theta \\ 0 & \text{Otherwise} \end{cases}.$$

$$\text{Then, } L(\theta) = \begin{cases} \frac{1}{\theta^n} & \text{if } \max x_i \le \theta \\ 0 & \text{Otherwise} \end{cases}.$$

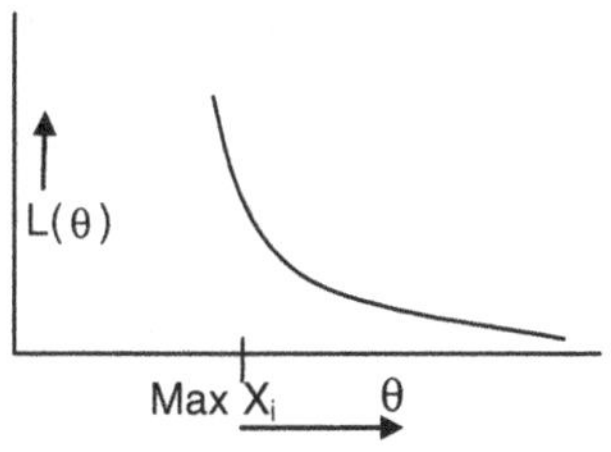

From the figure, it is clear that the likelihood $L(\theta)$ will be the largest when θ = Max X_i. Therefore Max X_i will be an MLE of θ. Note that $E(\text{Max}\,X_i) = \frac{n}{n+1}\theta \neq \theta$. Therefore, here MLE is a biased estimator.

(g) An MLE may be worthless.

Example 2.6

$$f(x,\pi) = \pi^x(1-\pi)^{1-x};\ x=0,1,\pi \in \left(\frac{1}{4},\frac{3}{4}\right)$$

Then, $L(\pi) = \begin{cases} \pi & \text{if } x = 1 \\ 1-\pi & \text{if } x = 0 \end{cases}$ i.e. $L(\pi)$ will be maximized at $\begin{cases} \pi = \frac{3}{4} & \text{if } x = 1 \\ \pi = \frac{1}{4} & \text{if } x = 0 \end{cases}$

Thus, $T = \frac{2X+1}{4}$ will be an MLE of θ.
Now, $E(T) = \frac{2\pi+1}{4} \neq \pi$. Thus, T is a biased estimator of π.

$$\begin{aligned} &\text{MSE of } T = E(T-\pi)^2 \\ &= E\left(\frac{2x+1}{4} - \pi\right)^2 = \frac{1}{16}E\{2(x-\pi)+1-2\pi\}^2 \\ &\qquad = \frac{1}{16}E\left\{4(x-\pi)^2 + (1-2\pi)^2 + 4(x-\pi)(1-2\pi)\right\} \\ &\qquad = \frac{1}{16}\left\{4\pi(1-\pi) + (1-2\pi)^2\right\} = \frac{1}{16} \end{aligned}$$

Now, we consider a trivial estimator $\delta(x) = \frac{1}{2}$.
MSE of $\delta(x) = \left(\frac{1}{2} - \pi\right)^2 \leq \frac{1}{16}$ = MSE of T $\forall \pi \in \left(\frac{1}{4}, \frac{3}{4}\right)$
Thus, in the sense of mean square error MLE is meaningless.
(h) An MLE may not be consistent

Example 2.7

$$f(x,\theta) = \begin{cases} \theta^x(1-\theta)^{1-x} & \text{if } \theta \text{ is rational} \\ (1-\theta)^x\theta^{1-x} & \text{if } \theta \text{ is rational} \quad 0<\theta<1, x=0,1. \end{cases}$$

An MLE of θ is $\hat{\theta}_n = \bar{X}$. Here, $\hat{\theta}_n$ is not a consistent estimator of θ.
(i) The regularity conditions in (d) are not necessary conditions.

Example 2.8

$$f(x,\theta) = \frac{1}{2}e^{-|x-\theta|}, \quad \begin{matrix} -\infty<x<\infty \\ -\infty<\theta<\infty \end{matrix}$$

Here, regularity conditions do not hold. However, the MLE (=sample median) is asymptotically normal and efficient.

Example 2.9 Let $X_1, X_2, \ldots, X_n$ be a random sample from $f(x,\alpha,\beta) = \beta e^{-\beta(x-\alpha)};\ \alpha \leq x < \infty$ and $\beta > 0$.
Find MLE's of α, β.

Solution

$$L(\alpha,\beta)=\beta^n e^{-\beta\sum_{i=1}^{n}(x_i-\alpha)}$$

$$\log_e L(\alpha,\beta)=n\log_e\beta-\beta\sum_{i=1}^{n}(x_i-\alpha)$$

$\frac{\partial \log L}{\partial \beta}=\frac{n}{\beta}-\sum(x_i-\alpha)$ and $\frac{\partial \log L}{\partial \alpha}=n\beta$.

Now, $\frac{\partial \log L}{\partial \alpha}=0$ gives us $\beta=0$ which is nonadmissible. Thus, the method of differentiation fails here.

Now, from the expression of $L(\alpha, \beta)$, it is clear that for fixed $\beta(>0)$, $L(\alpha, \beta)$ becomes maximum when α is the largest. The largest possible value of α is $X_{(1)}$ = Min x_i.

Now, we maximize $L\{X_{(1)},\beta\}$ with respect to β. This can be done by considering the method of differentiation.

$$\frac{\partial \log L\{x_{(1)},\beta\}}{\partial\beta}=0\Rightarrow\frac{n}{\beta}-\sum(x_i-\min x_i)=0\ \Rightarrow\beta=\frac{n}{\sum(x_i-\min x_i)}$$

So, the MLE of (α, β) is $\left\{\min x_i,\frac{n}{\sum(x_i-\min x_i)}\right\}$.

Example 2.10 Let $X_1,X_2,\ldots,X_n$ be a random sample from $f(x,\alpha,\beta)=\begin{cases}\frac{1}{\beta-\alpha}, & \alpha\le x\le\beta\\ 0, & \text{Otherwise}\end{cases}$

(a) Show that the MLE of (α, β) is (Min X_i, Max X_i).

(b) Also find the estimators of α and β by the method of moments.

Proof

$$(a)L(\alpha,\beta)=\frac{1}{(\beta-\alpha)^n}\quad \text{if } \alpha\le \text{Min}x_i<\text{Max}x_i\le\beta \tag{2.1}$$

It is evident from (2.1), that the likelihood will be made as large as possible when $(\beta-\alpha)$ is made as small as possible. Clearly, α cannot be larger than Min x_i and β cannot be smaller than Max x_i; hence, the smallest possible value of $(\beta-\alpha)$ is (Max x_i − Min x_i). Then the MLE'S of α and β are $\hat{\alpha}=\text{Min}\,x_i$ and $\hat{\beta}=\text{Max}\,x_i$, respectively.

(b) We know $E(x)=\mu_1^1=\frac{\alpha+\beta}{2}$ and $V(x)=\mu_2=\frac{(\beta-\alpha)^2}{12}$

Hence, $\frac{\alpha+\beta}{2}=\bar{x}$ and $\frac{(\beta-\alpha)^2}{12}=\frac{1}{n}\sum_{i=1}^{n}(x_i-\bar{x})^2$

By solving, we get $\hat{\alpha} = \bar{x} - \sqrt{\frac{3\sum(x_i-\bar{x})^2}{n}}$ and $\hat{\beta} = \bar{x} + \sqrt{\frac{3\sum(x_i-\bar{x})^2}{n}}$

Successive approximation for the estimation of parameter

It frequently happens that the likelihood equation is by no means easy to solve. A general method in such cases is to assume a trial solution and correct it by an extra term to get a more accurate solution. This process can be repeated until we get the solution to a sufficient degree of accuracy.

Let L denote the likelihood and θ^* be the MLE.

Then $\left.\frac{\partial \log L}{\partial \theta}\right|_{\theta=\theta^*} = 0$. Suppose θ_0 is a trial solution of $\frac{\partial \log L}{\partial \theta} = 0$

Then

$0 = \left.\frac{\partial \log L}{\partial \theta}\right|_{\theta=\theta^*} = \left.\frac{\partial \log L}{\partial \theta}\right|_{\theta=\theta_0} + (\theta^* - \theta_0)\left.\frac{\partial^2 \log L}{\partial \theta^2}\right|_{\theta=\theta_0}$ + terms involving $(\theta^* - \theta_0)$ with powers higher than unity.

$\Rightarrow 0 \simeq \left.\frac{\partial \log L}{\partial \theta}\right|_{\theta=\theta_0} + (\theta^* - \theta_0)\left.\frac{\partial^2 \log L}{\partial \theta^2}\right|_{\theta=\theta_0}$, neglecting the terms involving $(\theta^* - \theta_0)$ with powers higher than unity.

$\Rightarrow 0 \simeq \left.\frac{\partial \log L}{\partial \theta}\right|_{\theta=\theta_0} - (\theta^* - \theta_0)\mathrm{I}(\theta_0)$, where $\mathrm{I}(\theta) = -E\left(\frac{\partial^2 \log L}{\partial \theta^2}\right)$.

Thus, the first approximate value of θ is

$$\theta^{(1)} = \theta_0 + \left\{ \frac{\left.\frac{\partial \log L}{\partial \theta}\right|_{\theta=\theta_0}}{\mathrm{I}(\theta_0)} \right\}.$$

Example 2.11 Let $X_1, X_2, \ldots, X_n$ be a random sample from $f(x, \theta) = \frac{1}{\pi\{1 + (x-\theta)^2\}}$

Here, $\frac{\partial \log f(x,\theta)}{\partial \theta} = \frac{2(x-\theta)}{1+(x-\theta)^2}$; and so the likelihood equation is $\sum_{i=1}^{n} \frac{(x_i-\theta)}{1+(x_i-\theta)^2} = 0$; clearly it is difficult to solve for θ.

So, we consider successive approximation method.

In this case, $\mathrm{I}(\theta) = \frac{n}{2}$.

Here, the first approximation is $\theta^{(1)} = \theta_0 + \frac{4}{n}\sum_{i=1}^{n} \frac{(x_i-\theta_0)}{1+(x_i-\theta_0)^2}$,

θ_0 being a trial solution.

Usually, we take θ_0 = sample median.

2.4 Method of Minimum χ^2

This method may be used when the population is grouped into a number of mutually exclusive and exhaustive class and the observations are given in the form of frequencies.

Suppose there are k classes and $\pi_i(\theta)$ is the probability of an individual belonging to the ith class. Let f_i denote the sample frequency. Clearly, $\sum_{i=1}^{k}\pi_i(\theta)=1$ and $\sum_{i=1}^{k}f_i=n$.

The discrepancy between observed frequency and the corresponding expected frequency is measured by the Pearsonian χ^2, which is given by $\chi^2=\sum_{i=1}^{k}\frac{\{f_i-n\pi_i(\theta)\}^2}{n\pi_i(\theta)}=\sum\frac{f_i^2}{n\pi_i(\theta)}-n.$

The principle of the method of minimum χ^2 consists of choosing an estimate of θ, say $\hat{\theta}$, we first consider the minimum χ^2 equations $\frac{\partial\chi^2}{\partial\theta_i}=0$, i = 1, 2,…,r and θ_i = ith component of θ.

It can be shown that for large n, the min χ^2 equations and the likelihood equations are identical and provides identical estimates.

The method of minimum χ^2, is found to be more troublesome to apply in many cases, and has no improvement on the maximum likelihood method. This method can be used when maximum likelihood equations are difficult to solve. In particular situations, this method may be simple. To avoid the difficulty in minimum χ^2 method, we consider another measure of discrepancy, which is given by $\chi'^2=\sum_{i=1}^{k}\frac{\{f_i-n\pi_i(\theta)\}^2}{f_i}$, χ'^2 is called modified Pearsonian χ^2. Now, we minimize, instead of χ^2, with respect to θ.

It can be shown that for large n the estimates obtained by min χ^2 would also be approximately equal to the MLE's. Difficulty arises if some of the classes are empty. In this case, we minimize

$$\chi''^2=\sum_{i:f_i\neq 0}\frac{\{f_i-n\pi_i(\theta)\}^2}{f_i}+2\text{M},$$

where M = sum of the expected frequencies of the empty classes.

Example 2.12 Let $(x_1,x_2,\ldots,x_n)$ be a given sample of size n. It is to be tested whether the sample comes from some Poisson distribution with unknown mean μ. How do you estimate μ by the method of modified minimum chi-square?

Solution

Let $x_1,x_2,\ldots,x_n$ be arranged in k groups such that there are

n_i observations with $x=i, i=r+1,\ldots,r+k-2$

n_L observations $x\leq r$

n_u observations with $x \geq r+k-1$ so that the smallest and the largest values of x, which are fewer, are pooled together and$n_L + \sum_{i=r+1}^{r+k-2} n_i + n_u = n$.

Let $\pi_i(\mu) = P(x=i) = \frac{e^{-\mu}\mu^i}{i!}$, $\pi_L(\mu) = P(x \leq r) = \sum_{i=0}^{r} \pi_i(\mu)$ and $\pi_u(\mu) = P(x \geq r+k-1) = \sum_{i=r+k-1}^{\infty} \pi_i(\mu)$.

Now using $\sum_{i=1}^{k} \frac{n_i}{\pi_i(\theta)} \frac{\partial \pi_i(\theta)}{\partial \theta_j} = 0$, $j = 1, 2, \ldots p$ we have $n_L \frac{\sum_{i=0}^{r} \left(\frac{i}{\mu}-1\right)\pi_i(\mu)}{\sum_{i=0}^{r} \pi_i(\mu)} + \sum_{i=r+1}^{r+k-2} n_i\left(\frac{i}{\mu}-1\right) + n_u \frac{\sum_{i=r+k-1}^{\infty}\left(\frac{i}{\mu}-1\right)\pi_i(\mu)}{\sum_{i=r+k-1}^{\infty} \pi_i(\mu)} = 0$.

Since there is only one parameter, i.e. $p = 1$ we get the only above equation. By solving, we get

$$n\hat{\mu} = n_L \frac{\sum\limits_{i=0}^{r} i\pi_i(\mu)}{\sum\limits_{i=0}^{r} \pi_i(\mu)} + \sum_{i=r+1}^{r+k-2} in_i + n_u \frac{\sum\limits_{i=r+k-1}^{\infty} i\pi_i(\mu)}{\sum\limits_{i=r+k-1}^{\infty} \pi_i(\mu)}$$

= sum of all x's

Hence, $\hat{\mu}$ is approximately the sample mean $\bar{x}$.

2.5 Method of Least Square

In the method of least square , we consider the estimation of parameters using some specified form of the expectation and second moment of the observations. For fitting a curve of the form $y = f(x, \beta_0, \beta_1, \ldots, \beta_p)$ to the data (x_i, y_i), i = 1, 2,…n, we may use the method of least squares. This method consists of minimizing the sum of squares.

$S = \sum_{i=1}^{n} \varepsilon_i^2$, where $\varepsilon_i = y_i - f(x_i, \beta_0, \beta_1, \ldots, \beta_p)$, i = 1, 2,…,n with respect to $\beta_0, \beta_1, \ldots, \beta_p$. Sometimes, we minimize $\sum w_i\varepsilon_i^2$ instead of $\sum \varepsilon_i^2$. In that case, it is called a weighted least square method.

To minimize S, we consider (p + 1) first order partial derivatives and get (p + 1) equations in (p + 1) unknowns. Solving these equations, we get the least square estimates of β_i's.

In general, the least square estimates do not have any optimum properties even asymptotically. However, in case of linear estimation this method provides good estimators. When $f(x_i, \beta_0, \beta_1, \ldots, \beta_p)$ is a linear function of the parameters and the

x-values are known, least square estimators will be BLUE. Again, if we assume that ε_i's are independently and identically normally distributed, then a linear estimator of the form $\underset{\sim}{a}' \underset{\sim}{\beta}$ will be MVUE for the entire class of unbiased estimators. In general, we consider n uncorrelated observations $y_1, y_2, \ldots y_n$ such that $E(y_i) = \beta_1 x_{1i} + \beta_2 x_{2i} + \cdots + \beta_k x_{ki}$.

$$V(y_i) = \sigma^2,\ i = 1, 2, \ldots\ldots, n,\ x_{1i} = 1 \forall i,$$

where $\beta_1, \beta_2 \ldots\ldots\ldots \beta_k$ and σ^2 are unknown parameters. If Y and β^* stand for column vectors of the variables y_i and parameters β_j and if $X = (x_{ji})$ be an $(n \times k)$ matrix of known coefficients x_{ji} then the above equation can be written as

$$E(Y) = X\beta^*$$

$$V(e) = E(ee') = \sigma^2 I$$

where $e = Y - X\beta^*$ is an $(n \times 1)$ vector of error random variable with $E(e) = 0$ and I is an $(n \times n)$ identity matrix. The least square method requires that β's be such calculated that $\phi = e'e = (Y - X\beta^*)'(Y - X\beta^*)$ be the minimum. This is satisfied when

$$\frac{\partial \phi}{\partial \beta^*} = 0$$

$$\text{Or, } 2X'(Y - X\beta^*) = 0.$$

The least square estimators β's is thus given by the vector $\hat{\beta}^* = (X'X)^{-1}X'Y$.

Example 2.13 Let $y_i = \beta_1 x_{1i} + \beta_2 x_{2i} + e_i$, $i = 1, 2, \ldots\ldots, n$ or $E(y_i) = \beta_1 x_{1i} + \beta_2 x_{2i}$, $x_{1i} = 1$ for all i.

Find the least square estimates of β_1 and β_2. Prove that the method of maximum likelihood and the method of least square are identical for the case of normal distribution.

Solution

In matrix notation we have

$$E(Y) = X\beta^*, \text{ where } X = \begin{pmatrix} 1 & x_{21} \\ 1 & x_{22} \\ \vdots & \vdots \\ 1 & x_{2n} \end{pmatrix},\ \beta^* = \begin{pmatrix} \beta_1 \\ \beta_2 \end{pmatrix} \text{ and } Y = \begin{pmatrix} y_1 \\ y_2 \\ \vdots \\ y_n \end{pmatrix}$$

Now,

$$\hat{\beta}^* = (X'X)^{-1}X'Y$$

Here, $$X'X = \begin{pmatrix} 1 & 1 & \ldots & 1 \\ x_{21} & x_{22} & \ldots & x_{2n} \end{pmatrix} \begin{pmatrix} 1 & x_{21} \\ 1 & x_{22} \\ \vdots & \vdots \\ 1 & x_{2n} \end{pmatrix} = \begin{pmatrix} n & \sum x_{2i} \\ \sum x_{2i} & \sum x_{2i}^2 \end{pmatrix}$$

$$X'Y = \begin{pmatrix} \sum y_i \\ \sum x_{2i}y_i \end{pmatrix}$$

$$\begin{aligned} \therefore \hat{\beta}^* &= \frac{1}{n\sum x_{2i}^2 - (\sum x_{2i})^2} \begin{pmatrix} \sum x_{2i}^2 & -\sum x_{2i} \\ -\sum x_{2i} & n \end{pmatrix} \begin{pmatrix} \sum y_i \\ \sum x_{2i}y_i \end{pmatrix} \\ &= \frac{1}{n\sum x_{2i}^2 - (\sum x_{2i})^2} \begin{pmatrix} \sum x_{2i}^2 \sum y_i - \sum x_{2i} \sum x_{2i}y_i \\ -\sum x_{2i} \sum y_i + n\sum x_{2i} \sum y_i \end{pmatrix} \end{aligned}$$

Hence,

$$\begin{aligned} \hat{\beta}_2 &= \frac{n\sum x_{2i} \sum y_i - \sum x_{2i} \sum y_i}{n\sum x_{2i}^2 - (\sum x_{2i})^2} = \frac{\sum x_{2i} \sum y_i - n\bar{x}_2\bar{y}}{\sum x_{2i}^2 - n\bar{x}_2^2} \\ &= \frac{\sum (x_{2i} - \bar{x}_2)(y_i - \bar{y})}{\sum (x_{2i} - \bar{x}_2)^2} \end{aligned}$$

$$\begin{aligned} \hat{\beta}_1 &= \frac{\sum x_{2i}^2 \sum y_i - \sum x_{2i} \sum x_{2i}y_i}{n\sum x_{2i}^2 - (\sum x_{2i})^2} \\ &= \frac{\bar{y}\sum x_{2i}^2 - \bar{x}_2 \sum x_{2i}y_i}{\sum x_{2i}^2 - n\bar{x}^2} \\ &= \bar{y} + \frac{\bar{y}n\bar{x}_2^2 - \bar{x}_2 \sum x_{2i}y_i}{\sum x_{2i}^2 - n\bar{x}_2^2} \\ &= \bar{y} - \bar{x}_2\hat{\beta}_2 \end{aligned}$$

Let y_i be an independent $N(\beta_1 + \beta_2 x_i, \sigma^2)$ variate, $i = 1, 2, \ldots\ldots, n$ so that $E(y_i) = \beta_1 + \beta_2 x_i$. The estimators of β_1 and β_2 are obtained by the method of least square on minimizing

$$\phi = \sum_{i=1}^{n} (y_i - \beta_1 - \beta_2 x_i)^2$$

The likelihood estimate is

$$L = \left(\frac{1}{\sqrt{2\pi}\sigma}\right)^n e^{-\frac{1}{2\sigma^2}\sum (y_i - \beta_1 - \beta_2 x_i)^2}$$

L is maximum when $\sum_{i=1}^{n} (y_i - \beta_1 - \beta_2 x_i)^2$ is minimum. By the method of maximum likelihood, we choose β_1 and β_2 such that $\sum_{i=1}^{n} (y_i - \beta_1 - \beta_2 x_i)^2 = \phi$ is minimum. Hence, both the methods of least square and maximum likelihood estimator are identical.

Example 2.14 Let $X_1, X_2, \ldots X_n$ be a random sample from p.d.f. $f(x; \theta, r) = \frac{1}{\theta^r \Gamma(r)} e^{-x/\theta} x^{r-1},\ x > 0;\ \theta > 0,\ r > 0.$

Find estimator of θ and r by

(i) Method of moments
(ii) Method of maximum likelihood

Answer

(i) Here, $E(x) = \mu_1^1 = r\theta,\ E(x^2) = \mu_2^1 = r(r+1)\theta^2$

$$m_1^1 = \bar{x},\ m_2^1 = \frac{1}{n}\sum_{i=1}^{n} x_i^2$$

Hence, $r\theta = \bar{x},\ r(r+1)\theta^2 = \frac{1}{n}\sum_{i=1}^{n} x_i^2$

By solving, we get $\hat{r} = \frac{n\bar{x}^2}{\sum_{i=1}^{n} (x_i - \bar{x})^2}$ and $\hat{\theta} = \frac{\sum_{i=1}^{n} (x_i - \bar{x})^2}{n\bar{x}}$

(ii) $L = \frac{1}{\theta^{nr}(\Gamma(r))^n} e^{-\frac{1}{\theta}\sum_{i=1}^{n} x_i} \prod_{i=1}^{n} x_i^{r-1}$

$\log L = -nr\log\theta - n\log\Gamma(r) - \frac{1}{\theta}\sum_i^n x_i + (r-1)\sum_{i=1}^{n} \log x_i$

Now, $\frac{\partial \log L}{\partial \theta} = -\frac{nr}{\theta} + \frac{n\bar{x}}{\theta^2} = 0 \Rightarrow \hat{\theta} = \frac{\bar{x}}{r}$

$$\frac{\partial \log L}{\partial r} = -n\log\theta - n\frac{\partial \log \Gamma(r)}{\partial r} + \sum_{i=1}^{n}\log x_i$$
$$= n\log r - n\frac{\Gamma'(r)}{\Gamma(r)} - n\log\bar{x} + \sum_{i}^{n}\log x_i$$

It is, however, difficult to solve the equation $\frac{\partial \log L}{\partial r} = 0$ and to get the estimate of r. Thus, for this example estimators of θ and r are more easily obtained by the method of moments than the method of maximum likelihood.

Example 2.15 If a sample of size one is drawn from the p.d.f $f(x,\beta) = \frac{2}{\beta^2}(\beta - x), 0 < x < \beta$.

Find $\hat{\beta}$, the MLE of β and β^*, the estimator of β based on method of moments. Show that $\hat{\beta}$ is biased, but β^* is unbiased. Show that the efficiency of $\hat{\beta}$ w.r.t. β^* is 2/3.

Solution

$$L = \frac{2}{\beta^2}(\beta - x)$$

$$\log L = \log 2 - 2\log\beta + \log(\beta - x)$$

$$\frac{\partial \log L}{\partial \beta} = -\frac{2}{\beta} + \frac{1}{\beta - x} = 0 \Rightarrow \beta = 2x$$

Thus, the MLE of β is given by $\widehat{\beta} = 2x$.
Now, $E(x) = \frac{2}{\beta^2}\int_0^\beta (\beta x - x^2)\mathrm{d}x = \frac{\beta}{3}$
Hence, $\frac{\beta}{3} = x \Rightarrow \beta = 3x$
Thus, the estimator of β based on method of moment is given by $\beta^* = 3x$.
Now,

$$E\left(\hat{\beta}\right) = 2 \times \frac{\beta}{3} = \frac{2\beta}{3} \neq \beta$$
$$E(\beta^*) = 3 \times \frac{\beta}{3} = \beta$$

Hence, $\hat{\beta}$ is biased but β^* is unbiased.

Again,

$$E(x^2) = \frac{2}{\beta^2}\int_0^{\beta}(\beta x^2 - x^3)\,\mathrm{d}x = \frac{\beta^2}{6}$$

$$\therefore V(x) = \frac{\beta^2}{6} - \frac{\beta^2}{9} = \frac{\beta^2}{18}$$

$$V(\beta^*) = 9V(x) = \frac{\beta^2}{2}$$

$$V\left(\hat{\beta}\right) = 4V(x) = \frac{2}{9}\beta^2$$

$$\begin{aligned} M\left(\hat{\beta}\right) &= V\left(\hat{\beta}\right) + \left[E\left(\hat{\beta}\right) - \beta\right]^2 \\ &= \frac{2}{9}\beta^2 + \left(\frac{2}{3}\beta - \beta\right)^2 \\ &= \frac{1}{3}\beta^2 \end{aligned}$$

Thus, the efficiency of $\hat{\beta}$ with respect to β^* is $\frac{2}{3}$.

Chapter 3
Theory of Testing of Hypothesis

3.1 Introduction

Consider a random sample from an infinite or a finite population. From such a sample or samples we try to draw inference regarding population. Suppose the form of the distribution of the population is F_θ which is assumed to be known but the parameter θ is unknown. Inferences are drawn about unknown parameters of the distribution. In many practical problems, we are interested in testing the validity of an assertion about the unknown parameter θ. Some hypothesis is made regarding the parameters and it is tested whether it is acceptable in the light of sample observations. As for examples, suppose we are interested in introducing a high yielding rice variety. We have at our disposal a standard variety having average yield x quintal per acre. We want to know whether the average yield for the new variety is higher than x. Similarly, we may be interested to check the claim of a tube light manufacturer about the average life hours achieved by a particular brand. A problem of this type is usually referred to as a problem of testing of hypothesis. Testing of hypothesis is closely linked with estimation theory in which we seek the best estimator of unknown parameter. In this chapter, we shall discuss the problem of testing of hypothesis.

3.2 Definitions and Some Examples

In this section, some aspects of statistical hypotheses and tests of statistical hypothesis will be discussed.

Let $\rho = \{p(x)\}$ be a class of all p.m.f or p.d.f. In testing problem $p(x)$ is unknown, but ρ is known. Our objective is to provide more information about $p(x)$ on the basis of $X = x$. That is, to know whether $p(x) \in \rho^* \subset \rho$.

P.K. Sahu et al., *Estimation and Inferential Statistics*,
DOI 10.1007/978-81-322-2514-0_3

Definition 1 A hypothesis is a conjecture or assertion about $p(x)$. It is of two types, viz., Null hypothesis (*H*) and alternative hypothesis (*K*).

Null hypothesis (*H*): A hypothesis that is tentatively set up is called null hypothesis. Alternative to H is called Alternative hypothesis.

H and K are such that $H \cap K = \varphi$ and $H \cup K \subseteq \rho$. We also write H as

$$\left.\begin{array}{r} H : p(x) \in \rho_H \subset \rho \\ \text{and } K \text{ as } K : p(x) \in \rho_K \subset \rho \end{array}\right\} \rho_H \cap \rho_K = \varphi \text{ and } \rho_H \cup \rho_K \subseteq \rho$$

Labeling of the distribution

Write $\rho = \{p(x) = p(^x/_\theta), \theta \in \Theta\}$. Then '$\theta$' is called the labelling parameter of the distribution and 'Θ' is called the parameter space.

Example 3.1 $X \sim \text{bin}(m, p) \Leftrightarrow X_1, X_2, \ldots X_m$ are i.i.d Bernoulli (p) $\Rightarrow X = \sum_{i=1}^{m} X_i \sim \text{bin}(m, p)$, m is known, $\theta = p$, $\Theta = [0, 1]$, outcome space $\mathcal{X} = \{0, 1, 2, \ldots m\} \equiv \{0, 1\}X\{0, 1\}X \ldots X\{0, 1\}$

$$p(x/\theta) = \binom{m}{x} p^x (1-p)^{m-x} \text{ Or } p\left(\underset{\sim}{x}/\theta\right) = p^{\sum_{i=1}^{m} x_i} (1-p)^{m - \sum_{i=1}^{m} x_i}$$

$\rho = \left\{\binom{m}{x} p^x (1-p)^{m-x}, p \in [0, 1]\right\}$ is known but $\binom{m}{x} p^x (1-p)^{m-x}$ is unknown if p is unknown.

Example 3.2 Let $X_1, X_2, \ldots X_{n_1}$ are i.i.d $P(\lambda_1)$ and $Y_1, Y_2, \ldots Y_{n_2}$ are i.i.d $P(\lambda_2)$. Also they are independent and n_1 and n_2 are known.
Now,

$$X = (X_1, X_2, \ldots X_{n_1}, Y_1, Y_2, \ldots Y_{n_2}),\ n = n_1 + n_2$$

$$\mathcal{X} = [\{0, 1, \ldots \infty\}]^{n_1} X [\{0, 1, \ldots \infty\}]^{n_2}$$

$$\theta = (\lambda_1, \lambda_2); \Theta = (0, \infty)X(0, \infty) = \{(\lambda_1, \lambda_2) : 0 < \lambda_1, \lambda_2 < \infty\}$$

$$p(x/\theta) = \prod_{i=1}^{n_1} p(x_i/\lambda_1) \prod_{j=1}^{n_2} p(y_j/\lambda_2) = \frac{\lambda_1^{\sum x_i} \lambda_2^{\sum y_j}}{\prod x_i! \prod y_j!} e^{-(n_1\lambda_1 + n_2\lambda_2)}$$

$\rho = \{p(^x/_\theta), 0 < \lambda_1, \lambda_2 < \infty\}$ is known but $p(^x/_\theta)$ is unknown if θ is unknown.

Example 3.3 $X_1, X_2, \ldots X_n$ are i.i.d $N(\mu, \sigma^2)$. $X = (X_1, X_2, \ldots X_n), n \geq 1, \theta = (\mu, \sigma^2)$ or $\{\mu\}$ (if σ^2 is known) or $\{\sigma^2\}$ (if μ is known), $\Theta = \{(\mu, \sigma^2) : -\infty < \mu < \infty, \sigma^2 > 0\}$ or $\{\mu : -\infty < \mu < \infty\} \equiv R'$ or $\{\sigma^2 : \sigma^2 > 0\}$.

$\mathcal{X} = R^n$: n-dimensional Euclidean space.

$$p(x/\theta) = (2\pi)^{-n/2}\sigma^{-n}e^{-\frac{1}{2\sigma^2}\sum_1^n (x_i-\mu)^2} \quad \text{or}$$

$$= (2\pi)^{-n/2}e^{-\frac{1}{2}\sum_1^n (x_i-\mu)^2}; \sigma^2 = 1 \text{ or}$$

$$= (2\pi)^{-n/2}\sigma^{-n}e^{-\frac{1}{2\sigma^2}\sum_1^n x_i^2}; \mu = 0. \text{ or}$$

$$\rho = \left\{p(x/\theta); -\infty < \mu < \infty, \sigma^2 > 0\right\} \text{ or}$$

$$\left\{p(x/\theta); -\infty < \mu < \infty\right\} \text{ or}$$

$\left\{p(x/\theta); \sigma^2 > 0\right\}$ all are known but unknown is $p(x/\theta)$ for fixed θ (Unknown).

Parametric set up

$p(x) = p(x/\theta)$; $\theta \in \Theta$. Then we can find $\Theta_H(\subset \Theta)$ and $\Theta_K(\subset \Theta)$ such that

$$\Theta_H \cap \Theta_K = \phi \text{ and } p_H = \{p(x/\theta);\ \theta \in \Theta_H\},\ p_K = \{p(x/\theta);\ \theta \in \Theta_K\}$$

So,

$$H : p \in p_H \Leftrightarrow H : \theta \in \Theta_H$$
$$K : p \in p_K \Leftrightarrow K : \theta \in \Theta_K.$$

Definition 2 Now a hypothesis H^* is called

i. Simple if H^* contains just one parametric point, i.e. H^* specifies the distribution $\{p(x/\theta)\}$ completely.
ii. Composite if H^* contains more than one parametric point, i.e. H^* cannot specify the distribution $\{p(x/\theta)\}$ completely.

Example 3.4 $X_1, X_2, \ldots X_n$ are i.i.d $N(\mu, \sigma^2)$. Consider the following hypothesis (H^*):

1. $H^* : \mu = 0, \sigma^2 = 1 : H^* \Rightarrow H \sim N(0,1)$
2. $H^* : \mu \leq 0, \sigma^2 = 1$
3. $H^* : \mu = 0, \sigma^2 > 0$
4. $H^* : \sigma^2 = \sigma_0^2$
5. $H^* : \mu + \sigma = 0$

The first one is a simple hypothesis and the remaining are composite hypotheses.

Definition 3 Let x be the observed value of the random variable X with probability model $p(x/\theta)$; θ unknown. Wherever $X = x$ is observed, $p(x/\theta)$ is a function of θ only and is called the likelihood of getting such a sample. It is simply called the likelihood function and often denoted by $L(\theta)$ or $L(\theta/x)$.

Definition 4 Test It is a rule for the acceptance or the rejection of the null hypothesis (*H*) on the basis of an observed value of *X*.

Definition 5 Non-randomized test

Let ω be a subset of $\mathcal{X}$ such that

$$X \in \omega \Rightarrow \text{The rejection of } H$$
$$X \in \mathcal{X} - \omega \Rightarrow \text{The acceptance of } H.$$

Then ω is called the critical region or a test for *H* against *K*. Test 'ω' means a rule determined by ω. Note that ω does not depend on the random experiment (that is on *X*). So it is called a non-randomized test.

Definition 6 Randomized test:

It consists in determining a function $\phi(x)$
such that

(i) $0 \leq \phi(x) \leq 1 \, \forall x \in \mathcal{X}$
(ii) *H* is rejected with probability $\phi(x)$ whenever $X = x$ is observed.

Such a '$\phi(x)$' is called 'Critical function' or 'test function' or simply 'test' for *H* against *K*. Here the function $\phi(x)$ depends on the random experiment (that is on *X*). So that name 'randomised' is justified.

e.g. (i) and (ii) $\Rightarrow$ whenever $X = x$ is observed, perform a Bernoullian trial with probability of success $\phi(x)$. If the trial results in success, reject *H*; otherwise *H* is accepted. Thus $\phi(x)$ represents the probability of rejection of *H*.

If $\phi(x)$ is non-randomized with critical region 'ω', then we have
$\omega = \{x : \phi(x) = 1\}$
$\mathcal{X} - \omega = \{x : \phi(x) = 0\}$ (Acceptance region).

Detailed study on Non-randomized test

If ω is Non-randomized test then it implies *H* is rejected iff $X \in \omega$. In many cases, we get a statistic $T = T(X)$ such that for some *C* or C_1 and C_2,

$[X \in \omega] \Leftrightarrow [X : T > C]$ or $[X : T < C]$ or $[X : T < C_1 \text{ or } : T > C_2]$, $C_1 < C_2$.
Such a '*T*' is called 'test statistic'.

The event $[T > C]$ is called right tail test based on *T*.
The event $[T < C]$ is called left tail test based on *T*.
The event $[T < C_1 \text{or } T > C_2]$ is called two tailed test based on '*T*'.

Sometimes C_1 and C_2 are such that $P\{T < C_1/\theta\} = P\{T > C_2/\theta\} \forall \theta \in \Theta_H$ then the test $[T < C_1 \text{ or } T > C_2]$ is called equal-tail test based on *T*.

Definition 7 Power Function

Let X be a random variable with $p(x/\theta)$ as p.d.f or p.m.f of X, $\theta \in \Theta$, $x \in \mathcal{X}$

Testing problem

$$H : \theta \in \Theta_H \text{ versus } K : \theta \in \Theta_K\{\Theta_H \cap \Theta_K = \emptyset\}$$

Let ω be a test for H against K.
Then the function given by

$$\begin{aligned} P_\omega(\theta) &= \text{Probability}\{\text{rejecting}\, H\, \text{under}\, \theta\}. \\ &= P\{X \in \omega/\theta\}, \theta \in \Theta \end{aligned}$$

is called power function (a function of θ) of the test 'ω'

For a given $\theta \in \Theta_K$, $P_\omega(\theta)$ is called the power of 'ω' at θ. For continuous case, we have $P_\omega(\theta) = \int_\omega p(x/\theta)\mathrm{d}x$ and for discrete case we have $P_\omega(\theta) = \sum_\omega p(x/\theta)$.

A test 'ω' is called size-α if

$$P_\omega(\theta) \le \alpha\ \forall \theta \in \Theta_H[\alpha : 0 < \alpha < 1] \tag{3.1}$$

and it is called strictly size-α if

$$P_\omega(\theta) \le \alpha\ \forall \theta \in \Theta_H \text{ and } P_\omega(\theta) = \alpha \,\text{for some}\, \theta \in \Theta_H \tag{3.2}$$

(3.1) $\Leftrightarrow \underset{\theta \in \Theta_H}{\text{Sup}}\ P_\omega(\theta) \le \alpha$ and (3.2) $\Leftrightarrow \underset{\theta \in \Theta_H}{\text{Sup}}\ P_\omega(\theta) = \alpha$.

The quantity $\text{Sup}\{P_\omega(\theta), \theta \in \Theta_H\}$ is called the size of the test. Sometimes 'α' is called the level of the test 'ω'

Some Specific cases

(i) θ: Real-valued; testing problem $H : \theta = \theta_0$ (Simple) or $H : \theta \le \theta_0$ (Composite) against $K : \theta > \theta_0$; ω: A test; $P_\omega(\theta)$: Power function; Size of the test: $P_\omega(\theta_0)$ or $\underset{\theta \le \theta_0}{\text{Sup}}\ P_\omega(\theta)$

(ii) $\theta = (\theta_1, \theta_2)$: 2 component vector

Testing problem: H: $\theta_1 = \theta_1^0$ (given) against $K : \theta_1 > \theta_1^0$ (composite)

ω: A test

$P_w(\theta)$: power function = $P_w(\theta_1, \theta_2) = P_w(\theta_1^0, \theta_2)$ (at H) = A function of θ_2.

Thus, the power function (under H) is still unknown. The quantity sup $\{P_w(\theta_1^0, \theta_2), \theta_2 \in \text{Space of } \theta_2\}$ is known and is called the size of the test. For, e.g. take $N(\mu, \sigma^2)$ distribution and consider the problem of testing H: $\mu = 0$ against K: $\mu > 0$, then the size of the test is

$$\text{Sup}\left\{P_w(\mu,\sigma^2)/_{\mu}=0, 0<\sigma^2<\infty\right\}.$$

Example 3.5 $X_1, X_2, \ldots, X_n$ are i.i.d $N(\mu, \sigma_0^2)$; $H : \mu \leq \mu_0$ against $K : \mu > \mu_0$.

$$\omega \equiv \left\{(X_1, X_2, \ldots, X_n) : \bar{X} > \mu_0 + \frac{\sigma_0}{\sqrt{n}}\right\}$$

$$\begin{aligned}
P_w(\theta) = P_w(\mu) &= P\left\{\bar{X} > \mu_0 + \tfrac{\sigma_0}{\sqrt{n}}/_{\mu}\right\} \\
&= P\left\{\frac{\sqrt{n}(\bar{X}-\mu)}{\sigma_0} > -\frac{\sqrt{n}(\mu-\mu_0)}{\sigma_0} + 1|\mu\right\} \\
&= P\left\{Z > 1 - \frac{\sqrt{n}(\mu-\mu_0)}{\sigma_0}|Z \sim N(0,1)\right\} \\
&= \Phi\left\{\frac{\sqrt{n}(\mu-\mu_0)}{\sigma_0} - 1\right\}
\end{aligned}$$

$$\begin{aligned}
\text{Size of } \omega &= \underset{\mu\leq\mu_0}{\text{Sup}}\ P_w(\mu) = \underset{\mu\leq\mu_0}{\text{Sup}}\left[\Phi\left\{\frac{\sqrt{n}(\mu-\mu_0)}{\sigma_0} - 1\right\}\right] \\
&= \Phi(-1) = \text{size of } \omega \text{ for testing } H : \mu = \mu_0.
\end{aligned}$$

Example 3.6

$X_1, X_2, \ldots, X_n$ are i.i.d $N(\mu, \sigma_0^2)$.
$H : \mu = \mu_0$ against $K : \mu > \mu_0$.

$$\omega = \left\{(X_1, X_2, \ldots, X_n) : \bar{X} > \mu_0 + \frac{\sigma_0}{\sqrt{n}}\tau_\alpha\right\}; \begin{array}{c}\alpha \in (0,1) \\ \Phi(-\tau_\alpha) = \alpha\end{array}$$

$$\begin{aligned}
P_w(\mu_0) &= \text{size of } \omega \text{ for testing } H \\
&= P\left\{\bar{X} > \mu_0 + \frac{\sigma_0}{\sqrt{n}}\tau_\alpha|\mu_0\right\} = P\left\{\frac{\sqrt{n}(\bar{X}-\mu_0)}{\sigma_0} > \tau_\alpha|\mu_0\right\} \\
&= P\{Z > \tau_\alpha|Z \sim N(0,1)\} = \alpha. \\
&\Rightarrow \text{Test is exactly size } '\alpha'.
\end{aligned}$$

Example 3.7 $X_1, X_2, \ldots, X_n$ are i.i.d. $N(\mu, \sigma^2)$
$H : \mu = \mu_0$ against $K : \mu > \mu_0$

$$\omega : \{(X_1, X_2, \ldots, X_n); \bar{X} > c\} \tag{3.3}$$

where 'c' is such that the test is of size 0.05.

$$P_w(\mu_0) = \text{size of } \omega \text{ for testing } H = P\left\{\overline{X} > {c}/{\mu_0}\right\}$$
$$= P\left\{\frac{\sqrt{n}(\overline{X} - \mu_0)}{\sigma_0} > \frac{(c - \mu_0)\sqrt{n}}{\sigma_0} / \mu_0\right\}$$
$$= P\left\{Z > \frac{(c - \mu_0)\sqrt{n}}{\sigma_0} / Z \sim N(0, 1)\right\} = 0.05(\text{given})$$
$$\Rightarrow \frac{(c - \mu_0)\sqrt{n}}{\sigma_0} = \tau_{0.05} \simeq 1.645 \Rightarrow c = \mu_0 + \frac{1.645\sigma_0}{\sqrt{n}} \tag{3.4}$$

Test given (3.3) and (3.4) is strictly (exactly) of size 0.05.
(or, level of significance of the test is 0.05).

Example 3.8 X_1 and X_2 are i.i.d. according to ($\Leftrightarrow$ Bernoulli (1, p)).

$$f\left({x}/{p}\right) = p^x(1 - p)^x; x = 0, 1$$

Testing problem, $H : p = \frac{1}{2}$ against $K : p > \frac{1}{2}$.
Consider the test $\omega = \{(X_1, X_2) : X_1 + X_2 = 2\}$
Accept H if $(X_1, X_2) \notin \omega$
Test statistic: $T = X_1 + X_2 \sim \text{bin}(2, p)$

$$\text{Size of the test is } P\left\{(X_1, X_2) \in {\omega}/{p = \tfrac{1}{2}}\right\} = P\left\{T = {2}/{p = \tfrac{1}{2}}\right\} = \left(\frac{1}{2}\right)^2 = 0.25$$

If we take $\omega = \{(X_1, X_2) : X_1 + X_2 = 1, 2\}$ i.e. accept H if $(X_1, X_2) \notin \omega$. We get size $= 2.\left(\frac{1}{2}\right)^2 + \left(\frac{1}{2}\right)^2 = 0.75$.

Let us take another test of the form:

ω : Reject H if $X_1 + X_2 = 2$
ω_B : Reject H if $X_1 + X_2 = 1$ with probability $\frac{1}{2}$
A: Accept H if $X_1 + X_2 = 0$

Sample space $= \{0, 1, 2\} = \omega + \omega_B + A$

$$\text{Size} = 1.\, P\{(X_1 + X_2) = 2\} + \frac{1}{2}P(X_1 + X_2 = 1) + 0.\, P(X_1 + X_2 = 0)$$
$$= 0.25 + 0.25 = 0.50$$

The test given above is called a randomized test.

Definition 8 Power function of a randomized test:

Consider $\phi(x)$ as a randomized test which is equivalent to probability of rejection of H when the observed value of $(X = x)$ and E as an Event of rejection of H. Then $P(E|X = x) = \phi(x)$. Power function of ϕ is

$$
\begin{aligned}
P_\phi(\theta) &= \text{Probability } \{\text{Rejection of } H \text{ under } \theta \text{ using the function } \phi\} \\
&= P\left\{{}^{E}\!/\!{}_{\theta}\right\} \\
&= \int_{*} P\left\{{}^{E}\!/\!{}_{x,\theta}\right\} \cdot p\{{}^{x}\!/\!{}_{\theta}\}\mathrm{d}x; \text{ when } X \text{ is continuous} \qquad (3.5) \\
&= \sum_{*} P\left\{{}^{E}\!/\!{}_{x,\theta}\right\} \cdot p\{{}^{x}\!/\!{}_{\theta}\}; \text{ when } X \text{ is discrete} \qquad (3.6)
\end{aligned}
$$

In case of (3.5), we get:

$$
\begin{aligned}
P_\phi(\theta) &= \int_{*} \phi(x)\, p\{{}^{x}\!/\!{}_{\theta}\}\mathrm{d}x \quad \left(\text{As } P\left({}^{E}\!/\!{}_{x,\theta}\right) = P\left({}^{E}\!/\!{}_{x}\right) = \phi(x)\right) \\
&= E_\theta \phi(x)
\end{aligned}
$$

In case of (3.6), we get: $P_\phi(\theta) = \sum_{*} \phi(x).p({}^{x}\!/\!{}_{\theta}) = E_\theta \phi(x)$

In either case we have $P_\phi(\theta) = E_\theta \phi(x) \forall \theta \in \Theta$.

Special cases

1. Suppose $\phi(x)$ takes only two values, viz. 0 and 1. In that case, we say $\phi(x)$ is non-randomized with critical region $\omega = \{x : \phi(x) = 1\}$.
   In that case
   $$
   \begin{aligned}
   P_\phi(\theta) &= 1.P_\theta\{\phi(x) = 1\} + 0.\, P_\theta\{\phi(x) = 0\} \\
   &= P_\theta\{X \in \omega\} = P_\omega(\theta).
   \end{aligned}
   $$
   $\therefore \phi$ is generalization of ω.
2. Suppose $\phi(x)$ takes three values, viz 0, a and I according as $x \in A$, $x \in w_B$ and $x \in \omega$. In that case $\phi(x)$ is called randomized test having the boundary region W_B. The power function of this test is $P_\phi(\theta) = P_\theta\{X \in \omega\} + aP_\theta\{X \in w_B\}$.

(1) $\Rightarrow$ no need of post randomization: Non-randomised test.
(2) $\Rightarrow$ requires post randomization: randomized test.

Example 3.9 $X_1, X_2, \ldots, X_n$ are i.i.d. Bernoulli (1, p), n = 25. Testing problem: $H : p = \frac{1}{2}$ against $K : p \neq \frac{1}{2}$.

Consider the following tests:

$$(1)\quad \left.\begin{aligned}\phi(x) &= 1 \text{ if } \sum_1^{25} x_i > 12 \\ &= 0 \text{ if } \sum_1^{15} x_i \le 12\end{aligned}\right\} \text{ Non-randomized}$$

$$(2)\quad \left.\begin{aligned}\phi(\mathrm{x}) &= 1 \text{ if } \sum_1^{25} x_i > c \\ &= a \text{ if } \sum_1^{25} x_i = c \\ &= 0 \text{ if } \sum_1^{25} x_i < c\end{aligned}\right\}$$

Find c and a such that $E_{p=\frac{1}{2}}\phi(x) = 0.05$. Randomized if $a \in (0,1)$ and Non-randomized if $a = 0 \text{ or } 1$. In case of (1), size $=$ $E_{p=\frac{1}{2}}\phi(x) = P\left\{\sum_1^{25} x_i > 12 | p = \frac{1}{2}\right\} = 0.50001$.

In case of (2), we want to get (c, a) such that $E_{p=\frac{1}{2}}\phi(x) = 0.05$.

$$\Leftrightarrow P_{p=\frac{1}{2}}\left\{\sum_1^{25} x_i > c\right\} + aP_{p=\frac{1}{2}}\left\{\sum_1^{25} x_i = c\right\} = 0.05$$

By inspection we find that $P_{p=\frac{1}{2}}\left\{\sum_1^{25} x_i > 17\right\} = 0.02237$ and $P_{p=\frac{1}{2}}\left\{\sum_1^{25} x_i > 16\right\} = 0.0546$. Hence, c = 17.

Now, $a = \frac{0.05 - P_{p=\frac{1}{2}}\left\{\sum_1^{15} x_i > c\right\}}{P\left\{\sum_1^{25} x_i = c\right\}} = \frac{0.05 - 0.02237}{0.03223} = 0.8573$.

Thus the test given by

$$\begin{aligned}\phi(x) &= 1 \text{ if } \sum_1^{25} x_i > 17 \\ &= 0.8573 \text{ if } \sum_1^{25} x_i = 17 \\ &= 0 \text{ if } \sum_1^{25} x_i < 17\end{aligned}$$

is randomized and of size 0.05.

But the test given by

$$\phi(x) = 1 \quad \text{if} \sum_{1}^{25} x_i \geq 17$$
$$= 0 \quad \text{if} \sum_{1}^{25} x_i < 17$$

is non-randomized and of size 0.0546 (at the level 0.06).

Performance of ω

Our object is to choose ω such that $P_\omega(\theta)\forall\theta \in \Theta_H$ and $(1 - P_\omega(\theta))\forall\theta \in \Theta_K$ are as small as possible. While performing a test ω we reach any of the following decisions:

I. Observe $X = x$, Accept H when θ actually belongs to Θ_H: A correct decision.
II. Observe $X = x$, Reject H when θ actually belongs to Θ_H: An incorrect decision.
III. Observe $X = x$, Accept H when θ actually belongs to Θ_K: An incorrect decision.
IV. Observe $X = x$, Reject H when θ actually belongs to Θ_K: A correct decision.

An incorrect decision of the type as stated in II above is called type-I error and an incorrect decision of the type as stated in III above is called type-II error. Hence, the performance of ω is measured by the following:

(a) Size of type-I error = Probability {Type-I error} $= \underset{\theta\in\Theta_H}{\text{Sup}}\, P\{X \in \omega/\theta\} =$

$$\underset{\theta\in\Theta_H}{\text{Sup}}\, P_\omega(\theta)$$

(b) Size of type-II error = Probability {Type-II error } $= P\{X \in \mathcal{X} - \omega\}\ \forall\theta \in \Theta_K$

$$= 1 - P_\omega(\theta)\ \forall\theta \in \Theta_K.$$

So we want to minimize simultaneously both the errors. In practice, it is not possible to minimize both of them simultaneously, because the minimization of one leads to the increase of the other.

Thus the conventional procedure: Choose 'ω' such that, for a given $\alpha \in (0, 1)$, $P_\omega(\theta) \leq \alpha \quad \forall\theta \in \Theta_H$ and $1 - P_\omega(\theta)\ \forall\theta \in \Theta_K$ is as low as possible, i.e., $P_\omega(\theta)\ \forall\theta \in \Theta_K$ is as high as possible. 'ω' satisfying above (if it exists) is called an optimum test at the level α.

Suppose $\Theta_H = \{\theta_0\}$ a single point set and $\Theta_K = \{\theta_1\}$ a single point set.

The above condition thus reduces to: $P_\omega(\theta_1)$ = maximum subject to $P_\omega(\theta_0) \leq \alpha$.

Definition 9

1. For testing $H : \theta \in \Theta_H$ against K: $\theta = \theta_1 \notin \Theta_H$, a test '$\omega_0$' is said to be most powerful (MP) level 'α' $\in (0, 1)$ if

$$P_{\omega_0}(\theta) \le \alpha \forall \theta \in \Theta_H \tag{3.7}$$

and

$$P_{\omega_0}(\theta_1) \ge P_{\omega}(\theta_1)\ \forall \omega \text{ satisfying (3.7)} \tag{3.8}$$

In particular, if $H: \theta = \theta_0$, (3.7) and (3.8) reduce to $P_{\omega_0}(\theta_0) \le \alpha$ and $P_{\omega_0}(\theta_1) \ge P_{\omega}(\theta_1)\ \forall \omega$ satisfying first condition.

2. A test 'ω_0' is said to be MP size-α, if $\text{Sup}_{\theta \in \Theta_H} P_{\omega_0}(\theta) = \alpha$ and $P_{\omega_0}(\theta_1) \ge P_{\omega}(\theta_1)\ \forall \omega$ satisfying $P_{\omega}(\theta) \le \alpha \forall \theta \in \Theta_H$. Again if $\Theta_H = \{\theta_0\}$, we get the above condition as $P_{\omega_0}(\theta_0) = \alpha$ and $P_{\omega_0}(\theta_1) \ge P_{\omega}(\theta_1) \forall \omega$ satisfying $P_{\omega}(\theta_0) \le \alpha$.
3. For testing $H: \theta \in \Theta_H$ against $K: \theta \in \Theta_K$, $\Theta_K \cap \Theta_H = \phi$, a test '$\omega_0$' is said to be Uniformly Most Powerful (UMP) level 'α' if

$$P_{\omega_0}(\theta) \le \alpha \forall \theta \in \Theta_H \tag{3.9}$$

$P_{\omega_0}(\theta_1) \ge P_{\omega}(\theta_1) \forall \theta_1 \in \Theta_K$ and $\forall \omega$ satisfying (3.9). i.e. 'ω_0'is said to be UMP size-α if $\underset{\theta \in \Omega_H}{\text{Sup}}\, P_{\omega_0}(\theta) = \alpha$ and $P_{\omega_0}(\theta_1) \ge P_{\omega}(\theta_1)\ \forall \theta_1 \in \Theta_K$ and $\forall \omega$ satisfying $\underset{\theta \in \Omega_H}{\text{Sup}}\, P_{\omega}(\theta) \le \alpha$. Again if $\Theta_H = \{\theta_0\}$, the aforesaid conditions reduce to

(a) $P_{\omega_0}\{\theta_0\} \le \alpha$ and $P_{\omega_0}\{\theta_1\} \ge P_{\omega}\{\theta_1\}\ \forall \theta_1 \in \Theta_K$ and $\forall \omega$ satisfying $P_{\omega}\{\theta_0\} \le \alpha$.
(b) $P_{\omega_0}\{\theta_0\} = \alpha$ and $P_{\omega_0}\{\theta_1\} \ge P_{\omega}\{\theta_1\}\ \forall \theta_1 \in \Theta_K$ and $\forall \omega$ satisfying $P_{\omega}\{\theta_0\} \le \alpha$.

4. A test ω^* is said to be unbiased if (under testing problem: $H: \theta = \theta_0$ against $K: \theta = \theta_1$, $(\theta_1 \ne \theta_0)$)
$P_{\omega^*}(\theta_1) \ge P_{\omega^*}(\theta_0)$ (⇒power ≥ size), i.e. it is said to be unbiased size-α if $P_{\omega^*}(\theta_0) = \alpha$ and $P_{\omega^*}(\theta_1) \ge \alpha$. If $K: \theta \in \Theta_K$ is composite, the above relation reduces to (A) $P_{\omega^*}(\theta_1) \ge P_{\omega^*}(\theta_0)\ \forall \theta_1 \in \Theta_K$ (B) $P_{\omega^*}(\theta_1) \ge \alpha \forall \theta_1 \in \Theta_K$ where $\alpha = P_{\omega^*}(\theta_0)$.
5. For testing $H: \theta = \theta_0$ against $K: \theta \in \Theta_K \not\ni \theta_0$, a test ω^* is said to be Uniformly Most Powerful Unbiased (UMPU) size-α if
(i) $P_{\omega^*}(\theta_0) = \alpha$; (ii) $P_{\omega^*}(\theta_1) \ge \alpha\ \forall \theta_1 \in \Theta_K$ and (iii) $P_{\omega^*}(\theta_1) \ge P_{\omega}(\theta_1)\ \forall \theta_1 \in \Theta_K\ \forall \omega$ satisfying (i) and (ii).

3.3 Method of Obtaining BCR

The definition of most powerful critical region, i.e. best critical region (BCR) of size α does not provide a systematic method of determining it. The following lemma, due to Neyman and Pearson, provides a solution of the problem if we, however, test a simple hypothesis against a simple alternative.

The Neyman–Pearson Lemma maybe stated as follows:

For testing $H: \theta = \theta_0$ against $K: \theta = \theta_1,\ \theta_0,\ \theta_1 \in \Theta, \quad \theta_1 \neq \theta_0,$
for some $\alpha \in (0,1)$, let ω_0 be a subset of $\mathcal{X}$. Suppose ω_0 satisfies the following conditions:

(i) If $x \in \omega_0,\ p\left({}^{x}/_{\theta_1}\right) \geq \lambda p\left({}^{x}/_{\theta_0}\right)$ (Inside ω_0)

(ii) If $x \in \mathcal{X} - \omega_0,\ p\left({}^{x}/_{\theta_1}\right) < \lambda p\left({}^{x}/_{\theta_0}\right)$ (Outside ω_0)

(x: observed value of X) where $\lambda(>0)$ is such that $P_{\omega_0}(\theta_0) = \alpha$. Then $P_{\omega_0}(\theta_1) \geq P_{\omega}\{\theta_1\} \forall \omega$ satisfying $P_{\omega}(\theta_0) \leq \alpha$. That means '$\omega_0$' is a MP size-$\alpha$ test.

Proof (Continuous case)

$$\begin{aligned}
P_{\omega_0}(\theta_1) - P_{\omega}(\theta_1) &= \int\limits_{\omega_0} p\left({}^{x}/_{\theta_1}\right)\mathrm{d}x - \int\limits_{\omega} p\left({}^{x}/_{\theta_1}\right)\mathrm{d}x \\
&= \int\limits_{\omega_0 - \omega} p\left({}^{x}/_{\theta_1}\right)\mathrm{d}x + \int\limits_{\omega_0 \cap \omega} p\left({}^{x}/_{\theta_1}\right)\mathrm{d}x - \int\limits_{\omega - \omega_0} p\left({}^{x}/_{\theta_1}\right)\mathrm{d}x - \int\limits_{\omega \cap \omega_0} p\left({}^{x}/_{\theta_1}\right)\mathrm{d}x \\
&= \int\limits_{\omega_0 - \omega} p\left({}^{x}/_{\theta_1}\right)\mathrm{d}x - \int\limits_{\omega - \omega_0} p\left({}^{x}/_{\theta_1}\right)\mathrm{d}x
\end{aligned} \tag{3.10}$$

□

Now, $x \in \omega_0 - \omega \Leftrightarrow x \in$ inside $\omega_0 \Rightarrow p\left({}^{x}/_{\theta_1}\right) \geq \lambda p\left({}^{x}/_{\theta_0}\right)$

$$\Rightarrow \int\limits_{\omega_0 - \omega} p\left({}^{x}/_{\theta_1}\right)\mathrm{d}x \geq \lambda \int\limits_{\omega_0 - \omega} p\left({}^{x}/_{\theta_0}\right)\mathrm{d}x$$

$x \in \omega - \omega_0 \Leftrightarrow x \in$ outside $\omega_0 \Rightarrow p\left({}^{x}/_{\theta_1}\right) < \lambda P\left({}^{x}/_{\theta_0}\right)$

$$\Rightarrow \int\limits_{\omega - \omega_0} p\left({}^{x}/_{\theta_1}\right)\mathrm{d}x < \lambda \int\limits_{\omega - \omega_0} P\left({}^{x}/_{\theta_0}\right)\mathrm{d}x$$

Hence R.H.S of (3.10)

$$\begin{aligned}
&\geq \lambda\left[\int\limits_{\omega_0 - \omega} p\left({}^{x}/_{\theta_0}\right)\mathrm{d}x - \int\limits_{\omega - \omega_0} p\left({}^{x}/_{\theta_0}\right)\mathrm{d}x\right] \\
&= \lambda\left[\int\limits_{\omega_0} p\left({}^{x}/_{\theta_0}\right)\mathrm{d}x - \int\limits_{\omega} p\left({}^{x}/_{\theta_0}\right)\mathrm{d}x\right] \\
&= \lambda\left[\alpha - \int\limits_{\omega} p\left({}^{x}/_{\theta_0}\right)\mathrm{d}x\right] = \lambda[\alpha - P_{\omega}(\theta_0)] \\
&\geq \lambda(\alpha - \alpha) = 0 \text{ as } P_{\omega}(\theta_0) \leq \alpha.
\end{aligned}$$

Hence we get $P_{\omega_0}(\theta_1) - P_{\omega}(\theta_1) \geq 0$

$$\Leftrightarrow P_{\omega_0}(\theta_1) \geq P_{\omega}(\theta_1)$$

(Similar result can be obtained for the discrete case replacing $\int$ by Σ)

Notes

1. Define $Y = \frac{p(x|\theta_1)}{p(x|\theta_0)}$. If the random variable Y is continuous, we can **always** find a λ such that, for $\alpha \in (0, 1)$ $P[Y \geq \lambda] = \alpha$. If the random variable Y is discrete, we **sometimes** find λ such that $P[Y \geq \lambda] = \alpha$.
   But, in most of the cases, we have (assuming that $P[Y \geq \lambda] \neq \alpha$) $P_{\theta_0}(Y \geq \lambda_1) < \alpha$ and $P_{\theta_0}(Y \geq \lambda_2) > \alpha$, $\lambda_1 > \lambda_2 (\Rightarrow P(Y \geq \lambda) = \alpha$ has no solution).
   In that case we get a non-randomized test $'\omega_0'$ of level α given by

$$\omega_0 = \left\{x : \frac{p(x|\theta_1)}{p(x|\theta_0)} \geq \lambda_1\right\}; \; P_{\omega_0}(\theta_0) \leq \alpha.$$

   In order to get a size-α test, we proceed as follows:

   (i) Reject H if $Y \geq \lambda_1$
   (ii) Accept H if $Y < \lambda_2$
   (iii) Acceptance (or Rejection) depends on the random experiment whenever $Y = \lambda_2$.

   Random experiment: when $Y = \lambda_2$ is observed, perform a random experiment with probability of success

$$P = a = \frac{\alpha - P_{\theta_0}\{Y \geq \lambda_1\}}{P\{Y = \lambda_2\}}.$$

   If the experiment results in success reject H; otherwise accept H. Hence, we get the following randomized test:

$$\begin{aligned}
\phi^0(x) &= 1 \text{ if } \frac{p(x|\theta_1)}{p(x|\theta_0)} \geq \lambda_1 \\
&= a = \frac{\alpha - P_{\theta_0}\{Y \geq \lambda_1\}}{P_{\theta_0}\{Y = \lambda_2\}} \text{ if } \frac{p(x/\theta_1)}{p(x/\theta_0)} = \lambda_2 \\
&= 0 \text{ if } \frac{p(x/\theta_1)}{p(x/\theta_0)} < \lambda_2.
\end{aligned}$$

   Test $\phi^0(x)$ is obviously of size-α.
2. $\lambda = 0 \Rightarrow P_{\omega_0}(\theta_1) = 1 \Rightarrow \omega_0$ is a trivial MP test.
3. If the test (ω_0) given by N–P lemma is independent of $\theta_1 \in \Theta_k$ that does not include θ_0, the test is UMP size-α.
4. Test (ω_0) is unbiased size-α.

Proof $\omega_0 = \{X : p(x|\theta_1) > \lambda p(x|\theta_0)\}$ we want to show $P_{\omega_0}(\theta_1) \geq \alpha$. Take $\lambda = 0$. Then $\omega_0 = \{X : p(x/\theta_1) > 0\}$. In that case $P_{\omega_0}(\theta_1) = \int_{\omega_0} p(x|\theta_1)\mathrm{d}x =$

$\int_{\{x:p(x|\theta_1)>0\}} p(x|\theta_1)\mathrm{d}x = \int_{*} p(x|\theta_1)\mathrm{d}x = 1 > \alpha.$

$\therefore$ Test is trivially unbiased.

So throughout we assume that $\lambda > 0$.

Now

$$
\begin{aligned}
& p(x|\theta_1) > \lambda p(x|\theta_0) \text{ [As inside } \omega_0 : p(x|\theta_1) > \lambda p(x|\theta_0)] \\
& \Rightarrow \int_{\omega_0} p(x|\theta_1)\mathrm{d}x \geq \lambda \int_{\omega_0} p(x|\theta_0)\mathrm{d}x = \lambda\alpha \\
& \Leftrightarrow P_{\omega_0}(\theta_1) \geq \lambda\alpha
\end{aligned} \tag{3.11}
$$

Again

$$
\begin{aligned}
& p(x|\theta_1) \leq \lambda p(x|\theta_0) \text{ [As outside } \omega_0 : p(x|\theta_1) \leq \lambda p(x|\theta_0)] \\
& \Rightarrow \int_{\omega_0^c} p(x|\theta_1)\mathrm{d}x \leq \lambda \int_{\omega_0^c} p(x|\theta_0)\mathrm{d}x \\
& \Leftrightarrow 1 - P_{\omega_0}(\theta_1) \leq \lambda(1-\alpha)
\end{aligned} \tag{3.12}
$$

(3.11) $\div$ (3.12) $\Rightarrow \frac{P_{\omega_0}(\theta_1)}{1-P_{\omega_0}(\theta_1)} \geq \frac{\alpha}{1-\alpha} \Leftrightarrow P_{\omega_0}(\theta_1) \geq \alpha$.

$\Rightarrow$ Test is unbiased.

Conclusion MP test is unbiased. Let ω_0 be a MP size-α test. Then, with probability one, the test is equivalent to (assuming that $\frac{p(x|\theta_1)}{p(x|\theta_0)}$ has continuous distribution under θ_0 and θ_1) $\omega_0 = \{x : p(x|\theta_1) > \lambda p(x|\theta_0)\}$ where λ is such that $P_{\omega_0}(\theta_0) = \alpha \in (0, 1)$. □

Example 3.10 $X_1, X_2, \ldots X_n$ are i.i.d. $N(\mu, \sigma_0^2)$, $-\infty < \mu < \infty$, $\sigma_0 =$ known. (without any loss of generality take $\sigma_0 = 1$).

$X = (X_1, X_2, \ldots X_n)$ observed value of $X = x = (x_1, x_2, \ldots, x_n)$. To find UMP size-$\alpha$ test for $H : \mu = \mu_0$ against $K : \mu > \mu_0$. Take any $\mu_1 > \mu_0$ and find MP size-α test for

$H : \mu = \mu_0$ against $K : \mu = \mu_1$;

Solution

$$
p\left({}^{x}\!/\!_{\mu}\right) = \left(\frac{1}{\sqrt{2\pi}}\right)^n e^{-\frac{1}{2}\sum_{1}^{n}(x_i-\mu)^2}.
$$

Then

$$\frac{p\left(x/\mu_1\right)}{p\left(x/\mu_0\right)} = \frac{e^{\frac{1}{2}\sum_1^n (x_i-\mu_0)^2}}{e^{\frac{1}{2}\sum_1^n (x_i-\mu_1)^2}} = e^{\frac{1}{2}\sum_1^n (\mu_1-\mu_0)(2x_i-\mu_1-\mu_0)}$$

$$= e^{n\bar{x}(\mu_1-\mu_0)-\frac{n}{2}\left(\mu_1^2-\mu_0^2\right)} \qquad \left[\because \bar{x} = \frac{1}{n}\sum x_i\right]$$

Hence, by N–P lemma, the MP size-α test is given by

$$\omega_0 = \left\{x : p\left(x/\mu_1\right) > \lambda p\left(x/\mu_0\right)\right\} \tag{3.13}$$

where λ is such that

$$P_{\omega_0}(\mu_0) = \alpha \tag{3.14}$$

$$(3.13) \Leftrightarrow \left\{x : e^{n\bar{x}(\mu_1-\mu_0)-\frac{n}{2}\left(\mu_1^2-\mu_0^2\right)} > \lambda\right\} \tag{3.15}$$

$$\Leftrightarrow \left\{x : \bar{x} > \frac{\log_e \lambda}{n(\mu_1 - \mu_0)} + \frac{1}{2}(\mu_1 + \mu_0)\right\} \text{ as } \mu_1 > \mu_0$$

$$\Leftrightarrow \{x : \bar{x} > c\}, \text{ say} \tag{3.16}$$

By (3.16),

$$(3.14) \Leftrightarrow P\left(\bar{x} > c/\mu_0\right) = \alpha$$

$$\Leftrightarrow P\left\{\frac{\sqrt{n}(\bar{x} - \mu_0)}{1} > \frac{\sqrt{n}(c - \mu_0)}{1}\bigg|\mu_0\right\} = \alpha$$

($X_1, X_2, \ldots X_n$ are i.i.d $N(\mu_0, 1)$ under $H \Rightarrow \bar{X} \sim N\left(\mu_0, \frac{1}{n}\right)$ under H)

$$\Leftrightarrow P\{Z > \sqrt{n}(c - \mu_0)|Z \sim N(0,1)\} = \alpha$$

$$\Rightarrow \sqrt{n}(c - \mu_0) = \tau_\alpha \left[\int_{\tau_\alpha}^{\infty} N(Z|(0,1))dz = \alpha\right]$$

$$\Leftrightarrow c = \mu_0 + \frac{1}{\sqrt{n}}\tau_\alpha \tag{3.17}$$

Test given by (3.16) and (3.17) is MP size-α for $H : \mu = \mu_0$ against $K : \mu = \mu_1(> \mu_0)$.

The test is independent of any $\mu_1(>\mu_0)$. Hence it is UMP size-α for $H : \mu = \mu_0$ against $K : \mu > \mu_0$.

Observations

1. Power function of the test given by (3.16) and (3.17) is

$$\begin{aligned} P_{\omega_0}(\mu) = P(X \in \omega_0|\mu) &= \Pr.\left\{\bar{X} > \mu_0 + \frac{\tau_\alpha}{\sqrt{n}}\middle|\mu\right\} \\ &= P\{Z > \sqrt{n}(\mu_0 - \mu) + \tau_\alpha | Z \sim N(0,1)\} \\ &= \int_{\tau_\alpha - \sqrt{n}(\mu-\mu_0)}^{\infty} N(Z|(0,1))dz \end{aligned}$$

(Under any $\mu : (X_1, X_2, \ldots, X_n)$ are i.i.d. $N(\mu, 1) \Rightarrow \sqrt{n}(\bar{x} - \mu) \sim N(0,1)$)

$$= 1 - \Phi\left(\tau_\alpha - \sqrt{n}(\mu - \mu_0)\right).$$

Hence, for any fixed $\mu(> \mu_0)$

$$P_{\omega_0}(\mu) \to 1 \text{ as } n \to \infty \tag{3.18}$$

and for any fixed $\mu(<\mu_0)$

$$P_{\omega_0}(\mu) \to 0 \text{ as } n \to \infty \tag{3.19}$$

(3.18) $\Rightarrow$ test is consistent against any $\mu > \mu_0$.

Definition 10

1. For testing $H : \theta = \theta_0$ against $K : \theta = \theta_1$, a test ω (based on n observations) is said to be consistent if the power $P_\omega(\theta_1)$ of the test tends to '1' as $n \to \infty$.
2. $P_{\omega_0}(\mu) = 1 - \Phi(\tau_\alpha - \sqrt{n}(\mu - \mu_0))$ which increases as μ increases for fixed n.

$$\begin{aligned} \Rightarrow P_{\omega_0}(\mu) &> 1 - \Phi(\tau_\alpha) \text{ for all } \mu > \mu_0 \\ &= 1 - (1 - \alpha) = \alpha \end{aligned}$$

   $\Rightarrow \omega_0$ is unbiased.
3. $P_{\omega_0}(\mu) < P_{\omega_0}(\mu_0)$ for all $\mu < \mu_0$

   $= \alpha$

   $\Rightarrow$ Power $< \alpha$ for any $\mu < \mu_0$
   That is, test ω_0 is biased for testing $H : \mu = \mu_0$ against $K : \mu < \mu_0$.
4. From (3.15), if $\mu_1 < \mu_0$, we get ω_0 to be equivalent to

$$\{x : \bar{x} < c'\} \tag{3.20}$$

and $P_{\omega_0}(\mu_0)$ is equivalent to $P\{\bar{X} < c' | \mu_0\} = \alpha$

$$\Rightarrow c' = \mu_0 - \frac{\tau_\alpha}{\sqrt{n}} \tag{3.21}$$

(by the same argument as before while finding c)
Test given by (3.20) and (3.21) is independent of any $\mu_1 < \mu_0$. Hence it is UMP size-α for $H : \mu = \mu_0$ against $K : \mu < \mu_0$.

5. (i) UMP size-α for $H : \mu = \mu_0$ against $K : \mu > \mu_0$ is $\omega_0 = \left\{x : \bar{x} > \mu_0 + \frac{\tau_\alpha}{\sqrt{n}}\right\}$

   (ii) UMP size-α test for $H : \mu = \mu_0$ against $K : \mu < \mu_0$ is $\omega_0' = \left\{x : \bar{x} < \mu_0 - \frac{\tau_\alpha}{\sqrt{n}}\right\}$
   Clearly, $\omega_0 \neq \omega_0'$ (ω_o is biased for H against $\mu < \mu_0$ and ω_0' is biased for H against $\mu > \mu_0$).
   There does not exist any test which is UMP for $H : \mu = \mu_0$ against $K : \mu \neq \mu_0$.

Example 3.11 $X_1, X_2, \ldots X_n$ are i.i.d. $N(\mu_0, \sigma^2)$, $\sigma^2 > 0$ and μ_0 is known (without any loss of generality we take $\mu_0 = 0$)
$X = (X_1, X_2, \ldots, X_n)$, observed value = $x = (x_1, x_2, \ldots, x_n)$
Testing problem: $H : \sigma = \sigma_0$ against $K : \sigma > \sigma_0$.
To find UMP size-α test for H against $K : \sigma > \sigma_0$ we take any $\sigma_1 > \sigma_0$.

Solution

Here $p(x/\sigma) = \left(\frac{1}{\sigma\sqrt{2x}}\right)^n e^{\frac{-1}{2\sigma^2}\sum_i^n x_i^2}$
Hence

$$\frac{p(x/\sigma_1)}{p(x/\sigma_0)} = \left(\frac{\sigma_0}{\sigma_1}\right)^n e^{\frac{1}{2}\sum_i^n x_i^2\left(\frac{1}{\sigma_0^2} - \frac{1}{\sigma_1^2}\right)} \tag{3.22}$$

By N–P lemma MP size-α test is given by

$$w_0 = \left\{x : \frac{p(x/\sigma_1)}{p(x/\sigma_0)} > \lambda\right\} \tag{3.23}$$

where $\lambda(> 0)$
is such that

$$P_{w_0}(\sigma_0) = \alpha \tag{3.24}$$

$$\text{Now, } \frac{p\left({}^{x}\!/_{\sigma_1}\right)}{p\left({}^{x}\!/_{\sigma_0}\right)} > \lambda \Leftrightarrow \left(\frac{\sigma_0}{\sigma_1}\right)^n e^{\frac{1}{2}\sum_i^n x_i^2\left(\frac{1}{\sigma_0^2}-\frac{1}{\sigma_1^2}\right)} > \lambda \text{ [from (3.22)]}$$

$$\Leftrightarrow \sum_i^n x_i^2 > \frac{2\log_e \lambda}{\left(\frac{1}{\sigma_0^2}-\frac{1}{\sigma_1^2}\right)} - \frac{n\log_e\left(\frac{\sigma_0}{\sigma_1}\right)^2}{\frac{1}{\sigma_0^2}-\frac{1}{\sigma_1^2}} \quad [\text{As } \sigma_1 > \sigma_0] \tag{3.25}$$

$$= c\,(\text{say})$$

Hence (3.23) and (3.24) are equivalent to

$$w_0 = \left\{x : \sum_i^n x_i^2 > c\right\} \tag{3.26}$$

$$\text{and } P\left\{\sum_i^n x_i^2 > {}^{c}\!/_{\sigma_0}\right\} = \alpha \tag{3.27}$$

Under any $\sigma^2, X_1, X_2, \ldots, X_n$ are i.i.d. $N(0, \sigma^2)$

$$\Rightarrow \frac{\sum_i^n x_i^2}{\sigma^2} \sim \chi_n^2$$

Hence (3.27)

$$\Rightarrow \frac{c}{\sigma_0^2} \sim \chi_{n,\alpha}^2 \left[\int_{\chi_{n,\alpha}^2}^{\infty} \left(\frac{1}{\Gamma(n/2)2^{n/2}}\right) e^{\frac{-y}{2}} y^{\frac{n}{2}-1} \mathrm{d}y = \alpha\right]$$

$$\Leftrightarrow c = \sigma_0^2 \chi_{n,\alpha}^2 \tag{3.28}$$

Thus the test given by

$$w_0 = \left\{x : \sum_i^n x_i^2 > \sigma_0^2 \chi_{n,\alpha}^2\right\} \tag{3.29}$$

is MP size-α for $H : \sigma = \sigma_0$ against $K : \sigma = \sigma_1$. Test is independent of any $\sigma_1 > \sigma_0$. Hence it is UMP size-α for $H : \sigma = \sigma_0$ against $K : \sigma_1 > \sigma_0$

Observations

1. Under any σ_0^2,

$$\frac{1}{\sigma_0^2}\sum_i^n x_i^2 = Y_n \sim \chi_n^2$$
$$\Rightarrow E(Y_n) = n, V(Y_n) = 2n$$

Hence, from the asymptotic theory of χ^2, for large n under H
$\frac{Y_n - n}{\sqrt{2n}}$ is asymptotically $N(0,1)$.
So, for large n, $w_0 = \left\{x : \frac{Y_n - n}{\sqrt{2n}} > \frac{\chi_{n,\alpha}^2 - n}{\sqrt{2n}}\right\}$
and $\frac{\chi_{n,\alpha}^2 - n}{\sqrt{2n}} \simeq \tau_\alpha$ i.e. $\chi_{n,\alpha}^2 \simeq \tau_\alpha\sqrt{2n} + n$
Thus, (3.29) can be approximated by

$$\omega_0 = \left\{x : \sum_{i=1}^n x_i^2 > \sigma_0^2\left(\tau_\alpha\sqrt{2n} + n\right)\right\}$$

2. UMP size-α test for $H : \sigma^2 = \sigma_0^2$ against $K : \sigma^2 > \sigma_0^2$ is

$$w_0 = \left\{x : \sum_i^n x_i^2 > \sigma_0^2\chi_{n,\alpha}^2\right\}$$

UMP size-α test for $H : \sigma^2 = \sigma_0^2$ against $K : \sigma^2 < \sigma_0^2$ is

$$w_* = \left\{x : \sum_i^n x_i^2 < \sigma_0^2\chi_{n,1-\alpha}^2\right\} \quad \left[\int_{\chi_{n,(1-\alpha)}^2}^{\infty} f(\chi_n^2)d\chi_n^2 = 1 - \alpha\right]$$

Clearly, $w_0 \neq w_*$. Hence there does not exist UMP test for $H : \sigma^2 = \sigma_0^2$ against $K : \sigma^2 \neq \sigma_0^2$.

The power function of the test w_0 is

$$P_{w_0}(\sigma^2) = P\left\{\sum_i^n x_i^2 > \sigma_0^2\chi_{n,\alpha}^2 / \sigma^2\right\} = \int_{\frac{\sigma_0^2}{\sigma^2}\chi_{n,\alpha}^2}^{\infty} f(\chi_n^2)d\chi_n^2$$

Clearly, $P_{w_0}(\sigma^2)$ increases as σ^2 increases.

Also $P_{w_0}(\sigma^2) \leq P_{w_0}(\sigma_0^2) = \alpha \ \forall \sigma^2 : \sigma^2 \leq \sigma_0^2$

Test is biased $\Rightarrow w_0$ cannot be recommended for $H : \sigma^2 = \sigma_0^2$ against $K : \sigma^2 < \sigma_0^2$.

Similarly w_* is biased (Here $Pw_*(\sigma^2)$ increases as σ^2 decreases) and hence it cannot be recommended for $H : \sigma^2 = \sigma_0^2$ against $K : \sigma^2 > \sigma_0^2$.

Next observe that $\frac{1}{n}\sum_{i}^{n} x_i^2$ is a consistent estimator of σ^2. That means, for fixed σ^2, as $n \to \infty \frac{1}{n}\sum_{i}^{n} x_i^2 \to \sigma^2$ in probability and $\frac{\sigma_0^2 \chi_{n,\alpha}^2}{n} \to \sigma_0^2$. Thus if $\sigma^2 > \sigma_0^2$, we get $\underset{n\to\infty}{Lt}\ P\left\{\sum_{i}^{n} x_i^2 > \sigma_0^2 \chi_{n,\alpha}^2 \big/ \sigma^2\right\} = 1$ implying that the test w_0 is consistent against $K: \sigma^2 > \sigma_0^2$.

Similarly the test w_* is consistent against $K: \sigma^2 < \sigma_0^2$

Example 3.12 Find the MP size-α test for $H: X \sim \frac{1}{\sqrt{2\pi}} e^{-X^2/2}$ against $K: X \sim \frac{1}{2} e^{-|X|}$

Answer MP size-α test is given by (Using N–P lemma)

$$\omega_0 = \{x : p(x/K) > \lambda p(x/H)\} \tag{3.30}$$

where λ is such that

$$P_{\omega_0}(H) = \alpha \tag{3.31}$$

Now,

$$\begin{aligned}
&\frac{p(x/K)}{p(x/H)} = \sqrt{\frac{\pi}{2}} e^{\frac{x^2}{2} - |x|} > \lambda \\
&\Leftrightarrow \log_e \sqrt{\frac{\pi}{2}} + \frac{x^2}{2} - |x| > \log_e \lambda \\
&\Leftrightarrow x^2 - 2|x| + \left\{\log_e\left(\frac{\pi}{2}\right) - 2\log_e \lambda\right\} > 0 \\
&\Leftrightarrow x^2 - 2|x| + C > 0
\end{aligned} \tag{3.32}$$

Using (3.32), (3.31) is equivalent to

$$P\{x^2 - 2|x| + C > 0/H\} = \alpha \tag{3.33.}$$

Test given by (3.32) and (3.33.) is MP size-α.
To find 'C' we proceed as follows:

$$\begin{aligned}
P\{x^2 - 2|x| + C > 0/H\} &= P_H\{x^2 - 2|x| + C > 0 \cap x < 0\} + P_H\{x^2 - 2|x| + C > 0 \cap x > 0\} \\
&= P_H\{x^2 + 2x + C > 0 \cap x < 0\} + P_H\{x^2 - 2x + C > 0 \cap x > 0\}
\end{aligned}$$

Now, under H, $X \sim N(0, 1)$

$$\Rightarrow P_H\{x^2+2x+C>0 \cap x<0\} = P_H\{x^2-2x+C>0 \cap x>0\}$$

Thus (3.33) is equivalent to

$$P_H\{x^2-2x+C>0 \cap x>0\} = \frac{\alpha}{2} \tag{3.34}$$

Writing $g(x) = x^2 - 2x + C \Rightarrow g''(x) = 2$ and $g'(x) = 0$ at $x = 1$
$\therefore g(x)$ is minimum at $x = 1$

$$\Rightarrow [x^2-2x+C>0 \cap x>0] \Leftrightarrow x<x_1(c) \text{ or } x>x_2(c)$$

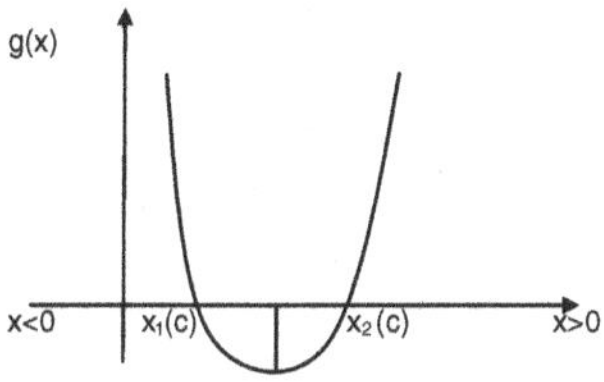

where $x_1(c)<x_2(c)$ are the roots of

$$x^2-2x+C=0$$
$$\Rightarrow x = \frac{2 \pm \sqrt{4-4c}}{2} = 1 \pm \sqrt{1-c}$$

So, $x_1(c) = 1-\sqrt{1-c}$ and $x_2(c) = 1+\sqrt{1-c}$
Hence (3.34)

$$\Leftrightarrow P_H\left\{0<x<1-\sqrt{1-c}\right\} + P_H\left\{x>1+\sqrt{1-c}\right\} = \frac{\alpha}{2}$$
$$\Leftrightarrow \Phi\left(1-\sqrt{1-c}\right) - \frac{1}{2} + 1 - \Phi\left(1+\sqrt{1-c}\right) = \frac{\alpha}{2}$$
$$\Leftrightarrow \Phi\left(1+\sqrt{1-c}\right) - \Phi\left(1-\sqrt{1-c}\right) = 1 - \frac{\alpha}{2} - \frac{1}{2} = \frac{1-\alpha}{2} \tag{3.35}$$

Test given by (3.32) and (3.35) is MP size-α.

Example 3.13 Let X be a single observation from the p.d.f. $p\left(x/\theta\right) = \frac{\theta}{\pi}\cdot\frac{1}{\theta^2+x^2}, \theta>0$. Find the UMP size-$\alpha$ test for $H:\theta=\theta_0$ against $K:\theta>\theta_0$

Answer Take any $\theta_1 > \theta_0$ and consider the ratio

$$\frac{p(x/\theta_1)}{p(x/\theta_0)} = \frac{\theta_1}{\theta_0} \cdot \frac{\theta_0^2 + x^2}{\theta_1^2 + x^2} = \frac{\theta_1}{\theta_0} \cdot \frac{\theta_0^2 + x^2}{(\theta_1^2 - \theta_0^2) + (\theta_0^2 + x^2)}$$

$$= \frac{\theta_1}{\theta_0} \cdot \frac{1}{1 + \left(\frac{\theta_1^2 - \theta_0^2}{\theta_0^2 + x^2}\right)},$$ which is a strictly increasing function of x^2 (i.e., $|x|$).

Since $\theta_1 > \theta_0$, hence we can find a 'C' such that

$$\frac{p(x/\theta_1)}{p(x/\theta_0)} > \lambda \Leftrightarrow |x| > C \tag{3.36}$$

where C is such that

$$P[|x| > C/\theta_0] = \alpha \tag{3.37}$$

$$\Leftrightarrow \int_C^\infty \frac{\theta_0}{\pi} \cdot \frac{dx}{\theta_0^2 + x^2} = \frac{\alpha}{2} \Leftrightarrow \frac{1}{\pi}\left[\tan^{-1}\left(\frac{x}{\theta_0}\right)\right]_C^\infty = \frac{\alpha}{2}$$

$$\Leftrightarrow \frac{1}{\pi}\left[\frac{\pi}{2} - \tan^{-1}\left(\frac{C}{\theta_0}\right)\right] = \frac{\alpha}{2} \Leftrightarrow 1 - \frac{2}{\pi}\tan^{-1}\left(\frac{C}{\theta_0}\right) = \alpha \tag{3.38}$$

Test given by (3.36) and (3.38) is MP size-α. As the test is independent of any $\theta_1 > \theta_0$, it is UMP size-α for $H : \theta = \theta_0$ against $K : \theta > \theta_0$. Power function is given by

$$P_{\omega_0}(\theta) = P\{|X| > C/\theta\} = 1 - \int_{-C}^{C} \frac{\theta}{\pi(\theta^2 + x^2)} dx$$

Example 3.14 X is a single observation from Cauchy p.d.f $f(x/\theta) = \frac{1}{\pi\{(x-\theta)^2 + 1\}}$, we are to find MP size-α test for $H : \theta = \theta_0$ against $K : \theta = \theta_1 (> \theta_0)$.

Answer $X \sim \text{Couchy}(\theta) \Rightarrow Y = X - \theta_0 \sim \text{Couchy}(\theta - \theta_0 = \delta)$. Hence $H : \theta = \theta_0 \Leftrightarrow H : \delta = 0$ using Y-observation. So, without any loss of generality we take $H : \theta = 0$ and for the sake of simplicity we take $\theta_1 = 1$.

Here, by N–P lemma, MP test has the critical region $\omega = \{x : p(x/\theta_1) > \lambda p(x/\theta_0)\}$ with $P_{\theta_0}(X \in \omega) = \alpha \in (0, 1)$

Here

$$\frac{p(x/\theta_1)}{p(x/\theta_0)} > \lambda \Leftrightarrow \frac{1+x^2}{1+(x-1)^2} > \lambda$$
$$\Leftrightarrow 1+x^2 > \lambda(1+x^2-2x+1)$$
$$\Leftrightarrow x^2(1-\lambda)+2\lambda x+1-2\lambda > 0 \quad (3.39)$$

Several cases

(a) $\lambda = 1 \Leftrightarrow x > 0$, hence the size of the test is $P(X > 0/\theta = 0) = \frac{1}{2}$.

(b) $0<\lambda<1$ if we write $g(x) = (1-\lambda)x^2 + 2\lambda x + (1-2\lambda)$,
we have, $g'(x) = 2(1-\lambda)x + 2\lambda = 0 \Rightarrow x = -\frac{\lambda}{1-\lambda}$
$g''(x) = 2(1-\lambda) > 0$, this means that the curve $y = g(x)$ has a minimum at $x = -\frac{\lambda}{1-\lambda}$.

Shape of the curve is:

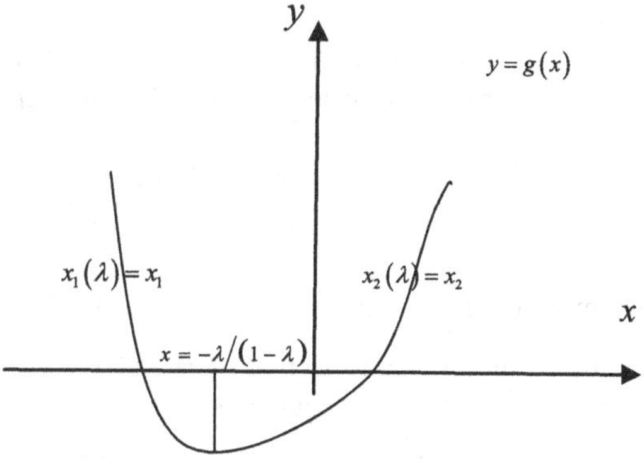

Here $x_1 < x_2$ are the roots of $g(x) = 0$. Clearly, test is given by $x < x_1$ or $x > x_2$ such that

$$P\{X < x_1/\theta = 0\} + P\{X > x_2/\theta = 0\} = \alpha \quad (3.40)$$

We take those values of x_1, x_2 that satisfies (3.40). Eventually, it is not possible to get x_1, x_2 for any given α. It exists for some specific values of α.

(c) If $\lambda > 1$, in that case $g''(x) = 2(1-\lambda) < 0$, thus $y = g(x)$ has the maximum at $x = -\left(\frac{\lambda}{1-\lambda}\right) > 0$. As shown in (b) above here also we can find x_1 and x_2 the two roots of $g(x) = 0$ and the test will be given by $x > x_1$ or $x < x_2$ with $P\{x_1 < X < x_2/\theta = \theta\} = \alpha$. Taking $\theta_1 = 2$, it can be shown that the MP test for $H : \theta = 0$ against $\theta = 2$ is completely different. Hence based on single observation there does not exist UMP test for $H : \theta = 0$ against $K : \theta > 0$

Randomized Test Testing problem $H : \theta = \theta_0$ against $K : \theta = \theta_1$. If the random variable $Y = \frac{p(X/\theta_1)}{p(X/\theta_0)}$ is continuous under $\theta = \theta_0$, we can always find $\lambda(>0)$ such that for a given $\alpha \in (0,1)$, $P_{\theta_0}(Y > \lambda) = \alpha$.
On the other hand, if the random variable Y is discrete under $\theta = \theta_0$, it may not be always possible to find λ such that, for a given $\alpha \in (0,1)$ $P_{\theta_0}(Y > \lambda) = \alpha$. In that case, we modify the non-randomized test $\omega_0 = \{x : p(x/\theta_1) > \lambda p(x/\theta_0)\}$ by using following functions:

$$\left.\begin{aligned} &= 1, \text{ if } p(x/\theta_1) > \lambda p(x/\theta_0) \\ \phi^0(x) &= a, \text{ if } p(x/\theta_1) = \lambda p(x/\theta_0) \\ &= 0, \text{ if } p(x/\theta_1) < \lambda p(x/\theta_0) \end{aligned}\right\} \Leftrightarrow \left\{\begin{aligned} Y > \lambda \\ Y = \lambda \\ Y < \lambda \end{aligned}\right\} \tag{3.41}$$

where 'a' and 'λ' are such that

$$P_{\theta_0}\{Y > \lambda\} + aP_{\theta_0}\{Y = \lambda\} = \alpha \tag{3.42}$$

The function given by (3.41) and (3.42) is called the randomized test corresponding to non-randomized test ω_0. It states that, after observing Y(i.e, X)

$$\begin{aligned} &\text{Reject } H \text{ if } Y > \lambda \\ &\text{Accept } H \text{ if } Y < \lambda \end{aligned}$$

Perform random experiment with probability of success = a, if $Y = \lambda$.

Occurrence of success ⇒ Rejection of H and
Occurrence of failure ⇒ Acceptance of H.

Now we can show that the test given by (3.41) and (3.42) is MP size-α among all tests ϕ satisfying $E_{\theta_0}\phi(x) \le \alpha$. Observe that $\phi^0(x) = 0 \Rightarrow [\phi^0(x) - \phi(x)] \ge 0 \forall x : p(x/\theta_1) > \lambda p(x/\theta_0)$ and $\phi^0(x) = 0 \Rightarrow [\phi^0(x) - \phi(x)] \le 0 \forall x : p(x/\theta_1) < \lambda p(x/\theta_0)$. Hence, for all x, we have,

$$\begin{aligned} &[\phi^0(x) - \phi(x)][p(x/\theta_1) - \lambda p(x/\theta_0)] \ge 0 \\ &\Rightarrow \int [\phi^0(x) - \phi(x)][p(x/\theta_1) - \lambda p(x/\theta_0)]dx \ge 0 \\ &\Leftrightarrow E_{\theta_1}\phi^0(x) - E_{\theta_1}\phi(x) - \lambda\alpha + \lambda E_{\theta_0}\phi(x) \ge 0 \\ &\Leftrightarrow E_{\theta_1}\phi^0(x) - E_{\theta_1}\phi(x) \ge \lambda(\alpha - E_{\theta_0}\phi(x)) \ge 0, \text{ As } \lambda > 0 \text{ and } E_{\theta_0}\phi(x) \le \alpha \\ &\Leftrightarrow P_{\phi^0}(\theta_1) \ge P_{\phi}(\theta_1) \end{aligned}$$

$\Rightarrow \phi^0$ is MP size-α among all $\phi : E_{\theta_0}\phi(x) \leq \alpha$.

Example 3.15 $X_1, X_2, \ldots\ldots, X_n$ are i.i.d according to $f(x/\theta) = \theta^x(1-\theta)^{1-x}, x = 0, 1$ To find UMP size-α test for $H : \theta = \theta_0$, against $K : \theta > \theta_0$.

Answer Take any $\theta_1 > \theta_0$. To get MP size-α test for $H : \theta = \theta_0$, against $K : \theta = \theta_1$, we consider the ratio

$$\begin{aligned} Y &= \frac{p(x/\theta_1)}{p(x/\theta_0)} = \frac{\prod_{i=1}^n f(x_i/\theta_1)}{\prod_{i=1}^n f(x_i/\theta_0)} = \frac{\theta_1^{\sum x_i}(1-\theta_1)^{n-\sum x_i}}{\theta_0^{\sum x_i}(1-\theta_0)^{n-\sum x_i}} \\ &= \left(\frac{1-\theta_1}{1-\theta_0}\right)^n \left\{\frac{\theta_1(1-\theta_0)}{\theta_0(1-\theta_1)}\right\}^s \end{aligned}$$

where $s = \sum x_i$. Observe that Y is a discrete r.v. under any θ.

Hence by the N–P lemma, MP size-α test is given by

$$\phi_0(x) = \left.\begin{array}{r} 1, \text{ if } Y > \lambda \\ a, \text{ if } Y = \lambda \\ 0, \text{ if } Y < \lambda \end{array}\right\}$$

$$\Leftrightarrow \left(\frac{1-\theta_1}{1-\theta_0}\right)^n \left\{\frac{\theta_1(1-\theta_0)}{\theta_0(1-\theta_1)}\right\}^s \leq \text{or} \geq \lambda, \tag{3.43}$$

where 'λ' and 'a' are such that $E_{\theta_0}\phi_0(x) = \alpha$

$$\Leftrightarrow P_{\theta_0}\{Y > \lambda\} + aP_{\theta_0}\{Y = \lambda\} = \alpha, \tag{3.44}$$

Now,

$$\left(\frac{1-\theta_1}{1-\theta_0}\right)^n \left\{\frac{\theta_1(1-\theta_0)}{\theta_0(1-\theta_1)}\right\}^s \leq \text{or} \geq \lambda$$

$$\Leftrightarrow n\log\frac{1-\theta_1}{1-\theta_0} + s\log\left\{\frac{\theta_1(1-\theta_0)}{\theta_0(1-\theta_1)}\right\} \leq \text{or} \geq \lambda' \quad \left[\lambda' = \log_e \lambda\right]$$

$$\begin{aligned} &\Leftrightarrow s \leq \text{or} \geq \frac{\lambda'}{\log\left\{\frac{\theta_1(1-\theta_0)}{\theta_0(1-\theta_1)}\right\}} - n\frac{\log\frac{1-\theta_1}{1-\theta_0}}{\log\left\{\frac{\theta_1(1-\theta_0)}{\theta_0(1-\theta_1)}\right\}} \\ &= C, \text{ (say)}, \quad \left[\text{As}, \theta_1 > \theta_0 \Rightarrow \log\left\{\frac{\theta_1(1-\theta_0)}{\theta_0(1-\theta_1)}\right\} > 0\right] \end{aligned}$$

Hence (3.43) and (3.44) are equivalent to

$$\phi_0(x) = \begin{Bmatrix} 1, \text{ if } s > C \\ a, \text{ if } s = C \\ 0, \text{ if } s < C \end{Bmatrix} \tag{3.45}$$

and

$$P_{\theta_0}\{s > C\} + aP_{\theta_0}\{s = C\} = \alpha \tag{3.46}$$

Under any θ, $s = \sum_1^n X_i \sim \text{bin}(n, \theta)$. Hence from (3.46) we have, either, $P_{\theta_0}\{s > C\} = \alpha \Leftrightarrow \sum\limits_{c+1}^{n} \binom{n}{s}\theta_0^s(1-\theta_0)^{n-s} = \alpha \Rightarrow a = 0$

or,

$$P_{\theta_0}\{s \geq C\} < \alpha < P_{\theta_0}\{s \geq C\}$$
$$\Rightarrow a = \frac{\alpha - \sum_{c+1}^{n} \binom{n}{s}\theta_0^s(1-\theta_0)^{n-s}}{\binom{n}{c}\theta_0^c(1-\theta_0)^{n-c}} \tag{3.47}$$

Test given by (3.45) and (3.47) is MP size-α for $H: \theta = \theta_0$ against $K: \theta = \theta_1 (> \theta_0)$. Test is independent of any $\theta_1 (> \theta_0)$. Hence it is UMP size-α for $H: \theta = \theta_0$ against $K: \theta > \theta_0$

Observation

1. For $\theta_1 < \theta_0 \Rightarrow \log\left\{\frac{\theta_1(1-\theta_0)}{\theta_0(1-\theta_1)}\right\} < 0$
   In that case (3.43) and (3.44) are equivalent to
   $$\phi_*(x) = \begin{Bmatrix} 1, \text{ if } s < C_* \\ a, \text{ if } s = C_* \\ 0, \text{ if } s > C_* \end{Bmatrix} \text{ and } P_{\theta_0}\{s < C_*\} + aP_{\theta_0}\{s = C_*\} = \alpha.$$
   We can get UMP for $H: \theta = \theta_0$ against $K: \theta < \theta_0$ by similar arguments. Obviously $\phi_0 \neq \phi_*$. So there does not exist a single test which is UMP for $H: \theta = \theta_0$ against $K: \theta \neq \theta_0$
2. By De Moivre–Laplace limit theorem, for large n, $\frac{S - n\theta}{\sqrt{n\theta(1-\theta)}}$ is approximately $N(0, 1)$.
   Hence, from (3.45) and (3.46), we get,
   $$\frac{C - n\theta_0}{\sqrt{n\theta_0(1-\theta_0)}} \simeq \tau_\alpha \Rightarrow C \simeq n\theta_0 + \tau_\alpha\sqrt{n\theta_0(1-\theta_0)}$$
   Then approximately size-α test is : Reject H if $s > n\theta_0 + \tau_\alpha\sqrt{n\theta_0(1-\theta_0)}$, Accept H otherwise.

3. Power function of test given by (3.45) and (3.46) is:

$$\begin{aligned}
P(\theta) &= E_\theta \phi_0(X) \\
&= P_\theta\{S > c\} + aP_\theta\{S = c\} \\
&= \sum_{S=c+1}^{n} \tbinom{n}{s}\theta^s(1-\theta)^{n-s} + a\tbinom{n}{c}\theta^c(1-\theta)^{n-c}
\end{aligned}$$

[Can be obtained using Biometrika table]

$$\begin{aligned}
&= (1-a)\sum_{S=c+1}^{n} \tbinom{n}{s}\theta^s(1-\theta)^{n-s} + a\sum_{S=c}^{n} \tbinom{n}{s}\theta^s(1-\theta)^{n-s} \\
&= (1-a)I_\theta(c+1, n-c) + aI_\theta(c, n-c+1),
\end{aligned}$$

[Can be obtained using incomplete Beta function table].

Observe, as $I_\theta(m,n)$ is an increasing function of θ, the Power function $P(\theta)$ increases with θ.

Example 3.16 Let X be a single observation. To find MP size-α test for $H: X \sim R(0,1)$ against $K: X \sim R\left(\frac{1}{2}, \frac{3}{2}\right)$

Answer $p(x/H) =^{1,\ \text{if}\ 0<x<1}_{0,\ \text{otherwise}}$

$$p(x/K) =^{1,\ \text{if}\ 1/2 < x < 3/2}_{0,\ \text{otherwise}}$$

As the ratio ${}^{p(x/K)}/_{p(x/H)}$ is discrete, MP test for H against K is given by:

$$\left.\begin{aligned}
&= 1 \text{ if}, \ p(x/K) > \lambda p(x/H) \\
\phi_0(x) &= a, \text{ if}\, p(x/K) = \lambda p(x/H) \\
&= 0, \text{ if}, \ p(x/K) < \lambda p(x/H)
\end{aligned}\right\} \tag{3.48}$$

where 'a' and 'λ' are such that

$$E_H\phi_0(x) = \alpha \tag{3.49}$$

Taking

$$\begin{aligned}
\lambda < 1; 0 < x \le \frac{1}{2} &\Rightarrow p(x/K) = 0 \text{ and}\, p(x/H) = 1 \\
&\Rightarrow p(x/k) < \lambda p(x/H) \Rightarrow \phi_0(x) = 0 \\
\frac{1}{2} < x < 1 &\Rightarrow p(x/K) = p(x/H) = {}^1\!/_2 \\
&\Rightarrow p(x/K) > \lambda p(x/H) \Rightarrow \phi_0(x) = 1 \\
1 \le x < \frac{3}{2} &\Rightarrow p(x/K) = 1 \text{ and}\, p(x/H) = 0 \\
&\Rightarrow p(x/K) > \lambda p(x/H) \Rightarrow \phi_0(x) = 1
\end{aligned}$$

So, for $\lambda < 1$, we get $E_H\phi_0(X) = 1.P_H(\frac{1}{2} < X < 1) + 1.P_H(X \geq 1) = \frac{1}{2}$. Thus it is a trivial test of size 0.5.

Taking $\lambda < 1$,

$$\left.\begin{array}{l} 0 < x \leq \frac{1}{2} \Rightarrow \phi_0(x) = 0 \\ \frac{1}{2} < x < 1 \Rightarrow \phi_0(x) = 0 \\ 1 \leq x \leq \frac{3}{2} \Rightarrow \phi_0(x) = 1 \end{array}\right\} E_H\phi_0(X) = 0 \text{ and it is a trivial test of size } 0.$$

Taking $\lambda = 1$,

$o < x \leq \frac{1}{2} \Rightarrow \phi_0(x) = 0$: we always accept H.
$1 \leq x < \frac{3}{2} \Rightarrow \phi_0(x) = 1$: We always reject H.

$\frac{1}{2} < x < 1 \Rightarrow p(x/K) = \lambda p(x/H) \Rightarrow$ We perform a random experiment with probability of success 'a' determined by $E_H\phi_0(x) = \alpha$.

$$\Leftrightarrow a.P_H\left(\frac{1}{2} < X < 1\right) = \alpha \Leftrightarrow a = 2\alpha$$

Thus the randomized test given by $\phi_0(x)$

$$\left.\begin{array}{l} = 0, \text{ if } 0 < x \leq \frac{1}{2} \\ = 2\alpha, \text{ if } \frac{1}{2} < x < 1 \\ = 1, \text{ if } 1 \leq x < \frac{3}{2} \end{array}\right\} \text{is MP size-}\alpha \text{ test.}$$

3.4 Locally MPU Test

The optimum region is obtained by the use of the following:

Generalization of N–P lemma.

Theorem 2 *Let* $g_0, g_1, g_2, \ldots g_m$ *be* $(m+1)$ *non-negative integrable functions on the sample space* $\mathcal{X}$. *Let* ω *be any region such that* $\int_\omega g_i(x)\mathrm{d}x = C_i, i = 1(1)m$ *where* C_i*'s are all known numbers.*

Suppose ω_0 *be a subset of* $\mathcal{X}$ *such that:*

Inside $\omega_0 : g_0(x) > \sum_1^m \lambda_i g_i(x)$,

Outside $\omega_0 : g_0(x) \leq \sum_1^m \lambda_i g_i(x)$, *where* $\lambda_1, \lambda_2, \ldots\ldots\lambda_m$ *are so chosen that* $\int\limits_{\omega_0} g_i(x)\mathrm{d}x = C_i, i = 1(1)m.$

Then we have $\int\limits_{\omega_0} g_0(x)\mathrm{d}x \geq \int\limits_{\omega} g_0(x)\mathrm{d}x.$

This is called generalized Neyman–Pearson Lemma.

Proof

$$\int\limits_{\omega_0} g_0(x)\mathrm{d}x - \int\limits_{\omega} g_0(x)\mathrm{d}x$$

$$= \int\limits_{\omega_0-\omega} g_0(x)\mathrm{d}x - \int\limits_{\omega-\omega_0} g_0(x)\mathrm{d}x.\ldots\ldots..(1) \begin{bmatrix} \omega_0 - \omega = \omega_0 - \omega \cap \omega_0 = \text{inside}\omega_0 \\ \omega - \omega_0 = \omega - \omega \cap \omega_0 = \text{outside}\omega_0 \end{bmatrix}$$

$$x \in \omega_0 - \omega \Rightarrow g_0(x) > \sum_1^m \lambda_i g_i(x)$$

$$\Rightarrow \int\limits_{\omega_0-\omega} g_0(x)\mathrm{d}x \geq \int\limits_{\omega_0-\omega} \left\{\sum_1^m \lambda_i g(x_i)\right\}\mathrm{d}x$$

$$= \sum_{i=1}^m \lambda_i \left\{\int\limits_{\omega_0-\omega} g_i(x)\mathrm{d}x\right\}$$

$$x \in \omega_0 - \omega \quad \Rightarrow g_0(x) \leq \sum_1^m \lambda_i g_i(x)$$

$$\Rightarrow \int\limits_{\omega-\omega_0} g_0(x)\mathrm{d}x \leq \int\limits_{\omega-\omega_0} \left\{\sum_1^m \lambda_i g_i(x)\right\}\mathrm{d}x = \sum_1^m \lambda_i \left\{\int\limits_{\omega-\omega_0} g_i(x)\mathrm{d}x\right\}$$

Hence L.H.S of (1)

$$\int\limits_{\omega_0-\omega} g_0(x)\mathrm{d}x - \int\limits_{\omega-\omega_0} g_0(x)\mathrm{d}x \geq \sum_i^m \lambda_i \left\{\int\limits_{\omega_0-\omega} g_i(x)\mathrm{d}x\right\} - \sum_i^m \lambda_i \left\{\int\limits_{\omega-\omega_0} g_i(x)\mathrm{d}x\right\}$$

$$= \sum_i^m \lambda_i \left[\int\limits_{\omega_0-\omega} g_i(x)\mathrm{d}x - \int\limits_{\omega-\omega_0} g_i(x)\mathrm{d}x\right]$$

$$= \sum_i^m \lambda_i \left[\int\limits_{\omega_0} g_i(x)\mathrm{d}x - \int\limits_{\omega} g_i(x)\mathrm{d}x\right] = \sum_i^m \lambda_i (C_i - C_i) = 0$$

$\Rightarrow$ Hence the proof. □

Locally Best Tests

1. One-sided case: For the family $\{p(x/\theta), \theta \in \Theta\}$, sometimes we cannot find UMP size-α test for $H: \theta = \theta_0$ against $K: \theta > \theta_0$ or $\theta < \theta_0$.
   For example, if $X_1, X_2, \ldots, X_n (n \geq 1)$ are i.i.d according to the p.d.f.

$$f(x/\theta) = \frac{1}{\pi} \frac{1}{1+(x-\theta)^2}, (-\infty < \theta < \infty, -\infty < x < \infty)$$

   we cannot find UMP size-α test for $H: \theta = \theta_0$ against $\theta > \theta_0$ or $\theta < \theta_0$.

In that case, we can find an $\varepsilon > 0$ for which there exists a critical region ω_0 such that $P_{\omega_0}(\theta_0) = \alpha$ and $P_{\omega_0}(\theta) \geq P_\omega(\theta) \forall \theta : \theta_0 < \theta < \theta_0 + \varepsilon$ and $\forall \omega : P_\omega(\theta_0) = \alpha$.

Construction Let $p(x/\theta)$ be such that, for every ω, $\frac{d}{d\theta} p_\omega(\theta)$ exists and is continuous in the neighborhood of θ_0. Then we have, by mean value theorem, for any $\theta > \theta_0$

$$P_\omega(\theta) = P_\omega(\theta_0) + (\theta - \theta_0) \frac{d}{d\theta} P_\omega(\theta) \Big]_{\theta = \theta^*}, \theta_0 < \theta^* < \theta$$

$$= P_\omega(\theta_0) + (\theta - \theta_0) P'_\omega(\theta^*), \text{(say)} \tag{3.50}$$

Similarly,

$$P_{\omega_0}(\theta) = P_{\omega_0}(\theta_0) + (\theta - \theta_0) P'_{\omega_0}(\theta^*), \text{(say)} \tag{3.51}$$

Let ω_0 be such that $P_{\omega_0}(\theta_0) = \alpha$ and $P'_{\omega_0}(\theta_0)$ is maximum, i.e. $P'_{\omega_0}(\theta_0) \geq P'_\omega(\theta_0) \forall \omega : P_{\omega_0}(\theta_0) = \alpha$. Then comparing (3.50) and (3.51), we get an $\varepsilon > 0$, such that $P_{\omega_c}(\theta) \geq P_\omega(\theta) \forall \theta : \theta_0 < \theta < \theta_0 + \varepsilon$. Such a ω_0 is called locally most powerful size-α test for $H: \theta = \theta_0$ against $\theta > \theta_0$.

Now our problem is to choose ω_0 such that

$$P_{\omega_0}(\theta_0) = \alpha \Leftrightarrow \int_{\omega_0} p(x/\theta_0) dx = \alpha \tag{3.52}$$

and

$$P'_{\omega_0}(\theta_0) \geq P'_\omega(\theta_0) \Leftrightarrow \int_{\omega_0} \frac{\delta p(x/\theta)}{d\theta_0} dx \geq \int_\omega \frac{\delta p(x/\theta)}{d\theta_0} dx$$
$$\Leftrightarrow \int_{\omega_0} p'(x/\theta_0) dx \geq \int_\omega p'(x/\theta_0) dx$$

where ω satisfies $P_\omega(\theta_0) = \alpha \Leftrightarrow \int_\omega p(x/\theta_0) dx = \alpha$

In the generalized N–P lemma, take $m = 1$ and set $g_0(x) = p'(x/\theta_0)$, $g_1(x) = p(x/\theta_0)$, $C_1 = \alpha$, $\lambda_1 = \lambda$.

Then we get,

$$\left.\begin{aligned}\text{Inside } \omega_0 : p'(x/\theta_0) > \lambda p(x/\theta_0) \\ \text{Outside } \omega_0 : p'(x/\theta_0) \leq \lambda p(x/\theta_0)\end{aligned}\right\} \tag{3.53}$$

Finally, $\int\limits_{\omega_0} p'(x/\theta_0)\mathrm{d}x \geq \int\limits_{\omega} p'(x/\theta_0)\mathrm{d}x$

where ω_0 and ω satisfy

$$P_{\omega_0}(\theta_0) = P_{\omega}(\theta_0) = \alpha \tag{3.54}$$

Thus the test given by (3.53) and (3.54) is locally most powerful size-α for $H : \theta = \theta_0$ against $\theta > \theta_0$.

Note If UMP test exists for $H : \theta = \theta_0$ against $\theta > \theta_0 \Rightarrow$ LMP test corresponding to the said problem must be identical to the UMP test. But the converse may not be true.

Example 3.17 $X_1, X_2, \ldots X_n$ are i.id $N(\theta, 1)$. $H : \theta = \theta_0$ against $\theta > \theta_0$.

LMP test is provided by

$$\omega_0 = \{x : p'(x/\theta_0) > \lambda p(x/\theta_0)\} \tag{3.55}$$

where λ is such that

$$\int\limits_{\omega_0} p(x/\theta_0)\mathrm{d}x = \alpha \tag{3.56}$$

It can be observed that

$$\begin{aligned} p'(x/\theta_0) &> \lambda p(x/\theta_0) \\ &\Leftrightarrow \frac{1}{p(x/\theta_0)} p'(x/\theta_0) > \lambda \\ &\Leftrightarrow \frac{\mathrm{d}}{\mathrm{d}\theta_0}[\log_e p(x/\theta_0)] > \lambda \end{aligned} \tag{3.57}$$

Here $p(x/\theta) = (2\pi)^{-n/2} e^{-\frac{1}{2}\sum(x_i-\theta)^2}$

$$\therefore \log p(x/\theta) = \text{const.} - \frac{1}{2}\sum_1^n (x_i - \theta)^2$$

$\therefore \frac{d\log(x/\theta_0)}{\mathrm{d}\theta_0} = \sum\limits_1^n (x_i - \theta_0)$, hence by (3.57), (3.55)

$$\Leftrightarrow \omega_0 = \{x : \bar{x} > \lambda'\}$$

and (3.56) $\Leftrightarrow P_{\theta_0}\{\bar{x} > \lambda'\} = \alpha$

$$\Leftrightarrow P_{\theta_0}\{\sqrt{n}(\bar{x} - \theta_0) > \sqrt{n}(\lambda' - \theta_0)\} = \alpha \Rightarrow \sqrt{n}(\lambda' - \theta_0) = \tau_\alpha$$

i.e, $\lambda' = \theta_0 + \frac{1}{\sqrt{n}}\tau_\alpha$. Thus $\omega_0 \Leftrightarrow \omega_0 = \left\{x : \bar{x} > \theta_0 + \frac{1}{\sqrt{n}}\tau_\alpha\right\}$
which is identical to the UMP test for $H : \theta = \theta_0$ against $\theta > \theta_0$.

General case: Let $X_1, X_2, \ldots X_n$ be i.i.d with p.d.f $f(x/\theta)$.
To find LMP for $H : \theta = \theta_0$ against $\theta > \theta_0$
Here $p(x/\theta) = \prod_{i=1}^{n} f(x_i/\theta)$;
LMP test is given by the critical region:
$\omega = \{x : p'(x/\theta_0) > \lambda p(x/\theta_0)\}$, where λ such that $P_\omega(\theta_0) = \alpha$
Now,

$$p'(x/\theta_0) > \lambda p(x/\theta_0) \Leftrightarrow \frac{p'(x/\theta_0)}{p(x/\theta_0)} > \lambda$$
$$\Leftrightarrow \frac{\delta \log p(x/\theta_0)}{\mathrm{d}\theta_0} > \lambda \quad [p(x/\theta) > 0]$$

$\Leftrightarrow \sum_1^n \frac{f'(x_i/\theta_0)}{f(x_i/\theta_0)} > \lambda$, (say) $\Leftrightarrow \sum_1^n y_i > \lambda$, where $y_i = \frac{f'(x_i/\theta_0)}{f(x_i/\theta_0)}$.
Now, under H, $y_i{'}s$ is i.i.d with

$$E_{\theta_0}\{y_i\} = \int \frac{f'(x_i/\theta_0)}{f(x_i/\theta_0)} f(x_i/\theta_0)\mathrm{d}x = \int f'(x/\theta_0)\mathrm{d}x$$
$$= \frac{\mathrm{d}}{\mathrm{d}\theta_0}\int f(x/\theta_0)\mathrm{d}x = \frac{d}{\mathrm{d}\theta_0}(1) = 0$$
$$V_{\theta_0}\{y_i\} = \int \left\{\frac{f'(x_i/\theta_0)}{f(x/\theta_0)}\right\}^2 f(x/\theta_0)\mathrm{d}x$$
$$= \int \left\{\frac{\partial \log f(x/\theta_0)}{\mathrm{d}\theta_0}\right\}^2 f(x/\theta_0)\mathrm{d}x$$
$$= I(\theta_0) \qquad [\text{Fisher's information}].$$

Hence, by Central Limit Theorem, for large n, $\frac{\sum_1^n y_i}{\sqrt{nI(\theta_0)}} \sim N(0,1)$, under H. So, for large n, the above test can be approximated by

$$\omega = \left\{ x : \sum_{i=1}^{n} \frac{f'(x_i/\theta_0)}{f(x_i/\theta_0)} > \tau_\alpha \sqrt{nI(\theta_0)} \right\}.$$

Locally Best test: Two-sided case

For testing $H : \theta = \theta_0$ against $\theta \neq \theta_0$ corresponding to the family $\{p(x/\theta), \theta \in \Theta\}$, it is being known that (expect some cases) there does not exist any test which is UMP for both sided alternatives. e.g. taking $\mu = 0$ against $\mu \neq 0$ for $N(\mu, 1)$ and taking $\sigma^2 = 1$ against $\sigma^2 \neq 1$ for $N(0, \sigma^2)$ etc.

In those cases, we can think of a test which is UMP in a neighbourhood of θ_0. Thus a test 'w_0' is said to be locally best (of size α) for $H : \theta = \theta_0$ against $K : \theta \neq \theta_0$ if there exists an $t > 0$ for which

(i) $P_{w_0}(\theta_0) = \alpha$
(ii) $P_w(\theta) \geq \alpha \; \forall \theta : |\theta - \theta_0| < t$ and $\forall w$ satisfying (i).

Let $p(^x/_\theta)$ be such that, for a chosen w

(i) $P'_w(\theta)$ exists in the neighbourhood of θ_0;
(ii) $P''_w(\theta)$ exists and is continuous at (in the neighbourhood) θ_0.

Then we have, by Taylor's Theorem

$$P_w(\theta) = P_{w_0}(\theta_0) + (\theta - \theta_0)P'_w(\theta_0) + \frac{(\theta - \theta_0)^2}{2!} P''_w(\theta^k);$$
$$|\theta^* - \theta_0| < |\theta - \theta_0|$$

Let w_0 be such that

(i) $P_{w_0}(\theta_0) = \alpha$ (size condition)
(ii) $P'_{w_0}(\theta_0) = 0$ (Locally unbiased condition)
(iii) $P''_{w_0}(\theta_0)$ is maximum

Then we can find an $t > 0$ such that $\forall \theta : |\theta - \theta_0| < t$, We have $P_{w_0}(\theta) \geq P_w(\theta) \forall w$ satisfying (i) and (ii).

Now $P_w(\theta) = P_w(\theta_0) + (\theta - \theta_0)P'_w(\theta_0) + \frac{(\theta-\theta_0)^2}{2!} P''_w(\theta_0^k) + \eta$ and $\eta \to 0$ as $\theta \to \theta_0$.

To get $P_{w_0}(\theta) \geq P_w(\theta) \forall \theta : |\theta - \theta_0| < t$ we must have $P''_{w_0}(\theta_0) \geq P''_w(\theta_0)$ [due to continuity of $P_w(\theta)$].

Then w_0 is called locally Most Powerful unbiased size-α test if

(i) $P_{w_0}(\theta_0) = \alpha$
(ii) $P'_{w_0}(\theta_0) = 0.$
(iii) $P''_{w_0}(\theta_0) \geq P''_w(\theta_0) \forall w$ satisfying (i) and (ii).

Construction

$$P_w(\theta_0) = \int_w p\left({}^x/_{\theta_0}\right)\mathrm{d}x, P'_w(\theta_0) = \int_w p'\left({}^x/_{\theta_0}\right)\mathrm{d}x,$$

$$P''_w(\theta_0) = \int_w p''\left({}^x/_{\theta_0}\right)\mathrm{d}x.$$

Let us set in generalized N–P lemma

$$g_0(x) = p''\left({}^x/_{\theta_0}\right), g_1(x) = p\left({}^x/_{\theta_0}\right), g_2(x) = p'\left({}^x/_{\theta_0}\right),$$

$$c_1 = \alpha,\ c_2 = 0$$

Then

$$w_0 = \left\{x : p''\left({}^x/_{\theta_0}\right) > \lambda_1 p\left({}^x/_{\theta_0}\right) + \lambda_2 p'\left({}^x/_{\theta_0}\right)\right\}$$

where λ_1 and λ_2 are such that $\int_{w_0} g_1(x)\mathrm{d}x = \alpha,\ \int_{w_0} g_2(x)\mathrm{d}x = 0.$

Then we have $\int_{w_0} g_0(x)\mathrm{d}x \geq \int_{w} g_0(x)\mathrm{d}x$ provided 'w' satisfies (i) and (ii).

$$\Leftrightarrow P''_{w_0}(\theta_0) \geq P''_w(\theta_0)$$

Example 3.18 $X_1, X_2, \ldots X_n$ are i.i.d. $N(\mu, 1)$. To find LMPU test for $H : \mu = \mu_0$ against K:$\mu \neq \mu_0$.

Answer Here $p\left({}^x/_\theta\right) = \left(\frac{1}{\sqrt{2\pi}}\right)^n e^{\frac{-1}{2}\sum_1^n (x_i-\mu)^2}$

$$p'\left({}^x/_\theta\right) = \left(\frac{1}{\sqrt{2\pi}}\right)^n n(\bar{x}-\mu)e^{\frac{-1}{2}\sum_1^n (x_i-\mu)^2} = n(\bar{x}-\mu)p\left({}^x/_\theta\right)$$

$$p''\left({}^x/_\theta\right) = [n(\bar{x}-\mu)]^2 p\left({}^x/_\theta\right) - np\left({}^x/_\theta\right)$$

LMPU size-α test is

$$w_0 = \left\{x : p''\left({}^x/_{\theta_0}\right) > \lambda_1 p\left({}^x/_{\theta_0}\right) + \lambda_2 p'\left({}^x/_{\theta_0}\right)\right\} \int_{\omega_0} p(x/\theta_0)\mathrm{d}x = \alpha \qquad (3.58)$$

and

$$\int_{\omega_0} p'(x/\theta_0)\mathrm{d}x = 0 \tag{3.59}$$

$$= \left\{x : [n(\bar{x} - \mu_0)]^2 - n > \lambda_1 + \lambda_2 n(\bar{x} - \mu_0)\right\}$$
$$= \left\{x : \{\sqrt{n}(\bar{x} - \mu_0)\}^2 > \lambda_1' + \lambda_2'\{\sqrt{n}(\bar{x} - \mu_0)\}\right\}$$
$$= \{x : y^2 > \lambda_1' + \lambda_2' y\};$$

$y = \sqrt{n}(\bar{x} - \mu_0) \sim N(0, 1)$ under H
(3.59) $\Longleftrightarrow$

$$\int_{y^2 > \lambda_1' + \lambda_2' y} yN({}^{y}/_{0}, 1)\mathrm{d}y = 0 \tag{3.60}$$

Now the LHS of (3.60) is zero irrespective of choice of any (λ_1', λ_2') since $N({}^{y}/_{0}, 1)$ is symmetrical about '0'.

Here, we can safely take $\lambda_2' = 0$ without affecting size condition. Then our test reduces to $w_0 : \{x : y^2 > \lambda_1'\} \equiv \{x : |y| > c\}$ and hence (3.58) is equivalent to $\int_{|y| > c} N({}^{y}/_{0}, 1)\mathrm{d}y = \alpha \Rightarrow c = \tau_{\alpha/2}$

Then we obtain LMPU test for $H : \mu = \mu_0$ against $\mu \neq \mu_0$.

A test which is locally most powerful and locally unbiased is called a Type A test and corresponding critical region 'w_0' is said to be Type-A critical region

3.5 Type A_1 (≡Uniformly Most Powerful Unbiased) Test

Let $p({}^{x}/_{\theta}), \theta \in \Theta$: Real parameter family of distributions.

Testing problem: $H : \theta = \theta_0$ against $K : \theta \neq \theta_0$.
$T(X) = T$: Test statistic.

(i) Right tail test based on T is UMP for $H : \theta = \theta_0$ against $\theta > \theta_0$ (in most of the cases)
(ii) Left tail test based on T is UMP for $H : \theta = \theta_0$ against $\theta < \theta_0$ (in most of the cases)

[As for example $N(\mu, 1)$, $N(0, \sigma^2)$ .... $T = \sum x_i$, $T = \sum x_i^2$ etc. and for $B(n, p), T = \bar{x}$ etc.]

There does not exist a single test which is UMP for $H : \theta = \theta_0$ against $\theta \neq \theta_0$.

If $p({}^{x}/_{\theta})$ has monotone likelihood ratio in $T(X)$; i.e.

$\frac{p\left(x/\theta_1\right)}{p\left(x/\theta_0\right)} \uparrow T(x)$ for $\theta_1 > \theta_0$; then (i) and (ii) are satisfied.

In that case, we try to choose a test w_0 for which

(i) $P_{w_0}(\theta_0) = \alpha$
(ii) $P_{w_0}(\theta) \geq \alpha \forall \theta \neq \theta_0$
(iii) $P_{w_0}(\theta) \geq P_w(\theta) \forall \theta \neq \theta_0 \forall w$ satisfying (i) and (ii)

Such a test is called UMPU size-α test for $H : \theta = \theta_0$ against $\theta \neq \theta_0$.
Let $p\left(x/\theta\right)$ be such that, for every test w,
$\frac{d}{d\theta}[P_w(\theta)]$ exists;
and

$$\frac{d}{d\theta}[P_w(\theta)] = \frac{d}{d\theta}\int\limits_w p(x/\theta)dx = \int\limits_w \frac{dp(x/\theta)}{d\theta}dx = \int\limits_w p'(x/\theta)dx \tag{3.61}$$

Then unbiasedness of a test

$$w \Rightarrow \frac{d}{d\theta_0}P_w(\theta) = 0 \tag{3.62}$$

Thus, if a test w_0 satisfies (i), (ii) and (iii); under (3.61), w_0 also satisfies (i) and (iii). Test satisfying (i), (iii) and (3.62) is called type-A_1 test.

For exponential distribution, if type-A_1 test exists, then it must be unbiased. But this is not true in general.

Construction Our problem is to get w_0 such that

(i) $\int\limits_{w_0} p\left(x/\theta_0\right)dx = \alpha,$

(ii) $\int\limits_{w_0} p'\left(x/\theta_0\right)dx = 0$

(iii) $\int\limits_{w_0} p\left(x/\theta\right)dx \geq \int\limits_{w} p\left(x/\theta\right)dx\ \forall w$ satisfying (i) and (ii) and $\forall \theta \neq \theta_0$

In generalized N–P Lemma, put $g_0 = p\left(x/\theta\right)$, $g_1 = p\left(x/\theta_0\right)$, $g_2 = p'\left(x/\theta_0\right)$, $c_1 = \infty$, $c_2 = 0$.

Then, define $w_0 = \left\{x : p\left(x/\theta\right) > \lambda_1 p\left(x/\theta_0\right) + \lambda_2 p'\left(x/\theta_0\right)\right\}$ and hence $\int\limits_{w_0} p\left(x/\theta\right)dx \geq \int\limits_{w} p\left(x/\theta\right)dx \forall w$ satisfying (i) and (ii) and $\forall \theta \neq \theta_0$.

For exponential distribution, it is always possible to have such region w_0 (which means type-A_1 test exists).

Example 3.19 $X_1, X_2, \ldots, X_n$ are i.i.d. $N(\mu, 1)$. We test $H : \mu = \mu_0$ against $K : \mu \neq \mu_0$

$$p(x/\theta) = (2\pi)^{-n/2} e^{\frac{-1}{2}\sum^{n}(x_i-\mu)^2}$$

$$p'(x/\theta) = (2\pi)^{-n/2} \sum_{i=1}^{n} (x_i - \mu) e^{\frac{-1}{2}\sum_{i}^{n}(x_i-\mu)^2} = \sum_{i}^{n} (x_i - \mu) p(x/\theta)$$

Then type-A_1 region (test) is given by

$$w_0 = \{x : p(x/\theta) > \lambda_1 p(x/\theta_0) + \lambda_2 n(\bar{x} - \mu_0) p(x/\theta_0)\}$$

$$\frac{p(x/\theta)}{p(x/\theta_0)} = \frac{e^{\frac{-1}{2}\sum(x_i-\mu)^2}}{e^{\frac{-1}{2}\sum(x_i-\mu_0)^2}} = \frac{e^{\frac{-n}{2}(\bar{x}-\mu)^2}}{e^{\frac{-n}{2}(\bar{x}-\mu_0)^2}} = e^{\frac{n}{2}(\mu-\mu_0)\{2\bar{x}-(\mu_0+\mu)\}}$$

$$\therefore w_0 = \{x : e^{(\mu-\mu_0)t} > \lambda_1' + \lambda_2' t\} \text{ where } t = \sqrt{n}(\bar{x} - \mu_0)$$
$$= \{x : e^{\delta_t} > \lambda_1' + \lambda_2' t\}$$

where $\lambda_{\prime 1}'$ and λ_1' are such that

$$\int_{w_0} p(x/\theta_0)\mathrm{d}x = \alpha, \quad \int_{w_0} n(\bar{x} - \mu)p(x/\theta_0)\mathrm{d}x = 0$$

$$\Leftrightarrow \int_{w_o} N(t/0, 1)\mathrm{d}t = \alpha \tag{3.63}$$

$$\Leftrightarrow \int_{w_0} tN(t/0, 1)\mathrm{d}t = 0 \tag{3.64}$$

Writing $g(t) = e^{\delta t} - \lambda_1' - \lambda_2' t$ we have $g'(t) = \delta e^{\delta t} - \lambda_2'$ and $g''(t) = \delta^2 e^{\delta t} > 0 \forall t$ $\Rightarrow y = g(t)$ has a single minimum (global minimum).

Now if we take $\alpha < 0.5$, because of (3.63) and since the distribution of t is symmetric about 0 under H_0 our shape of the curve will be like as shown below. From the graph, we observe that $c_1 < c_2$, $g(t) > 0$ for $t < c_1$ and $t > c_2$ and $g(t) \leq 0$ otherwise.

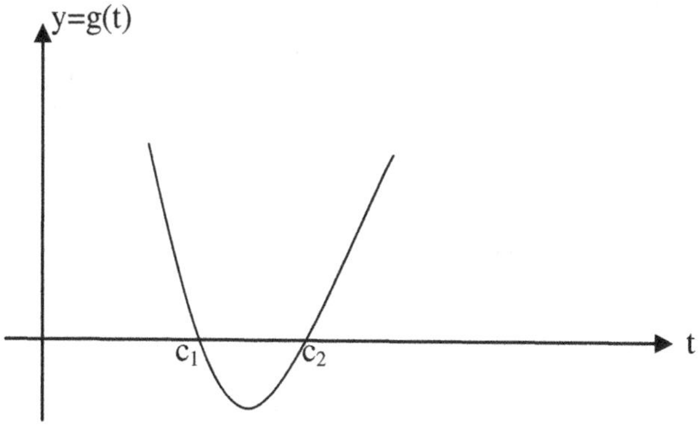

Hence w_0 is equivalent to $w_o = \{x : t < c_1 \,\text{or}\, t > c_2\}$
(3.63) $\Leftrightarrow \int\limits_{t<c_1, t>c_2} N(t/0,1)\mathrm{d}t = \alpha$ and (3.64)

$$\Leftrightarrow \int\limits_{t<c_1, t>c_2} tN(t/0,1)\mathrm{d}t = 0 \tag{3.65}$$

Now, as $T \sim N(0,1)$, we take w_0 as

$$w_0 = \{x : t < -c \,\text{and}\, t > c\} \tag{3.66}$$

where c is such that

$$\int\limits_{|t|>c} N(t/0,1)\mathrm{d}t = \alpha \Rightarrow c = \tau_{\alpha/2} \tag{3.67}$$

Here (3.65) is automatically satisfied. Hence test given by (3.66) and (3.67) is type-A_1 (which is UMPU).

Example 3.20

$$X_1, X_2, \ldots\ldots, X_n \text{ are i.i.d. } N(0, \sigma^2).$$

Testing Problem, $H : \sigma^2 = \sigma_0^2$ against $K : \sigma^2 \neq \sigma_0^2$

$$p(x/\theta) = \left(\frac{1}{\sigma\sqrt{2\Pi}}\right)^n e^{\frac{-1}{2\sigma^2}\sum_i^n x_i^2}$$

$$p'(x/\theta) = \left(\frac{\sum\limits_i^n x_i^2}{\sigma^2} - n\right)\frac{1}{2\sigma^2}p(x/\theta)$$

Thus,

$$w_0 = \left\{x : p(x/\theta) > \lambda_1 p(x/\theta_0) + \lambda_2\left(\frac{\sum_i^n x_i^2}{\sigma_0^2} - n\right)\frac{1}{2\sigma_0^2}p\left(x/\theta_0\right)\right\}$$

$$= \left\{x : \frac{p(x/\theta)}{p(x/\theta_o)} > \lambda_1' + \lambda_2' t\right\},\ t = \frac{\sum_i^n x_i^2}{\sigma_0^2}$$

$$\text{As } \frac{p(x/\theta)}{p(x/\theta_0)} = \left(\frac{\sigma_0}{\sigma}\right)^n e^{\frac{\sum\limits_i^n x_i^2}{2\sigma_0^2}\left(1-\frac{\sigma_0^2}{\sigma^2}\right)}$$

$$w_0 = \left\{x : \left(\frac{\sigma_0}{\sigma}\right)^n e^{\frac{\delta}{2}t} > \lambda_1' + \lambda_2' t\right\}$$

Now as before the curve $y = g(t) = \left(\frac{\sigma_0}{\sigma}\right)^n e^{\frac{\delta t}{2}} - \lambda_1' - \lambda_2' t$ has a single minimum.
Here $P\left\{T > {}^0/_\theta\right\} = 1$

$\therefore$ Shape of the curve $g(t)$ will be as shown below

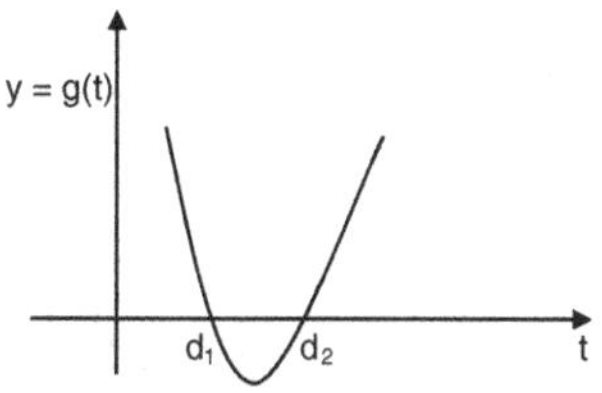

which means there exists d_1 and d_2
such that w_0 is equivalent to $w_0 = \{x : t < d_1 \text{ or } t > d_2\}$
Here d_1 and d_2 are such that

$$\int_{w_0} p\left({}^x/_{\theta_0}\right)\mathrm{d}x = \alpha \Leftrightarrow \int_{d_1}^{d_2} f_{\chi_n^2}(t)\mathrm{d}t = 1 - \alpha \tag{3.68}$$

and

$$\int_{w_0} p'\left({}^x/_{\theta_0}\right)\mathrm{d}x = 0 \Leftrightarrow \int_{t<d_1 \text{ or } t>d_2} (t-n) f_{\chi_n^2}(t)\mathrm{d}t = 0 \tag{3.69}$$

$$(3.69) \Leftrightarrow \int_{t<d_1 \text{ or } t>d_2} t f_{\chi_n^2}(t)\mathrm{d}t = n \int_{t<d_1 \text{ or } d_2} f_{\chi_n^2}(t)\mathrm{d}t = n\alpha, \text{ by } (3.68)$$

$$\Leftrightarrow \int_{d_1}^{d_2} t f_{\chi_n^2}(t)\mathrm{d}t = (1-\alpha)n$$

$$\Leftrightarrow \int_{d_1}^{d_2} f_{\chi_{n+2}^2}(t)\mathrm{d}t = (1-\alpha) \tag{3.70}$$

Thus UMPU (a type-A_1) size α test is
$\omega_0 = \{x : t < d_1 \text{ or } t > d_2\}$ such that

$$P\{d_1 < \chi_n^2 < d_2\} = 1 - \alpha \text{ and } P\{d_1 < \chi_{x+2}^2 < d_2\} = 1 - \alpha.$$

Note in this example $\Rightarrow$ type A_1 test $\Leftrightarrow$ type-A test.

Example 3.21 $X_1, X_2, \ldots, X_n$ are i.i.d with $p(x/\theta) = \theta e^{-\theta x}$. Find Type-A and Type-$A_1$ test for $H: \theta = \theta_0$ against $\theta \neq \theta_0$.

Answer proceed as Examples 3.19 and 3.20 and hence get

$$\omega_0 = \left\{ x : \sum_1^n X_i < c_1 \text{ or } \sum_1^n X_i > c_2 \right\}$$

where c_1 and c_2 are such that

$$P\left\{ \frac{c_1}{2\theta_0} - 1 < \chi^2_{2n} < \frac{c_2}{2\theta_0} - 1 \right\} = 1 - \alpha \text{ and}$$

$$\cdot\ P\left\{ \frac{c_1}{2\theta_0} - 1 < \chi^2_{2n+2} < \frac{c_2}{2\theta_0} - 1 \right\} = 1 - \alpha.$$

Chapter 4
Likelihood Ratio Test

4.1 Introduction

In the previous chapter we have seen that UMP or UMP-unbiased tests exist only for some special families of distributions, while they do not exist for other families. Further, computations of UMP-unbiased tests in K-parameter family of distribution are usually complex. Neyman and Pearson (1928) suggested a simple method for testing a general testing problem.

Consider $X \sim p(x|\theta)$, where θ is a real parameter or a vector of parameters, $\theta \in \Theta$.

A general testing problem is

$$H : \theta \in \Theta_0 \text{ Against } K : \theta \in \Theta_1.$$

Here, H and K may be treated as the subsets of Θ. These are such that $H \cap K = \phi$ and $H \cup K \subseteq \Theta$. Given that $X = x, p(\mathrm{x}|\theta)$ is a function of θ and is called likelihood function. Likelihood test for H against K is provided by the statistic

$$L(x) = \frac{\operatorname{Sup}_{\theta \in H} p(x|\theta)}{\operatorname{Sup}_{\theta \in H \cup K} p(x|\theta)},$$

which is called the likelihood ratio criterion for testing H against K. It is known that

(i) $p(x|\theta) \geq 0 \forall \theta$
(ii) $\operatorname{Sup}_{\theta \in H} p(x|\theta) \leq \operatorname{Sup}_{\theta \in H \cup K} p(x|\theta)$.

Obviously $0 \leq L(x) \leq 1$. The numerator in $L(x)$ measures the best explanation that the observation X comes from some population under H and the denominator

P.K. Sahu et al., *Estimation and Inferential Statistics*,
DOI 10.1007/978-81-322-2514-0_4

measures the best explanation of X to come from some population covered under $H \cup K$. Higher values of the numerator correspond to the better explanation of X given by H compared to the overall best possible explanation of X, which results in larger values in $L(x)$ leading to acceptance of H. That is, $L(x)$ would be larger under H than under K. Indeed, smaller values of $L(x)$ will lead to the rejection of H. Hence, our test procedure is:

Reject H iff $L(x) < C$

and accept H otherwise,

where C is such that $P\{L(x) < C|H\} = \alpha \in (0, 1)$.

If the distribution of $L(x)$ is continuous, then the size α is exactly attained and no randomization on the boundary is needed. If the distribution is discrete, the size may not attain α and one may require randomization. In this case, we have C from the relation

$$P\{L(x) < C|H\} \leq \alpha.$$

Here, we reject H if $L(x) < C$,

accept H if $L(x) > C$,

and reject with probability 'a' iff $L(x) = C$.

Thus, we have $P\{L(x) < C|H\} + aP\{L(x) = C|H\} = \alpha$.

The likelihood ratio tests are useful, especially when θ is a vector of parameters and the testing involves only some of them. This test criterion is very popular because of its computational simplicity. Moreover, this criterion proves to be a powerful alternative for testing vector valued parameters that involve nuisance parameters. Generally, the likelihood ratio tests result in optimal tests, whenever they exist. An LR test is generally UMP, if an UMP test at all exists. In many cases the LR tests are unbiased, although this is not universally true. However, it is difficult to compute the exact null distribution of the test statistic $L(x)$ in many cases. Therefore, a study of large sample properties of $L(x)$ becomes necessary where maximum likelihood estimators follow normal distribution under certain regularity conditions. We mention the following large sample property of the likelihood ratio test statistic without proof.

Under H, the asymptotic distribution of $-2\log_e L(x)$ is distributed as χ^2 with degrees of freedom equal to the difference between the number of independent parameters in Θ and the number in Θ_0.

Drawback: Likelihood ratio test is constructed completely by intuitive argument. So, it may not satisfy all the properties that are satisfied by a test obtained from N–P theory; it also may not be unbiased.

4.1.1 Some Selected Examples

Example 4.1 Let X be a binomial $b(n, \theta)$ random variable. Find the size-α likelihood ratio test for testing $H : \theta \leq \theta_0$ against $K : \theta > \theta_0$

Solution Here, $\Theta_0 = \{\theta : 0 \leq \theta \leq \theta_0\}$ and $\Theta = \{\theta : 0 \leq \theta \leq 1\}$.

The likelihood ratio test statistic is given as

$$L(x) = \frac{\operatorname{Sup}_{\theta \in H} p(x|\theta)}{\operatorname{Sup}_{H \cup K} p(x|\theta)} = \frac{\operatorname{Sup}_{\theta \leq \theta_0} p(x|\theta)}{\operatorname{Sup}_{\Theta} p(x|\theta)}$$

$$= \frac{\operatorname{Sup}_{\theta \leq \theta_0} \binom{n}{x} \theta^x (1-\theta)^{n-x}}{\operatorname{Sup}_{\Theta} \binom{n}{x} \theta^x (1-\theta)^{n-x}}$$

The MLE of θ for $\theta \in \Theta$ is $\widehat{\theta} = \frac{x}{n}$.

For, $\theta \in \Theta_0$, we have

$$\widehat{\theta}_H = \frac{x}{n} \text{ if } \frac{x}{n} \leq \theta_0$$
$$= \theta_0 \text{ if } \frac{x}{n} > \theta_0$$

Thus, we have

$$\operatorname{Sup}_{\Theta} \binom{n}{x} \theta^x (1-\theta)^{n-x} = \binom{n}{x} \left(\frac{x}{n}\right)^x \left(1 - \frac{x}{n}\right)^{n-x}$$

$$\operatorname{Sup}_{\theta \leq \theta_0} \binom{n}{x} \theta^x (1-\theta)^{n-x} = \begin{cases} \binom{n}{x} \left(\frac{x}{n}\right)^x \left(1 - \frac{x}{n}\right)^{n-x} & \text{if } \frac{x}{n} \leq \theta_0 \\ \binom{n}{x} \theta_0^x (1-\theta_0)^{n-x} & \text{if } \frac{x}{n} > \theta_0 \end{cases}$$

So, $L(x) = \begin{cases} 1 & \text{if } \frac{x}{n} \leq \theta_0 \\ \frac{\theta_0^x (1-\theta_0)^{n-x}}{\left(\frac{x}{n}\right)^x \left(1-\frac{x}{n}\right)^{n-x}} & \text{if } \frac{x}{n} > \theta_0 \end{cases}$

It can be observed that $L(x) \leq 1$ when $x > n\theta_0$ and $L(x) = 1$ when $x \leq n\theta_0$. This shows that $L(x)$ is the decreasing function of x. Thus, $L(x) < C$ iff $x > C'$ and the likelihood ratio test rejects H_0 if $x > C'$ where C' is obtained as

$P_{\theta_0}(X > C') = \alpha$. Since X is a discrete random variable, C' is obtained such that

$$P_{\theta_0}(X > C') \leq \alpha < P_{\theta_0}(X > C' - 1).$$

Example 4.2 Let $X_1, \ldots, X_n$ be a random sample from a normal distribution with mean μ and variance σ^2. Find out the likelihood ratio test of

(a) $H : \mu = \mu_0$ aganist $K : \mu \neq \mu_0$ when σ^2 is known.
(b) $H : \mu = \mu_0$ aganist $K : \mu \neq \mu_0$ when σ^2 is unknown.

Solution

(a) Here, $\Theta_0 = \{\mu_0\},\ \Theta = \{\mu : -\infty < \mu < \infty\}$

$$p(x|\theta) = p(x|\mu) = (2\pi)^{-n/2} (\sigma^2)^{-n/2} e^{-\frac{1}{2\sigma^2}\sum_{i=1}^{n}(X_i-\mu)^2}$$

The likelihood ratio test statistic is given as

$$L(x) = \frac{\operatorname*{Sup}_{H} p(x|\mu)}{\operatorname*{Sup}_{H\cup K} p(x|\mu)} = \frac{\operatorname*{Sup}_{\Theta_0} p(x|\mu)}{\operatorname*{Sup}_{\Theta} p(x|\mu)}$$

The maximum likelihood estimate of μ for $\mu \in \Theta$ is $\bar{x}$.

So, $\operatorname*{Sup}_{\Theta_0} p(x|\mu) = (2\pi)^{-n/2}(\sigma^2)^{-n/2} e^{-\frac{1}{2\sigma^2}\sum_{i=1}^{n}(X_i-\mu_0)^2}$

and $\operatorname*{Sup}_{\Theta} p(x|\mu) = (2\pi)^{-n/2}(\sigma^2)^{-n/2} e^{-\frac{1}{2\sigma^2}\sum_{i=1}^{n}(X_i-\bar{x})^2}$.

This gives

$$L(x) = \frac{e^{-\frac{1}{2\sigma^2}\sum_{i=1}^{n}(X_i-\mu_0)^2}}{e^{-\frac{1}{2\sigma^2}\sum_{i=1}^{n}(X_i-\bar{x})^2}} = e^{-\frac{n}{2\sigma^2}(\bar{x}-\mu_0)^2}$$

The rejection region $L(x) < C$ gives

$$-\frac{n}{2\sigma^2}(\bar{x}-\mu_0)^2 < C_1$$

$$\text{or,} \qquad \left|\frac{\sqrt{n}(\bar{x}-\mu_0)}{\sigma}\right| > C_2$$

Thus, the likelihood ratio test is given as

$$\phi(\bar{x}) = \begin{cases} 1 & \text{if } \left|\frac{\sqrt{n}(\bar{x}-\mu_0)}{\sigma}\right| > C_2 \\ 0 & \text{Otherwise} \end{cases}$$

where the constant C_2 is obtained by the size condition

$$E_{\mu_0}[\phi(\bar{x})] = \alpha$$

$$\text{or,} \qquad P_{\mu_0}\left[\left|\frac{\sqrt{n}(\bar{x}-\mu_0)}{\sigma}\right| > C_2\right] = \alpha$$

Now, under $H: \mu = \mu_0$, the statistic $\frac{\sqrt{n}(\bar{x}-\mu_0)}{\sigma}$ follows $N(0, 1)$ distribution. Since the distribution is symmetrical about 0, C_2 must be the upper $\alpha/2$—point of the distribution. Finally, the test is given as

$$\phi(\bar{x}) = \begin{cases} 1 & \text{if } \left|\frac{\sqrt{n}(\bar{x}-\mu_0)}{\sigma}\right| > \tau_{\alpha/2} \\ 0 & \text{Otherwise} \end{cases}$$

(b) Here, $\Theta_0 = \{(\mu, \sigma^2) : \mu = \mu_0, \sigma^2 > 0\}$

$$\Theta = \{(\mu, \sigma^2) : -\infty < \mu < \infty, \sigma^2 > 0\}$$

In this case,

$$\operatorname*{Sup}_{\Theta_0} p(x|\mu, \sigma^2) = \operatorname*{Sup}_{\Theta_0} \left(\frac{1}{2\pi\sigma^2}\right)^{n/2} e^{-\frac{1}{2\sigma^2}\sum_{i=1}^{n}(X_i-\mu)^2}$$

MLE of σ^2 given $\mu = \mu_0$ is given as

$$s_0^2 = \frac{1}{n}\sum_{i=1}^{n}(X_i - \mu_0)^2.$$

This gives $\operatorname*{Sup}_{\Theta_0} p(x|\mu_0, \sigma^2) = \left(\frac{1}{2\pi s_0^2}\right)^{n/2} e^{-\frac{n}{2}}$.

Further, $\operatorname*{Sup}_{\Theta} p(x|\mu, \sigma^2) = \operatorname*{Sup}_{\mu,\sigma^2} p(x|\mu, \sigma^2) = \operatorname*{Sup}_{\mu,\sigma^2} p\left(\frac{1}{2\pi\sigma^2}\right)^{n/2} e^{-\frac{1}{2\sigma^2}\sum_{i=1}^{n}(X_i-\mu)^2}$

The MLE of μ and σ^2 are given as $\bar{x}$ and $\frac{1}{n}\sum_{i=1}^{n}(X_i - \bar{X})^2 = \frac{(n-1)}{n}s^2$, where $s^2 = \frac{1}{n-1}\sum_{i=1}^{n}(X_i - \bar{X})^2$. We have,

$$\operatorname*{Sup}_{\mu,\sigma^2} p(x|\mu, \sigma^2) = \left(\frac{1}{2\pi\frac{(n-1)}{n}s^2}\right)^{n/2} e^{-\frac{n}{2}}$$

Hence, likelihood ratio test statistic is given as

$$L(x) = \frac{\left(\frac{1}{2\pi s_0^2}\right)^{-\frac{n}{2}} e^{-\frac{n}{2}}}{\left(\frac{1}{2\pi\frac{(n-1)}{n}s^2}\right)^{\frac{n}{2}} e^{-\frac{n}{2}}} = \left(\frac{(n-1)s^2}{ns_0^2}\right)^{n/2}$$

$$= \left(\frac{(n-1)s^2}{\sum_{i=1}^{n}(X_i - \mu_0)^2}\right)^{n/2} = \left[\frac{(n-1)s^2}{n(\bar{x}-\mu_0)^2 + \sum_{i=1}^{n}(X_i - \bar{X})^2}\right]^{n/2}$$

$$= \left[\frac{(n-1)s^2}{n(\bar{x}-\mu_0)^2 + (n-1)s^2}\right]^{n/2}$$

The LR critical region is given as

$$L(x) < C$$

$$\text{or,} \quad \frac{n(\bar{x} - \mu_0)^2}{s^2} > C_1$$

$$\text{or,} \quad \left| \frac{\sqrt{n}(\bar{x} - \mu_0)}{s} \right| > C_2.$$

The likelihood ratio test is given as

$$\phi(\bar{x}, s) = \begin{cases} 1 & \text{if} \left| \frac{\sqrt{n}(\bar{x} - \mu_0)}{s} \right| > C_2, \\ 0 & \text{otherwise} \end{cases}$$

where the constant C_2 is obtained by the size condition

$$P_{\mu_0}\left[\left| \frac{\sqrt{n}(\bar{x} - \mu_0)}{s} \right| > C_2\right] = \alpha.$$

Now under $H : \mu = \mu_0$, the statistic $\frac{\sqrt{n}(\bar{x} - \mu_0)}{s}$ is distributed as, t with $(n - 1)$ d.f which is symmetric about 0. Hence, $C_2 = t_{\frac{\alpha}{2}, n-1}$. Finally, the test is given as

$$\phi(\bar{x}, s) = \begin{cases} 1 & \text{if} \left| \frac{\sqrt{n}(\bar{x} - \mu_0)}{s} \right| > t_{\frac{\alpha}{2}, n-1} \\ 0 & \text{otherwise} \end{cases}$$

Example 4.3 $X_1, X_2 \ldots X_n$ are i.i.d $N(\mu, \sigma^2)$. Derive LR test for $H : \mu \leq \mu_0$ against $K : \mu > \mu_0$.

Answer $\theta = (\mu, \sigma^2)$, $\Theta = \{\theta : -\infty < \mu < \infty, \sigma^2 > 0\}$

Here, $p(x/\theta) = p(x/\mu, \sigma^2) = (2\pi)^{-\frac{n}{2}} (\sigma^2)^{-\frac{n}{2}} e^{-\frac{1}{2\sigma^2} \sum_{1}^{n} (X_i - \mu)^2}$

Likelihood ratio criterion

$$L(x) = \frac{\underset{H}{\operatorname{Sup}}(x/\mu, \sigma^2)}{\underset{H \cup K}{\operatorname{Sup}}(x/\mu, \sigma^2)} = \frac{\underset{\mu \leq \mu_0}{\operatorname{Sup}}(x/\mu, \sigma^2)}{\underset{\Theta}{\operatorname{Sup}}(x/\mu, \sigma^2)} \qquad [H \cup K = \Theta = (\mu \leq \mu_0) \cup (\mu > \mu_0)]$$

$$= \frac{p(x/\hat{\mu}_H, \hat{\sigma}_H^2)}{p(x/\hat{\mu}, \hat{\sigma}^2)}$$

where $(\hat{\mu}_H, \hat{\sigma}_H^2)$: MLE (μ, σ^2) under H

$(\hat{\mu}, \hat{\sigma}^2)$: MLE of (μ, σ^2) under $H \cup K$ (in the unrestricted case).

For $(\mu, \sigma^2) \in H \cup K$, i.e. Θ, we have

$$\widehat{\mu} = \bar{x}, \widehat{\sigma}^2 = \frac{1}{n}\sum_1^n (x_i - \bar{x})^2 = \frac{(n-1)}{n}s^2$$

For $(\mu, \sigma^2) \in H$, we have

$$\widehat{\mu}_H = \bar{x} \text{ if } \bar{x} \le \mu_0 \text{ and } \hat{\sigma}_H^2 = \frac{n-1}{n}s^2 \text{ if } \bar{x} \le \mu_0$$
$$= \mu_0 \text{ if } \bar{x} > \mu_0 \text{ and } \hat{\sigma}^2{}_H = s_0^2 = \frac{1}{n}\sum_1^n (x_i - \mu_0)^2 \text{ if } \bar{x} > \mu_0.$$

Thus, we have $p\left(x/\widehat{\mu}, \hat{\sigma}^2\right) = (2\pi)^{\frac{-n}{2}}\left(\frac{n-1}{n}s^2\right)^{\frac{-n}{2}}e^{\frac{-n}{2}}$

$$p\left(x/\widehat{\mu}_H, \hat{\sigma}^2 H\right) = (2\pi)^{-\frac{n}{2}}\left(\frac{n-1}{n}s^2\right)^{\frac{-n}{2}}e^{\frac{-n}{2}} \text{ if } \bar{x} \le \mu_0$$
$$= (2\pi)^{-\frac{n}{2}}\left(s_0^2\right)^{-\frac{n}{2}}e^{-\frac{n}{2}} \text{ if } \bar{x} > \mu_0$$

So, $L(x) = 1 \text{ if } \bar{x} \le \mu_0$

$$= \left(\frac{\frac{n-1}{n}s^2}{s_0^2}\right)^{n/2}, \text{ if } \bar{x} > \mu_0$$

Hence, we reject H if $L(x) < C$, where $C(<1)$ is such that

$$P\{L(x) < C/\mu = \mu_0\} = \alpha \in (0,1) \tag{4.1}$$

$$\Leftrightarrow \left(\frac{\frac{n-1}{n}s^2}{s_0^2}\right)^{n/2} < C \text{ and } \bar{x} > \mu_0$$

$$\Leftrightarrow \left[\frac{(n-1)s^2}{(n-1)s^2 + n(\bar{x} - \mu_0)^2}\right]^{n/2} < C \text{ and } \bar{x} > \mu_0$$

$$\Leftrightarrow 1 + \frac{n(\bar{x} - \mu_0)^2}{(n-1)s^2} > C' \text{ and } \bar{x} > \mu_0$$

$$\Leftrightarrow \frac{\sqrt{n}(\bar{x} - \mu_0)}{s} > C'' \tag{4.2}$$

Thus, (4.1) is $\Leftrightarrow P\left\{\frac{\sqrt{n}(\bar{x} - \mu_0)}{s} > C''/\mu = \mu_0\right\} = \alpha$

$$\Leftrightarrow P\left\{\frac{\sqrt{n}(\bar{x}-\mu_0)}{\sqrt{\frac{\sum_1^n (x_i-\bar{x})^2}{n-1}}} > C''/\mu = \mu_0\right\} = \alpha$$

$$\Rightarrow C'' = t_{\alpha,n-1}$$

Hence, reject H iff $\frac{\sqrt{n}(\bar{x}-\mu_0)}{s} > t_{\alpha,n-1}$

$\Rightarrow$ Test can be carried out by using students' t-statistic.

Example 4.4 $X_1, X_2 \ldots X_n$ are i.i.d $N(\mu, \sigma^2)$; $-\infty < \mu < \infty, \sigma^2 > 0$. Find the LR test for

I. $H : \sigma^2 = \sigma_0^2$ against $K : \sigma^2 > \sigma_0^2$
II. $H : \sigma^2 = \sigma_0^2$ against $K : \sigma^2 \neq \sigma_0^2$

Answer I. $\theta = (\mu, \sigma^2)$

$$p(x/\mu,\sigma^2) = \text{Likelihood function } = (2\pi)^{-n/2}(\sigma^2)^{-n/2}e^{-\frac{1}{2\sigma^2}\sum_{i=1}^{n}(x_i-\mu)^2}$$
$$= (2\pi)^{-n/2}(\sigma^2)^{-n/2}e^{-\frac{1}{2\sigma^2}\left[\sum(x_i-\bar{x})^2+n(\bar{x}-\mu)^2\right]}$$

Likelihood ratio is:

$$L(x) = \frac{\text{Sup}_{\mu,\sigma^2=\sigma_0^2}p(x/\mu,\sigma^2)}{\text{Sup}_{\mu,\sigma^2\geq\sigma_0^2}p(x/\mu,\sigma^2)} = \frac{p(x/\hat{\mu}_H,\sigma_0^2)}{p(x/\hat{\mu},\hat{\sigma}^2)},$$

where $\hat{\mu}$ = (MLE of μ overall $\theta : \sigma^2 \geq \sigma_0^2$) = $\bar{x}$

$$\hat{\sigma}^2 = \text{MLE of } \sigma^2 = \begin{cases} \frac{n-1}{n}s^2, \text{if } \frac{n-1}{n}s^2 \geq \sigma_0^2 \\ \sigma_0^2, \text{if } \frac{n-1}{n}s^2 < \sigma_0^2 \end{cases}$$

$\hat{\mu}_H$ = MLE of μ under H = $\bar{x}$

$$\text{Hence we get, } L(x) = \begin{cases} \frac{(\sigma_0^2)^{n/2}e^{-\frac{(n-1)s^2}{2\sigma_0^2}}}{\left(\frac{(n-1)}{n}s^2\right)^{-n/2}e^{-\frac{n}{2}}}, \text{if } \frac{n-1}{n}s^2 \geq \sigma_0^2 \\ 1, \text{if } \frac{n-1}{n}s^2 < \sigma_0^2 \end{cases}$$

Now we apply LR technique: reject H iff

$$L(x) < \mathrm{C}. \tag{4.3}$$

where C (<1) is such that

$$P\{L(x) < C/H\} = \alpha \in (0,1) \tag{4.4}$$

$$(1) \Leftrightarrow \left(\frac{\frac{n-1}{n}s^2}{\sigma_0^2}\right)^{\frac{n}{2}} e^{-\frac{(n-1)s^2}{2\sigma_0^2}} < C' \qquad \text{iff } \frac{(n-1)s^2}{\sigma_0^2} \geq n$$

$$\Leftrightarrow u^{\frac{n}{2}} e^{-\frac{u}{2}} < C^{**} \quad \text{if } u \geq n \tag{4.5}$$

Writing $g(u) = u^{\frac{n}{2}} e^{-\frac{u}{2}}, u \geq 0$

$$g'(u) = \frac{n}{2} u^{\frac{n}{2}-1} \cdot e^{-\frac{u}{2}} - \frac{u^{\frac{n}{2}}}{2} e^{-\frac{u}{2}} = 0$$

$$\Rightarrow n - u = 0 \Leftrightarrow u = n$$

The curve $y = g(u)$ has a maximum and the shape of the curve is

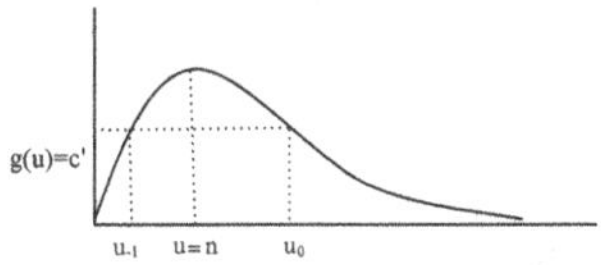

From the graph, it is clear that $g(u) < C^{**} \Leftrightarrow u < u_{-1}$ or $u > u_0$ where $0 < u_{-1} < n < u_0$.

Hence, (4.5) $\Leftrightarrow u > u_0$ and (4.4) $\Leftrightarrow P_H(U > u_0) = \alpha$

$$\Leftrightarrow P\{\chi^2_{n-1} > u_0\} = \alpha \begin{bmatrix} \text{As under } H, \\ U \sim \chi^2_{n-1} \end{bmatrix}$$

$$\Rightarrow u_0 = \chi^2_{n-1,\alpha}$$

Thus, LR test is: reject H if $\sum_{i=1}^{n} (x_i - \bar{x})^2 > \sigma_0^2 \chi^2_{n-1,\alpha}$.

II. $L(x) = \dfrac{\mathrm{Sup}_{\mu,\sigma^2=\sigma_0^2} p(x/\mu,\sigma^2)}{\mathrm{Sup}_{\mu,\sigma^2} p(x/\mu,\sigma^2)} = \dfrac{(\sigma_0^2)^{-n/2} e^{-\frac{(n-1)s^2}{2\sigma_0^2}}}{\left(\frac{n-1}{n}s^2\right)^{-n/2} e^{-n/2}} = K \cdot u^{\frac{n}{2}} e^{-\frac{u}{2}}$

Our test is to reject H if $u^{\frac{n}{2}} e^{-\frac{u}{2}} < C'$, where C' is such that $P_H\left\{U^{\frac{n}{2}} e^{-\frac{U}{2}} < C'\right\} = \alpha$.

From the graph, we observe that the line $y = C'$ cuts the curve $y = g(u)$ at two points: u_{-1} and u_0 such that $0 < u_{-1} < \mathrm{n} < u_0$. Hence, the test is equivalent to reject H iff $u < u_{-1}$ or $u > u_0$, where

$$P_H(\chi^2_{n-1} < u_{-1}) + P_H(\chi^2_{n-1} > u_0) = \alpha.$$

Although χ^2 is not symmetric, for the matter of simplicity, equal error probabilities $\alpha/2$ are attached to both left-and right-sided critical regions. Thus, $u_{-1} = \chi^2_{n-1,1-\frac{\alpha}{2}}$ and $u_0 = \chi^2_{n-1,\frac{\alpha}{2}}$.

Example 4.5 Let $X_1, X_2, \ldots X_{n_1}$ and $Y_1, Y_2, \ldots Y_{n_2}$ be two independent samples drawn from $N(\mu_1, \sigma_1^2)$ and $N(\mu_2, \sigma_2^2)$, respectively. Find out the likelihood ratio test of

(a) $H : \sigma_1^2 = \sigma_2^2$ against $K : \sigma_1^2 > \sigma_2^2$
(b) $H : \sigma_1^2 = \sigma_2^2$ against $K : \sigma_1^2 \neq \sigma_2^2$, when μ_1 and μ_2 are unknown

(a) Here, $\theta = (\mu_1, \mu_2, \sigma_1^2, \sigma_2^2)$

$$\Theta_0 = \left\{(\mu_1, \mu_2, \sigma_1^2, \sigma_2^2) : -\infty < \mu_1, \mu_2 < \infty, \sigma_1^2 = \sigma_2^2 = \sigma^2 > 0\right\}$$
$$\Theta = \left\{(\mu_1, \mu_2, \sigma_1^2, \sigma_2^2) : -\infty < \mu_i < \infty, \sigma_i^2 > 0, i = 1, 2\right\}$$

$$p(x, y|\theta) = (2\pi)^{-\frac{n_1+n_2}{2}} \sigma_1^{-n_1} \sigma_2^{-n_2} e^{-\frac{1}{2\sigma_1^2}\sum_{i=1}^{n_1}(X_i-\mu_1)^2 - \frac{1}{2\sigma_2^2}\sum_{i=1}^{n_2}(y_i-\mu_2)^2}$$

$$L(x, y) = \frac{\operatorname{Sup}_{\theta \in H} p(x, y|\theta)}{\operatorname{Sup}_{\theta \in H \cup K} p(x, y|\theta)} = \frac{p\left(x, y\middle|\widehat{\theta}_H\right)}{p\left(x, y\middle|\widehat{\theta}\right)}$$

where $\widehat{\theta}_H$ = MLE of θ under H

$\widehat{\theta}$ = MLE of θ under $H \cup K$.

Under H, we obtain MLEs

$$\widehat{\mu}_{1H} = \bar{x},\ \widehat{\mu}_{2H} = \bar{y},\ \widehat{\sigma}_H^2 = \frac{\sum (x_i - \bar{x})^2 + \sum (y_i - \bar{y})^2}{n_1 + n_2}$$

Under $H \cup K$, MLEs are

$$\begin{cases} \widehat{\mu}_1 = \bar{x}, \widehat{\mu}_2 = \bar{y}, \widehat{\sigma}_1^2 = \frac{1}{n_1}\sum (x_i - \bar{x})^2 \\ \widehat{\sigma}_2^2 = \frac{1}{n_2}\sum (y_i - \bar{y})^2 \quad \text{if} \quad \frac{\widehat{\sigma}_1^2}{\widehat{\sigma}_2^2} \geq 1 \\ \widehat{\mu}_1 = \bar{x}, \widehat{\mu}_2 = \bar{y}, \widehat{\sigma}_H^2 \quad \text{if} \quad \frac{\widehat{\sigma}_1^2}{\widehat{\sigma}_2^2} < 1 \end{cases}$$

Hence, $p\left(x, y\middle|\widehat{\theta}_H\right) = (2\pi)^{-\frac{n_1+n_2}{2}} \left(\widehat{\sigma}_H^2\right)^{-\frac{n_1+n_2}{2}} e^{-\frac{n_1+n_2}{2}}$

and $$p\left(x, y\middle|\widehat{\theta}\right) = \begin{cases} (2\pi)^{-\frac{n_1+n_2}{2}} \left(\widehat{\sigma}_1^2\right)^{-\frac{n_1}{2}} \left(\widehat{\sigma}_2^2\right)^{-\frac{n_2}{2}} e^{-\frac{n_1+n_2}{2}} & \text{if} \quad \frac{\widehat{\sigma}_1^2}{\widehat{\sigma}_2^2} \geq 1 \\ (2\pi)^{-\frac{n_1+n_2}{2}} \left(\widehat{\sigma}_H^2\right)^{-\frac{n_1+n_2}{2}} e^{-\frac{n_1+n_2}{2}} & \text{if} \quad \frac{\widehat{\sigma}_1^2}{\widehat{\sigma}_2^2} < 1 \end{cases}$$

$$\text{Therefore, } L(x,y) = \begin{cases} \dfrac{\left(\widehat{\sigma}_1^2\right)^{\frac{n_1}{2}}\left(\widehat{\sigma}_2^2\right)^{\frac{n_2}{2}}}{\left(\widehat{\sigma}_H^2\right)^{\frac{n_1+n_2}{2}}} & \text{if } \dfrac{\widehat{\sigma}_1^2}{\widehat{\sigma}_2^2} \geq 1 \\ 1 & \text{if } \dfrac{\widehat{\sigma}_1^2}{\widehat{\sigma}_2^2} < 1 \end{cases}$$

$$= \begin{cases} \dfrac{\left\{\frac{\sum (x_i-\bar{x})^2}{n_1}\right\}^{n_1/2}\left\{\frac{\sum (y_i-\bar{y})^2}{n_2}\right\}^{n_2/2}}{\left\{\frac{\sum (x_i-\bar{x})^2 + \sum (y_i-\bar{y})^2}{n_1+n_2}\right\}^{(n_1+n_2)/2}} & \text{if } \dfrac{\sum (x_i-\bar{x})^2 / n_1}{\sum (y_i-\bar{y})^2 / n_2} \geq 1 \\ 1 & \text{if } \dfrac{\sum (x_i-\bar{x})^2 / n_1}{\sum (y_i-\bar{y})^2 / n_2} < 1 \end{cases}$$

$$= \begin{cases} \dfrac{(n_1+n_2)^{\frac{n_1+n_2}{2}}}{n_1^{n_1/2}\, n_2^{n_2/2}} \cdot \dfrac{\left\{\frac{\sum (x_i-\bar{x})^2}{\sum (y_i-\bar{y})^2}\right\}^{n_1/2}}{\left\{1+\frac{\sum (x_i-\bar{x})^2}{\sum (y_i-\bar{y})^2}\right\}^{\frac{n_1+n_2}{2}}} & \text{if } \dfrac{\sum (x_i-\bar{x})^2 / n_1}{\sum (y_i-\bar{y})^2 / n_2} \geq 1 \\ 1 & \text{if } \dfrac{\sum (x_i-\bar{x})^2 / n_1}{\sum (y_i-\bar{y})^2 / n_2} < 1 \end{cases}$$

Now, under the null hypothesis $H : \sigma_1^2 = \sigma_2^2 = \sigma^2$, consider the statistic

$$F = \frac{\sum (x_i-\bar{x})^2 / (n_1-1)}{\sum (y_i-\bar{y})^2 / (n_2-1)} = \frac{s_1^2}{s_2^2} \sim F_{n_1-1, n_2-1}.$$

On writing $L(x)$ in terms of F, we have

$$L(x,y) = \begin{cases} \dfrac{(n_1+n_2)^{(n_1+n_2)/2}}{n_1^{n_1/2}\, n_2^{n_2/2}} \cdot \dfrac{\left(\frac{n_1-1}{n_2-1}F\right)^{n_1/2}}{\left(1+\frac{n_1-1}{n_2-1}F\right)^{(n_1+n_2)/2}} & \text{if } \mathrm{F} \geq \frac{n_1(n_2-1)}{n_2(n_1-1)} \\ 1 & \text{if } \mathrm{F} < \frac{n_1(n_2-1)}{n_2(n_1-1)} \end{cases}$$

Now we apply LR technique: reject

$$H \text{ iff } L(x,y) < C \tag{4.6}$$

where $C(<1)$ is such that

$$P\{L(x,y) < C|H\} = \alpha \in (0,1). \tag{4.7}$$

$$(4.6) \Rightarrow \frac{\left(\frac{n_1-1}{n_2-1}F\right)^{n_1/2}}{\left(1+\frac{n_1-1}{n_2-1}F\right)^{(n_1+n_2)/2}} < C_1 \quad \text{if} \quad \mathrm{F} \geq \frac{n_1(n_2-1)}{n_2(n_1-1)},$$

where C_1 is such that $P\left[\frac{\left(\frac{n_1-1}{n_2-1}F\right)^{n_1/2}}{\left(1+\frac{n_1-1}{n_2-1}F\right)^{(n_1+n_2)/2}} < C_1 \quad \text{and} \quad \mathrm{F} \geq \frac{n_1(n_2-1)}{n_2(n_1-1)}\right] = \alpha.$

Writing $g(F) = \frac{\left(\frac{n_1-1}{n_2-1}F\right)^{n_1/2}}{\left(1+\frac{n_1-1}{n_2-1}F\right)^{(n_1+n_2)/2}}$

$$\therefore g'(F) = \frac{n_1}{2}\left(\frac{n_1-1}{n_2-1}F\right)^{\frac{n_1}{2}-1} \cdot \frac{n_1-1}{n_2-1} \cdot \left(1+\frac{n_1-1}{n_2-1}F\right)^{-\frac{n_1+n_2}{2}} - \left(\frac{n_1-1}{n_2-1}F\right)^{\frac{n_1}{2}} \frac{n_1+n_2}{2} \cdot$$

$$\left(1+\frac{n_1-1}{n_2-1}F\right)^{-\frac{n_1+n_2}{2}-1} \frac{n_1-1}{n_2-1} = 0$$

$$\Rightarrow n_1\left(1+\frac{n_1-1}{n_2-1}F\right) - (n_1+n_2)\left(\frac{n_1-1}{n_2-1}\right)F = 0$$

$$\Rightarrow F = \frac{n_1(n_2-1)}{n_2(n_1-1)}$$

The curve $g(F)$ has single maximum at $F = \frac{n_1(n_2-1)}{n_2(n_1-1)}$ and the shape of the curve is

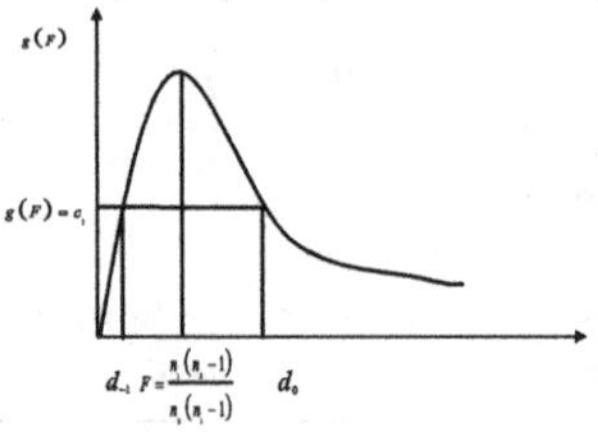

From the graph, we observe that $g(F) = C_1$ and $F \geq \frac{n_1(n_2-1)}{n_2(n_1-1)}$ $\Rightarrow F > d_0\left(> \frac{n_1(n_1-1)}{n_2(n_2-1)}\right)$. The constant d_0 is obtained by the size condition

$$P_{\sigma_1^2=\sigma_2^2}\{F > d_0\} = \alpha$$

This gives $d_0 = F_{n_1-1,n_2-1;\alpha}$

$$\therefore \text{LR test is given by } \phi(x,y) = \begin{cases} 1 & \text{if } \frac{s_1^2}{s_2^2} > F_{n_1-1,n_2-1;\alpha} \\ 0 & \text{otherwise} \end{cases}$$

(b) Similarly, for testing $H : \sigma_1^2 = \sigma_2^2$ against $K : \sigma_1^2 \neq \sigma_2^2$ the LR test is equivalent to

$$\frac{s_1^2}{s_2^2} < d\_1 \text{ or } \frac{s_1^2}{s_2^2} > d_0.$$

These constants d_1 and d_0 are obtained by the size condition

$$P_H\{F < d\_1\} = P_H\{F > d_0\} = \alpha/2$$

This gives $d\_1 = F_{n_1-1,n_2-1;1-\frac{\alpha}{2}}$ and $d_0 = F_{n_1-1,n_2-1;\alpha/2}$. The LR test is, therefore, given as

$$\phi(x,y) = \begin{cases} 1 & \text{if} \quad \frac{s_1^2}{s_2^2} < F_{n_1-1,n_2-1;1-\alpha/2} \\ & \text{or} \quad \frac{s_1^2}{s_2^2} > F_{n_1-1,n_2-1;\alpha/2} \\ 0 & \text{otherwise} \end{cases}$$

Example 4.6 Let $X_1, X_2, \ldots, X_{n_1}$ and $Y_1, Y_2, \ldots Y_{n_2}$ be two independent samples drawn from $N(\mu_1, \sigma_1^2)$ and $N(\mu_2, \sigma_2^2)$, respectively. Obtain the likelihood ratio test of

(a) $H : \mu_1 = \mu_2$ against $K : \mu_1 \neq \mu_2$ when σ_1^2 and σ_2^2 are known
(b) $H : \mu_1 = \mu_2$ against $K : \mu_1 \neq \mu_2$ when $\sigma_1^2 = \sigma_2^2 = \sigma^2$ but unknown
(c) $H : \mu_1 \geq \mu_2$ against $K : \mu_1 < \mu_2$ when $\sigma_1^2 = \sigma_2^2 = \sigma^2$ but unknown

Solution

(a) Here, $\theta = (\mu_1, \mu_2, \sigma_1^2, \sigma_2^2)$

$$\Theta_0 = \{(\mu_1 = \mu_2 = \mu); -\infty < \mu < \infty\}$$
$$\Theta = \{(\mu_1, \mu_2); -\infty < \mu_i < \infty, i = 1, 2\}$$

$$p(x, y|\theta) = (2\pi)^{-\frac{n_1+n_2}{2}} \sigma_1^{-n_1} \sigma_2^{-n_2} e^{-\frac{1}{2\sigma_1^2}\sum_{i=1}^{n_1}(X_i-\mu_1)^2 - \frac{1}{2\sigma_2^2}\sum_{i=1}^{n_2}(y_i-\mu_2)^2}$$

ML estimators of μ_1 and μ_2 under Θ are given as
$\widehat{\mu}_1 = \bar{x}$ and $\widehat{\mu}_2 = \bar{y}$

$$\sup_{(\mu_1,\mu_2)\in\Theta} p(x,y|\theta) = (2\pi)^{-\frac{n_1+n_2}{2}}\sigma_1^{-n_1}\sigma_2^{-n_2}e^{-\frac{1}{2\sigma_1^2}\sum_{i=1}^{n_1}(x_i-\bar{x})^2-\frac{1}{2\sigma_2^2}\sum_{i=1}^{n_2}(y_i-\bar{y})^2}$$

Under $\mu \in \Theta_0$,

$$p(x,y|\mu) = (2\pi)^{-\frac{n_1+n_2}{2}}\sigma_1^{-n_1}\sigma_2^{-n_2}e^{-\frac{1}{2\sigma_1^2}\sum_{i=1}^{n_1}(X_i-\mu)^2-\frac{1}{2\sigma_2^2}\sum_{i=1}^{n_2}(y_i-\mu)^2}$$

On taking log, we get

$$\log p(x,y|\mu) = k - \frac{1}{2\sigma_1^2}\sum(x_i-\mu)^2 - \frac{1}{2\sigma_2^2}\sum(y_i-\mu)^2,$$

where k is a constant which is independent of μ.

The ML estimator for μ is obtained as

$$\begin{aligned}
&\frac{\delta}{\delta\mu}\log p(x,y|\mu) = 0\\
&\Rightarrow \frac{1}{\sigma_1^2}\sum_1^{n_1}(x_i-\mu) + \frac{1}{\sigma_2^2}\sum(y_i-\mu) = 0\\
&\Rightarrow \frac{1}{\sigma_1^2}n_1\bar{x} + \frac{1}{\sigma_2^2}n_2\bar{y} = \left(\frac{n_1}{\sigma_1^2}+\frac{n_2}{\sigma_2^2}\right)\mu\\
&\Rightarrow \widehat{\mu}_H = \frac{\frac{n_1\bar{x}}{\sigma_1^2}+\frac{n_2\bar{y}}{\sigma_2^2}}{\frac{n_1}{\sigma_1^2}+\frac{n_2}{\sigma_2^2}} = \frac{\frac{\sigma_1^2}{n_1}\bar{y}+\frac{\sigma_2^2}{n_2}\bar{x}}{\frac{\sigma_1^2}{n_1}+\frac{\sigma_2^2}{n_2}}.
\end{aligned}$$

This gives

$$\sup_{(\mu_1,\mu_2)\in\Theta_0} p(x,y|\theta) = (2\pi)^{-\frac{n_1+n_2}{2}}\sigma_1^{-n_1}\sigma_2^{-n_2}e^{-\frac{1}{2\sigma_1^2}\sum_{i=1}^{n_1}\left(x_i-\widehat{\mu}_H\right)^2-\frac{1}{2\sigma_2^2}\sum_{i=1}^{n_2}\left(y_i-\widehat{\mu}_H\right)^2}$$

LR test $L(x, y)$ is given as

$$\begin{aligned}
L(x,y) &= \frac{e^{-\frac{1}{2\sigma_1^2}\left[\sum(x_i-\bar{x})^2+n_1\left(\bar{x}-\widehat{\mu}_H\right)^2\right]-\frac{1}{2\sigma_2^2}\left[\sum(y_i-\bar{y})^2+n_2\left(\bar{y}-\widehat{\mu}_H\right)^2\right]}}{e^{-\frac{1}{2\sigma_1^2}\sum(x_i-\bar{x})^2-\frac{1}{2\sigma_2^2}\sum(y_i-\bar{y})^2}}\\
&= e^{-\frac{n_1}{2\sigma_1^2}\left(\bar{x}-\widehat{\mu}_H\right)^2-\frac{n_2}{2\sigma_2^2}\left(\bar{y}-\widehat{\mu}_H\right)^2}
\end{aligned}$$

Now, $\left(\bar{x}-\widehat{\mu}_H\right)^2=\left[\frac{\frac{\sigma_1^2}{n_1}(\bar{x}-\bar{y})}{\frac{\sigma_1^2}{n_1}+\frac{\sigma_2^2}{n_2}}\right]^2$

$$\left(\bar{y}-\widehat{\mu}_H\right)^2=\left[\frac{\frac{\sigma_2^2}{n_2}(\bar{y}-\bar{x})}{\frac{\sigma_1^2}{n_1}+\frac{\sigma_2^2}{n_2}}\right]^2$$

$$\therefore \frac{n_1}{\sigma_1^2}(\bar{x}-\widehat{\mu}_H)^2+\frac{n_2}{\sigma_2^2}(\bar{y}-\widehat{\mu}_H)^2=(\bar{x}-\bar{y})^2\left(\frac{\sigma_1^2}{n_1}+\frac{\sigma_2^2}{n_2}\right)^{-1}$$

Thus, $L(x,y)=e^{-\frac{1}{2}\left(\frac{\sigma_1^2}{n_1}+\frac{\sigma_2^2}{n_2}\right)^{-1}(\bar{x}-\bar{y})^2}$
The rejection region $L(x,y)<C$ gives

$$-\frac{1}{2}\left(\frac{\sigma_1^2}{n_1}+\frac{\sigma_2^2}{n_2}\right)^{-1}(\bar{x}-\bar{y})^2<C_1$$

$$\text{or, }\left(\frac{(\bar{x}-\bar{y})^2}{\frac{\sigma_1^2}{n_1}+\frac{\sigma_2^2}{n_2}}\right)>C_2$$

$$\text{or, }\left|\frac{\bar{x}-\bar{y}}{\sqrt{\frac{\sigma_1^2}{n_1}+\frac{\sigma_2^2}{n_2}}}\right|>C_3$$

We know that under $H:\mu_1=\mu_2$, $\frac{\bar{x}-\bar{y}}{\sqrt{\frac{\sigma_1^2}{n_1}+\frac{\sigma_2^2}{n_2}}}\sim N(0,\,1)$. Hence, the likelihood ratio test has critical region

$$\omega=\left\{(x,y):\left|\frac{\bar{x}-\bar{y}}{\sqrt{\frac{\sigma_1^2}{n_1}+\frac{\sigma_2^2}{n_2}}}\right|>C_3\right\},$$

where C_3 is such that

$$P_H\left[\left|\frac{\bar{x}-\bar{y}}{\sqrt{\frac{\sigma_1^2}{n_1}+\frac{\sigma_2^2}{n_2}}}\right|>C_3\right]=\alpha$$

This gives $C_3=\tau_{\frac{\alpha}{2}}$.

Finally, the LR test is given as

$$\phi(\bar{x},\bar{y}) = \begin{cases} 1 & \text{if} \quad \frac{|\bar{x}-\bar{y}|}{\sqrt{\frac{\sigma_1^2}{n_1}+\frac{\sigma_2^2}{n_2}}} > \tau_{\frac{\alpha}{2}} \\ 0 & \text{Otherwise} \end{cases}$$

(b) Here $\theta = \left(\mu_1, \mu_2, \sigma_1^2, \sigma_2^2\right)$

$$\Theta_0 = \left\{\left(\mu, \sigma^2\right); -\infty < \mu < \infty, \sigma^2 > 0\right\}$$

$$\Theta = \left\{\left(\mu_1, \mu_2, \sigma^2\right); -\infty < \mu_i < \infty, \sigma^2 > 0, i = 1, 2\right\}$$

For $(\mu_1, \mu_2, \sigma^2) \in \Theta$,

$$p\left(x, y|\mu_1, \mu_2, \sigma^2\right) = \left(\frac{1}{2\pi\sigma^2}\right)^{\frac{n_1+n_2}{2}} e^{-\frac{1}{2\sigma^2}\left[\sum_1^{n_1}(x_i-\mu_1)^2+\sum_1^{n_2}(y_i-\mu_2)^2\right]}$$

On taking log, we get

$$\log p = -\frac{n_1+n_2}{2}\log\left(2\pi\sigma^2\right) - \frac{1}{2\sigma^2}\left[\sum_1^{n_1}(x_i-\mu_1)^2 + \sum_1^{n_2}(y_i-\mu_2)^2\right]$$

The ML estimators for $(\mu_1, \mu_2, \sigma^2) \in \Theta$ are given as

$$\frac{\delta \log p}{\delta \mu_1} = 0 \Rightarrow \hat{\mu}_1 = \bar{x}$$

$$\frac{\delta \log p}{\delta \mu_2} = 0 \Rightarrow \hat{\mu}_2 = \bar{y}$$

$$\frac{\delta \log p}{\delta \sigma^2} = 0 \Rightarrow \hat{\sigma}^2 = \frac{\sum(x_i-\bar{x})^2 + \sum(y_i-\bar{y})^2}{n_1+n_2}$$

$$\therefore \sup_{(\mu_1,\mu_2,\sigma^2)\in\Theta} p\left(x, y|\mu_1, \mu_2, \sigma^2\right) = \left(\frac{1}{2\pi}\right)^{\frac{n_1+n_2}{2}} \left(\hat{\sigma}^2\right)^{\frac{-(n_1+n_2)}{2}} e^{-\frac{1}{2}(n_1+n_2)}$$

For $(\mu, \sigma^2) \in \Theta_0$,

$$p\left(x, y|\mu, \sigma^2\right) = \left(\frac{1}{2\pi\sigma^2}\right)^{\frac{n_1+n_2}{2}} e^{-\frac{1}{2\sigma^2}\left[\sum_1^{n_1}(x_i-\mu)^2+\sum_1^{n_2}(y_i-\mu)^2\right]}$$

$$\therefore \log p = -\frac{n_1+n_2}{2}\log\left(2\pi\sigma^2\right) - \frac{1}{2\sigma^2}\left[\sum_1^{n_1}(x_i-\mu)^2 + \sum_1^{n_2}(y_i-\mu)^2\right]$$

Now,

$$\frac{\delta \log p}{\delta \mu} = 0 \Rightarrow \widehat{\mu}_H = \frac{n_1\bar{x} + n_2\bar{y}}{n_1 + n_2}$$

$$\frac{\delta \log p}{\delta \sigma^2} = 0 \Rightarrow \widehat{\sigma}_H^2 = \frac{1}{n_1+n_2}\left[\sum_1^{n_1}\left(x_i - \widehat{\mu}_H\right)^2 + \sum_1^{n_2}\left(y_i - \widehat{\mu}_H\right)^2\right]$$

$$= \frac{1}{n_1+n_2}\left[\sum_1^{n_1}(x_i-\bar{x})^2 + n_1\left(\bar{x} - \widehat{\mu}_H\right)^2 + \sum_1^{n_2}(y_i-\bar{y})^2 + n_2\left(\bar{y} - \widehat{\mu}_H\right)^2\right]$$

Here, $\left(\bar{x} - \widehat{\mu}_H\right)^2 = \left(\bar{x} - \frac{n_1\bar{x} + n_2\bar{y}}{n_1 + n_2}\right)^2 = \left\{\frac{n_2(\bar{x} - \bar{y})}{n_1 + n_2}\right\}^2$

$$\left(\bar{y} - \widehat{\mu}_H\right)^2 = \left(\bar{y} - \frac{n_1\bar{x} + n_2\bar{y}}{n_1 + n_2}\right)^2 = \left\{\frac{n_1(\bar{y} - \bar{x})}{n_1 + n_2}\right\}^2$$

This gives

$$\left(\widehat{\sigma}_H^2\right) = \frac{1}{n_1+n_2}\left[\sum_1^{n_1}(x_i-\bar{x})^2 + n_1\left\{\frac{n_2(\bar{x}-\bar{y})}{n_1+n_2}\right\}^2 + \sum_1^{n_2}(y_i-\bar{y})^2 + n_2\left\{\frac{n_1(\bar{y}-\bar{x})}{n_1+n_2}\right\}^2\right]$$

$$= \frac{1}{n_1+n_2}\left[\sum_1^{n_1}(x_i-\bar{x})^2 + \sum_1^{n_2}(y_i-\bar{y})^2 + \frac{n_1 n_2}{n_1+n_2}(\bar{x}-\bar{y})^2\right]$$

Therefore, $\underset{(\mu,\sigma^2)\in\Theta_0}{\text{Sup}}\ p(x,y|\mu,\sigma^2) = \left(\frac{1}{2\pi}\right)^{\frac{n_1+n_2}{2}}\left(\widehat{\sigma}_H^2\right)^{\frac{-(n_1+n_2)}{2}} e^{-\frac{1}{2}(n_1+n_2)}$

Hence we get,

$$L(x,y) = \frac{\underset{(\mu,\sigma^2)\in\Theta_0}{\text{Sup}}\ p(x,y|\mu,\sigma^2)}{\underset{(\mu_1,\mu_2,\sigma^2)\in\Theta}{\text{Sup}}\ p(x,y|\mu_1,\mu_2,\sigma^2)}$$

$$= \left(\frac{\widehat{\sigma}^2}{\widehat{\sigma}_H^2}\right)^{\frac{n_1+n_2}{2}} = \frac{\sum_1^{n_1}(x_i-\bar{x})^2 + \sum_1^{n_2}(y_i-\bar{y})^2}{\sum_1^{n_1}(x_i-\bar{x})^2 + \sum_1^{n_2}(y_i-\bar{y})^2 + \frac{n_1n_2}{n_1+n_2}(\bar{x}-\bar{y})^2}$$

$$= \left[\frac{1}{1 + \frac{n_1n_2(\bar{x}-\bar{y})^2}{(n_1+n_2)\left\{\sum_1^{n_1}(x_i-\bar{x})^2 + \sum_1^{n_2}(y_i-\bar{y})^2\right\}}}\right]$$

$$= \left[\frac{1}{1 + \frac{(\bar{x}-\bar{y})^2}{\frac{\left(\frac{1}{n_1}+\frac{1}{n_2}\right)(n_1+n_2-2)\left\{\sum_1^{n_1}(x_i-\bar{x})^2+\sum_1^{n_2}(y_i-\bar{y})^2\right\}}{(n_1+n_2-2)}}} \right]$$

We know, $\bar{X} \sim N\left(\mu_1, \frac{\sigma^2}{n_1}\right)$ and $\bar{Y} \sim N\left(\mu_2, \frac{\sigma^2}{n_2}\right)$

$$\bar{X} - \bar{Y} \sim N\left(\mu_1 - \mu_2, \sigma^2\left(\frac{1}{n_1} + \frac{1}{n_2}\right)\right)$$

Thus, $\frac{\bar{X}-\bar{Y}-(\mu_1-\mu_2)}{\sigma\sqrt{\left(\frac{1}{n_1}+\frac{1}{n_2}\right)}} \sim N(0,1)$

Again, $\frac{1}{\sigma^2}\sum (X_i - \bar{X})^2 \sim \chi^2_{n_1-1}$
and $\frac{1}{\sigma^2}\sum (Y_i - \bar{Y})^2 \sim \chi^2_{n_2-1}$.
Therefore, $\frac{1}{\sigma^2}\left[\sum (X_i - \bar{X})^2 + \sum (Y_i - \bar{Y})^2\right] \sim \chi^2_{n_1+n_2-2}$
Thus, under $H : \mu_1 = \mu_2$,

$$t = \frac{(\bar{X} - \bar{Y})\Big/\sigma\sqrt{\frac{1}{n_1} + \frac{1}{n_2}}}{\sqrt{\frac{1}{\sigma^2}\left[\sum (X_i - \bar{X})^2 + \sum (Y_i - \bar{Y})^2\right]\frac{1}{n_1+n_2-2}}} \sim t_{n_1+n_2-2},$$

$$\text{or, } t = \frac{(\bar{x} - \bar{y})}{\sqrt{\left(\frac{1}{n_1} + \frac{1}{n_2}\right)\cdot s^2}} \sim n_1 + n_2 - 2$$

where $s^2 = \frac{\sum (x_i - \bar{x})^2 + \sum (y_i - \bar{y})^2}{n_1 + n_2 - 2} = \frac{(n_1 - 1)s_1^2 + (n_2 - 1)s_2^2}{n_1 + n_2 - 2}$

So, $L(x,y) = \frac{1}{1 + \frac{t^2}{n_1+n_2-2}}$

Thus, the rejection region $L(x,y) < C$ gives

$$1 + \frac{t^2}{n_1 + n_2 - 2} > C_1$$
$$\text{or,} \quad t^2 > C_2$$
$$\text{or,} \quad |t| > C_3$$

Therefore, the LR test is given as $|t| > C_3$,where C_3 is obtained as $P_H[|t| > C_3] = \alpha$.

This gives $C_3 = t_{n_1+n_2-2,\alpha/2}$. Hence, LR test is given as

$$\phi(x,y) = \begin{cases} 1 & \text{if} \quad \dfrac{|\bar{x}-\bar{y}|}{s\sqrt{\left(\frac{1}{n_1}+\frac{1}{n_2}\right)}} > t_{n_1+n_2-2,\alpha/2} \\ 0 & \quad\quad \text{Otherwise} \end{cases}$$

(c) Proceeding similarly as in (b), for testing $H : \mu_1 \geq \mu_2$ against $K : \mu_1 < \mu_2$ the LR test is given as

$$\phi(x,y) = \begin{cases} 1 & \text{if} \quad \dfrac{\bar{x}-\bar{y}}{s\sqrt{\left(\frac{1}{n_1}+\frac{1}{n_2}\right)}} < -t_{n_1+n_2-2,\alpha} \\ 0 & \quad\quad \text{Otherwise} \end{cases}$$

Example 4.7 Suppose $x_{ij} \sim N(\mu_i, \sigma^2), j = 1(1)n_i, i = 1(1)k$ independently. This is one-way classified data.

We are to find LR test for $H : \mu_1 = \mu_2 = \cdots = \mu_k$ against K: μ_i' are not all equal.

Answer Here, $\theta = (\mu_1, \mu_2, \ldots \mu_k, \sigma^2)$ and $\Theta = \{\theta : -\infty < \mu_i < \infty, i = 1(1)k, \sigma^2 > 0\}$. Observe that $H \cup K = \Theta$. Likelihood functions $= p(x/\theta) = (2\pi)^{-n/2}\sigma^{-n}e^{-\frac{1}{2\sigma^2}\sum_1^k\sum_1^{n_i}(x_{ij}-\mu_i)^2}$, $n = \sum_1^k n_i$.

Likelihood ratio is $L(x) = \dfrac{\operatorname{Sup}_{\theta\in H} p(x/\theta)}{\operatorname{Sup}_{\theta\in\Theta} p(x/\theta)} = \dfrac{p\left(x/\theta_H\right)}{p(x/\theta)}$,

where θ and θ_H are, respectively, the MLEs of $\theta(\in \Theta)$ and $\theta(\in H)$.

Now, $\theta \in \Theta \Rightarrow$ MLEs are $\mu_i = \bar{x}_i = \frac{1}{n_i}\sum_1^{n_i} x_{ij}$

$$\left[\text{as } \frac{\partial \log p(x/\theta)}{\partial \mu_i} = 0 \Rightarrow \mu_i = \bar{x}_i\right]$$

$$\sigma^2 = \frac{1}{n}\sum_1^k\sum_1^{n_i}\left(x_{ij}-\bar{x}_i\right)^2 = \frac{\text{within S.S.}}{n} = \frac{W}{n}.(\text{say}).$$

$$\left[\text{Here } \frac{\partial \log p(x/\theta)}{\partial \sigma^2} = 0 \Rightarrow \sigma^2 = \frac{1}{n}\sum_1^k\sum_1^{n_i}\left(x_{ij}-\bar{x}_i\right)^2\right]$$

Again $\theta \in H \Rightarrow \theta = (\mu, \sigma^2)$, where μ is the common value of μ_i's.

Here, we have MLEs

$$\mu_H = \frac{1}{n}\sum_1^k \sum_1^{n_i} x_{ij} = \frac{1}{n}\sum_1^k n_i \bar{x}_i = \bar{\bar{x}}, \text{(say)}$$

$$\sigma_H^2 = \frac{1}{n}\sum_1^k \sum_1^{n_i} \left(x_{ij} - \bar{\bar{x}}\right)^2 = \frac{\text{Total S.S.}}{n} = \frac{T}{n}$$

$$= \frac{1}{n}\left[W + \sum_1^k n_i\left(\bar{x}_i - \bar{\bar{x}}\right)^2\right] = \frac{W+B}{n}$$

$$\left[B = \sum_1^k n_i\left(\bar{x}_i - \bar{\bar{x}}\right)^2 = \text{Between(means) S.S}\right].$$

Hence, we get $p\left(x/\hat{\theta}\right) = (2\pi)^{-n/2}(\sigma)^{-n}e^{-\frac{n}{2}}.$

$$p\left(x/\hat{\theta}_H\right) = (2\pi)^{-n/2}(\hat{\sigma}_H)^{-n}e^{-\frac{n}{2}}$$

So, $L(x) = \left(\frac{\hat{\sigma}^2}{\hat{\sigma}_H^2}\right)^{n/2}$ and therefore reject H iff $L(x) < c, P_H\{L(x) < c\} = \alpha \in (0,1)(0 < c < 1)$

$$\Leftrightarrow \frac{\hat{\sigma}_H^2}{\sigma^2} > c' \Leftrightarrow \frac{W+B}{W} > c' \Leftrightarrow \frac{B}{W} > c''$$

$$\Leftrightarrow T^* = \frac{B/k-1}{W/n-k} > c'''$$

The size condition now reduces to $P_H\{T^* > c'''\} = \alpha$ under H.
Under H, $T^* \sim F(k-1, n-k)$

$$\therefore c''' = F_{\alpha,(k-1,n-k)}$$

So, our LR test is $\frac{B/k-1}{W/n-k} > F_{\alpha,(k-1,n-k)}$ as rejection of H.

Note It is the same as ANOVA test.

Special case: (i) $\mu = \mu_0$ (given)

$$L(x) = \left(\frac{\hat{\sigma}^2}{\hat{\sigma}_H{}^2}\right)^{n/2} = \left[\frac{\sum_1^k \sum_1^{n_i}\left(x_{ij} - \bar{x}_i\right)^2}{\sum_1^k \sum_1^{n_i}\left(x_{ij} - \mu_0\right)^2}\right]^{n/2}$$

$$= \left[\frac{W}{W + \sum_1^k n_i(\bar{x}_i - \mu_0)^2}\right]^{n/2}$$

Test reduces to reject H iff

$$T^{**} = \frac{\frac{1}{k}\sum_1^k n_i(\bar{x}_i - \mu_0)^2}{W/(n-k)} > F_{\alpha,(k,n-k)}$$

(ii) Common value is unknown (μ) but $\sigma^2 = \sigma_0^2$ is known.

$$L(x) = \frac{\exp\left\{-\frac{1}{2\sigma_0^2}\sum_1^k\sum_1^{n_i}\left(x_{ij} - \bar{\bar{x}}\right)^2\right\}}{\exp\left\{-\frac{1}{2\sigma_0^2}\sum_1^k\sum_1^{n_i}\left(x_{ij} - \bar{x}_i\right)^2\right\}} = \frac{\exp\left\{-\frac{1}{2\sigma_0^2}(B+W)\right\}}{\exp\left\{-\frac{W}{2\sigma_0^2}\right\}}$$

$$= \exp\left\{-\frac{B}{2\sigma_0^2}\right\}$$

Hence LR test is: reject H iff

$$\frac{B}{\sigma_0^2} > \chi^2_{\alpha,k-1}.$$

(iii) If min $(n_1, n_2, \ldots, n_k)$ is large, we can approximate the distribution of $-2\log L(x)$ by χ^2—distribution with d.f. $k-1$.

Note The above hypothesis is equivalent to homogeneity of k univariate normal population.

Example 4.8

$$\text{Suppose } x_{ij} \sim N\left(\mu_i, \sigma_i^2\right),\ j = 1(1)n_i,\ i = 1(1)k \text{ independently.}$$

Obtain the likelihood ratio test of $H: \sigma_1^2 = \sigma_2^2 = \sigma_3^2 = \cdots = \sigma_k^2$ against K: not all σ_i's are equal.

Answer $\theta = \left(\mu_1, \mu_2, \ldots, \mu_k, \sigma_1^2, \sigma_2^2, \ldots, \sigma_k^2\right)$

$$\Theta = \left\{\theta : -\infty < \mu_i < \infty, \sigma_i^2 > 0, i = 1(1)k\right\}$$

$$\text{Likelihood function} = p\left({}^{x}/_{\theta}\right) = \frac{(2\pi)^{-n/2}}{\prod_{i=1}^k\left(\sigma_i^2\right)^{\frac{n_i}{2}}}\prod_{i=1}^k\left\{e^{-\frac{1}{2\sigma_i^2}\sum^{n_i}\left(x_{ij}-\mu_i\right)^2}\right\},\quad \left[n = \sum^k n_i\right]$$

Now, $\left[\frac{\partial \log p(x/\theta)}{\partial \mu_i} = 0 \Rightarrow \frac{-2}{2\sigma_i^2}\sum_{j=1}^{n_i}(x_{ij}-\mu_i)(-1) = 0 \Rightarrow \hat{\mu}_i = \bar{x}_i\right]$

and

$$\frac{\partial \log p(x/\theta)}{\partial \sigma_i^2} \Rightarrow \frac{-n_i}{2\sigma_i^2} + \frac{1}{2\sigma_i^4}\sum_{j=1}^{n_i}(x_{ij}-\mu_i)^2 = 0$$

$$\Rightarrow \hat{\sigma}_i^2 = \frac{1}{n_i}\sum_{j=1}^{n_i}(x_{ij}-\bar{x}_i)^2 = \frac{n_i - 1}{n_i}s_i^2$$

Hence, for $\theta \in \Theta$ we get $p\left(x/\hat{\theta}\right) = (2\pi)^{-n/2}\prod_{i=1}^{k}\left(\hat{\sigma}_i^2\right)^{-\frac{n_i}{2}}$

$$\left(= \operatorname*{Sup}_{\theta\in\Theta} p(x/\theta)\right)$$

Under H, $p(x/\theta)$ reduces to

$$p(x/\theta) = (2\pi)^{-n/2}\sigma^{-n}e^{-\frac{1}{2\sigma^2}\sum^{k}\sum^{n_i}(x_{ij}-\mu_i)^2},$$

where from we get $\widehat{\mu}_{iH} = \bar{x}_i$ and $\widehat{\sigma}_H^2 = \frac{1}{n}\sum^{k}\sum^{n_i}(x_{ij}-\bar{x}_i)^2 = \frac{1}{n}\sum^{k}(n_i-1)s_i^2$

Hence, $\operatorname*{Sup}_{\theta\in H} p(x/\theta) = p\left(x/\hat{\theta}_H\right) = (2\pi)^{-n/2}\left(\hat{\sigma}_H^2\right)^{-n/2}e^{-n/2}$

Hence, likelihood ratio is

$$L(x) = \frac{\left(\hat{\sigma}_H^2\right)^{-n/2}}{\prod_{i=1}^{k}\left(\hat{\sigma}_i^2\right)^{\frac{-n_i}{2}}} = \frac{\prod_{i=1}^{k}\left\{\frac{(n_i-1)s_i^2}{n_i}\right\}^{\frac{n_i}{2}}}{\left[\frac{1}{n}\sum_{i=1}^{k}(n_i-1)s_i^2\right]^{n/2}}.$$

The distribution of the statistic obtained in $L(x)$ is difficult to calculate. Therefore, we could only say about its asymptotic distribution, i.e. $-2\log_e L(x)$.

$$\text{So, } -2\log_e L(x) = n\log_e\frac{\sum_{i=1}^{k}(n_i-1)s_i^2}{n} - \sum_{i=1}^{k} n_i \log_e\frac{(n_i-1)}{n_i}s_i^2$$

is distributed as $\chi^2_{2k-(k+1)=k-1}$ for large n_i's.

It has been suggested by Bartlett (1937) that the above approximation to Chi-square for large n can be improved if we replace the ML estimators of σ^2's by unbiased estimators, i.e. if we replace n_i by $n_i - 1$ and n by $n - k$ in the above expression. So,

$$-2\log_e L(x) = (n-k)\log_e \frac{\sum_{i=1}^{k}(n_i-1)s_i^2}{n-k} - \sum_{i=1}^{k}(n_i-1)\log_e s_i^2$$

$$= \sum_{i=1}^{k}(n_i-1)\log_e \frac{s^2}{s_i^2}, \qquad \text{where } s^2 = \frac{\sum_{i=1}^{k}(n_i-1)s_i^2}{\sum_{i=1}^{k}(n_i-1)}$$

Bartlett has also suggested that Chi-square approximation will hold goof for n_i as low as four or five if the above statistic is divided by υ, where

$$\upsilon = 1 + \frac{1}{3(k-1)}\left[\sum_{i=1}^{k}\frac{1}{n_i-1} - \frac{1}{\sum_{i=1}^{k}(n_i-1)}\right]$$

Hence, $T = \frac{\sum_{i=1}^{K}(n_i-1)\log_e \frac{s^2}{s_i^2}}{\upsilon} \sim \chi^2_{k-1}$
So, we reject H approximately at level α iff

$$T > \chi^2_{k-1,\alpha}$$

It is noted that the rapidity of convergence for this statistic T towards χ^2 is greater than that of $-2\log_e L(x)$.

Example 4.9 $X_1, X_2 \ldots X_n$ are i.i.d. with density $\frac{1}{\sigma}e^{-\frac{1}{\sigma}(x-\mu)}$ for $x \geq \mu$. Find the LR test for testing

I. $H: \mu = \mu_0$ against K: $\mu \neq \mu_0$
II. $H: \sigma = \sigma_0$ against K: $\sigma \neq \sigma_0$

Solution

I. Likelihood function

$$p\left({}^{x}/_{\mu,\sigma}\right) = \frac{1}{\sigma^n}e^{-\frac{1}{\sigma}\sum_{i}^{n}(x_i-\mu)} \quad \text{if } x_i > \mu \forall i$$
$$= 0 \text{ otherwise}$$

MLEs of μ and σ are given as
$\hat{\mu} = y_1$, y_1 = 1st order statistic
$\hat{\sigma} = \frac{1}{n}\sum_{i=1}^{n}(y_i - y_1)$, $y_1 < y_2 \cdots < y_n$ are the order statistics of $x_1, x_2 \ldots, x_n$.
Then

$$\operatorname*{Sup}_{\mu,\sigma} p\left({}^{x}/_{\mu,\sigma}\right) = p\left({}^{x}/_{\hat{\mu},\hat{\sigma}}\right) = (\hat{\sigma})^{-n}e^{-n}$$

Under H, $p\left({}^{x}/_{\mu,\sigma}\right)$ reduces to

$$p\left({}^{x}/_{\mu_0,\sigma}\right) = \sigma^{-n} e^{-\frac{1}{\sigma}\sum_i^n (x_i - \mu_0)}$$

$\Rightarrow$ MLE of σ is $\hat{\sigma}_H = \frac{1}{n}\sum_i^n (x_i - \mu_0) = \frac{1}{n}\sum_i^n (y_i - \mu_0)$

Then $\sup_{\mu,\sigma \in H} p\left({}^{x}/_{\mu,\sigma}\right) = p\left({}^{x}/_{\mu_0,\hat{\sigma}_H}\right) = (\hat{\sigma}_H)^{-n} e^{-n}$

Then likelihood ratio is given as

$$L(x) = \frac{\sup_{\mu,\sigma \in H} p\left({}^{x}/_{\mu,\sigma}\right)}{\sup_{\mu,\sigma} p\left({}^{x}/_{\mu,\sigma}\right)} = \left(\frac{\hat{\sigma}}{\hat{\sigma}_H}\right)^n$$

Now, reject H iff

$$L(x) < C \Leftrightarrow \frac{\sum (y_i - y_1)}{\sum (y_i - \mu_0)} < c$$
$$\Leftrightarrow \frac{\sum (y_i - y_1)}{\sum (y_i - y_1) + n(y_1 - \mu_0)} < c \Leftrightarrow \frac{n(y_1 - \mu_0)}{\sum (y_i - y_1)} > c'$$

Under

$$H : \mu = \mu_0$$
$$\frac{n(y_1 - \mu_0)/2}{\sum (y_i - y_1)/2n - 2} \sim F_{2,2n-2}.$$

Hence, we reject H iff

$$T = \frac{n/2(y_1 - \mu_0)}{\sum (y_i - y_1)/(2n - 2)} > F_{\alpha;2,2n-2}$$

II. As earlier, it can be shown that the test has acceptance region as

$$c_1 < T = \frac{1}{\sigma_0}\sum_i^n (y_i - y_1) < c_2,$$

where c_1 and c_2 are determined that

$$P_H\{c_1 < \chi^2_{2n-2} < c_2\} = 1 - \alpha$$
$$P_H\{c_1 < \chi^2_{2n} < c_2\} = 1 - \alpha$$

Example 4.10 Let $(X_{11}, X_{21}), (X_{12}, X_{22}) \ldots, (X_{1n}, X_{2n})$ be a random sample from a bivariate normal distribution with means μ_1 and μ_2, variances σ_1^2 and σ_2^2 and correlation coefficient ρ. Find the likelihood ratio test of
$H : \rho = 0$ against $K : \rho \neq 0$

Solution

$$\text{Here, } \theta = \left(\mu_1, \mu_2, \sigma_1^2, \sigma_2^2, \rho\right)$$
$$\Theta = \left\{\left(\mu_1, \mu_2, \sigma_1^2, \sigma_2^2, \rho\right) : -\infty < \mu_i < \infty, \sigma_i^2 > 0, -1 < \rho < 1, i = 1, 2\right\}$$
$$\Theta_0 = \left\{\left(\mu_1, \mu_2, \sigma_1^2, \sigma_2^2, \rho\right) : -\infty < \mu_i < \infty, \sigma_i^2 > 0, \rho = 0, i = 1, 2\right\}$$

In Θ, ML estimators for $\mu_1, \mu_2, \sigma_1^2, \sigma_2^2$ and ρ are
$\widehat{\mu}_1 = \bar{x}_1, \widehat{\mu}_2 = \bar{x}_2, \widehat{\sigma}_1^2 = \frac{1}{n}\sum(x_{1i} - \bar{x}_1)^2, \widehat{\sigma}_2^2 = \frac{1}{n}\sum(x_{2i} - \bar{x}_2)^2.$ and $\widehat{\rho} = \frac{\sum(x_{1i}-\bar{x}_1)(x_{2i}-\bar{x}_2)}{\left\{\sum(x_{1i}-\bar{x}_1)^2\sum(x_{2i}-\bar{x}_2)^2\right\}^{1/2}} = r.$

Thus,

$$\sup_{\theta\in\Theta} p(x|\theta) = \left(2\pi\widehat{\sigma}_1\widehat{\sigma}_2\sqrt{1-r^2}\right)^{-n} e^{-\frac{1}{2(1-r^2)}\left[\frac{n\hat{\sigma}_1^2}{\hat{\sigma}_1^2}+\frac{n\hat{\sigma}_2^2}{\hat{\sigma}_2^2}-2r.n.r\right]}$$
$$= \left(2\pi\widehat{\sigma}_1\widehat{\sigma}_2\sqrt{1-r^2}\right)^{-n} e^{-n}$$

In Θ_o, ML estimators for μ_1, μ_2, σ_1^2 and σ_2^2 are

$$\widehat{\mu}_{1H} = \bar{x}_1, \widehat{\mu}_{2H} = \bar{x}_2, \widehat{\sigma}_{1H}^2 = \frac{1}{n}\sum(x_{1i} - \bar{x}_1)^2, \widehat{\sigma}_{2H}^2 = \frac{1}{n}\sum(x_{2i} - \bar{x}_2)^2$$

$$\text{Thus, } \sup_{\theta\in\Theta} p(x|\theta) = \left(2\pi\widehat{\sigma}_{1H}\widehat{\sigma}_{2H}\right)^{-n} e^{-\frac{1}{2}\left[\frac{n\hat{\sigma}_{1H}^2}{\hat{\sigma}_{1H}^2}+\frac{n\hat{\sigma}_{2H}^2}{\hat{\sigma}_{2H}^2}\right]}$$

$$= \left(2\pi\widehat{\sigma}_{1H}\widehat{\sigma}_{2H}\right)^{-n} e^{-n}$$

Hence, the LR is given as

$$L(x) = \frac{\sup_{\theta\in\Theta_0} p(x|\theta)}{\sup_{\theta\in\Theta} p(x|\theta)} = \left(1 - r^2\right)^{n/2}$$

The LR critical region is given as

$$\begin{aligned} & L(x) < C \\ \text{or,}\quad & \left(1 - r^2\right)^{n/2} < C \\ \text{or,}\quad & 1 - r^2 < C_1 \\ \text{or,}\quad & r^2 > C_2 \\ \text{or,}\quad & |r| > C_3, \end{aligned}$$

where C_3 is obtained as

$$P_H[|r| > C_3] = \alpha$$

Thus, the test of $H : \rho = 0$ against $K : \rho \neq 0$ is based on r, the distribution of the sample correlation coefficient and its distribution for $\rho = 0$ is symmetric about 0.

Thus, $P_H[r < -C_3] = P_H[r > C_3] = \alpha/2$

Equivalently, the critical region for $H : \rho = 0$ against $K : \rho \neq 0$ is

$$\frac{|r|\sqrt{n-2}}{\sqrt{1-r^2}} > k.$$

Since $\frac{r\sqrt{n-2}}{\sqrt{1-r^2}}$ has the t-distribution with $(n-2)$ d.f. when $\rho = 0$, the constant k is given as

$$P_H\left[\frac{|r|\sqrt{n-2}}{\sqrt{1-r^2}} > k\right] = \alpha.$$

This gives $k = t_{n-2,\alpha/2}$.

Note For example, if $n = 4$ and $\alpha = 0.05$ then

$$\int_{-1}^{-c_3} \frac{1}{2}\,\mathrm{d}r = \int_{c_3}^{1} \frac{1}{2}\,\mathrm{d}r = 0.025$$

gives $C_3 = 0.95$. Hence, H is rejected at 5 % level of significance if r based on a sample of size four is such that $|r| > 0.95$.

Example 4.11 Let $X_1, X_2, \ldots, X_n$ be a random sample form density $f(x) = \frac{1}{\lambda}e^{-x/\lambda}, x > 0, \lambda > 0$. Find the likelihood ratio test of $H : \lambda = \lambda_0$ against $K : \lambda \neq \lambda_0$.

Solution Here, $\theta = (\lambda), \Theta = \{\lambda : \lambda > 0\}$

$$\Theta_0 = \{\lambda : \lambda = \lambda_0\}$$

In Θ, MLE of λ is $\widehat{\lambda} = \bar{x}$

Thus, the LR test is

$$L(x) = \frac{\underset{\Theta_0}{Sup}\, p(x|\lambda)}{\underset{\Theta}{Sup}\, p(x|\lambda)} = \frac{\frac{1}{\lambda_o^n} e^{\frac{-n\bar{x}}{\lambda_0}}}{\frac{1}{\bar{x}^n}.e^{-n}} = \frac{\bar{x}^n}{\lambda_0^n} e^{\frac{-n\bar{x}}{\lambda_0}}.e^n$$

The rejection region $L(x) < C$ gives

$$\bar{x}^n e^{-n\bar{x}/\lambda_0} < C_1,$$

writing $g(\bar{x}) = \bar{x}^n e^{\frac{-n\bar{x}}{\lambda_0}}$.

It shows that the curve $y = g(\bar{x})$ has single maximum at $\bar{x} = \lambda_0$ and the shape of the curve is

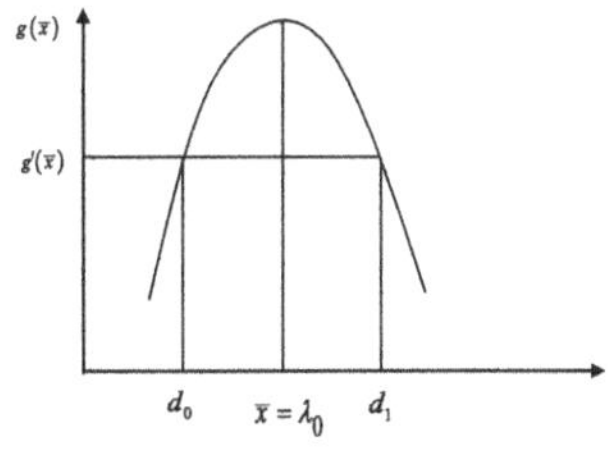

The graph shows the critical regions $0 < \bar{x} < d_0$ or $d_1 < \bar{x} < \infty$ corresponding to the critical region $L(x) < C$. The constants d_0 and d_1 are obtained by the size condition

$$P_H[d_0 < \bar{x} < d_1] = 1 - \alpha.$$

In this problem, $X \sim G(1, \lambda)$

$$M_x(t) = (1 - \lambda t)^{-1}$$

$$\therefore M_{\bar{x}}(t) = \left(1 - \frac{\lambda t}{n}\right)^{-n}$$

Thus, $\bar{X} \sim G\left(n, \frac{\lambda}{n}\right)$, i.e. $f(\bar{x}) = \frac{1}{\Gamma(n)}\left(\frac{n}{\lambda}\right)^n e^{-\frac{n\bar{x}}{\lambda}} \cdot \bar{x}^{n-1}$.

One can find the values of d_0 and d_1 from the gamma distribution table under H_0.

Chapter 5
Interval Estimation

5.1 Introduction

Inpoint estimation when a random sample $(X_1, X_2, \ldots, X_n)$ is drawn from a population having distribution function F_θ and θ is the unknown parameter (or the set of unknown parameter). We try to estimate the parametric function $\gamma(\theta)$ by means of a single value, say t, the value of a statistic T corresponding to the observed values $(x_1, x_2, \ldots, x_n)$ of the random variables $(X_1, X_2, \ldots, X_n)$. This estimate may differ from the exact value of $\gamma(\theta)$ in the given population. In other words, we take t as an estimate of $\gamma(\theta)$ such that $|t - \gamma(\theta)|$ is small with high probability. In the point estimate we try to choose a unique point in the parameter space which can reasonably be considered as the true value of the parameter. Instead of unique estimate of the parameter we are interested in constructing a family of sets that contain the true (unknown) parameter value with a specified (high) probability. In many problems of statistical inference we are not interested only in estimating the parameter or testing some hypothesis concerning the parameter, we also want to get a lower or an upper bound or both, for the real-valued parameter. Here two limits are computed from the set of observations, say t_1 and t_2 and it is claimed with a certain degree of confidence (measured in probabilistic terms) that the true value of $\gamma(\theta)$ lies between t_1 and t_2. Thus we get an interval (t_1, t_2) which we expect would include the true value of $\gamma(\theta)$. So this type of estimation is called intervalestimation. In this chapter we discuss the problem of interval estimation.

5.2 Confidence Interval

An interval depending on a random variable X is called a random interval. For example, (X, $2X$) is a random interval. Note that, $\frac{1}{2} \leq X \leq 1 \Leftrightarrow X \leq 1 \leq 2X$.

P.K. Sahu et al., *Estimation and Inferential Statistics*,
DOI 10.1007/978-81-322-2514-0_5

A confidence interval (CI) of θ is a random interval which covers the true value of the parameter θ with specified degrees of confidence (assurance). In other words, a random interval $I(X) = [\underline{\theta}(X), \overline{\theta}(X)]$ satisfying

$$\Pr_\theta\left\{\theta \in I\left(\underset{\sim}{X}\right)\right\} \geq 1 - \alpha \forall \theta \in \Theta \tag{7.1}$$

will be a confidence interval for θ at confidence level $(1 - \alpha)$. If equality in (7.1) holds then $(1 - \alpha)$ will be called confidence coefficient. $\underline{\theta}(X)$ and $\overline{\theta}(X)$ are the lower and upper confidence limits respectively.

Let $I(X) = [\underline{\theta}(X), \infty]$ be a random interval such that $\Pr_\theta\{\theta \in I(X)\} = \Pr_\theta\{\theta \geq \underline{\theta}(X)\} \geq 1 - \alpha \forall \theta \in \Theta$. Then $\underline{\theta}(X)$ is called the lower confidence bound of θ at confidence level $(1 - \alpha)$. Similarly we can define upper confidence bound $\overline{\theta}(X)$ such that $\Pr_\theta\{\theta \in I(X)\} = \Pr_\theta\{\theta \leq \overline{\theta}(X)\} \geq 1 - \alpha \forall \theta \in \Theta$, corresponding to a random interval $I(X) = [-\alpha, \overline{\theta}(X)]$.

Remark 1 In making the probability statement we do not mean θ is a random variable. Indeed, θ is a constant. All that is meant here is that the probability is $(1 - \alpha)$ that the random interval $[\underline{\theta}(X), \overline{\theta}(X)]$ will cover θ whatever the true value of θ may be. More specifically, it is asserted that about $100(1 - \alpha)\%$ statements of the form $\theta \in [\underline{\theta}(X), \overline{\theta}(X)]$ should be correct.

Remark 2 In thepoint estimation, we choose an estimate, say $\widehat{\theta}(x)$, on the basis of a sample $\underset{\sim}{x}$ such that the difference $\left|\widehat{\theta}\left(\underset{\sim}{x}\right) - \theta\right|$ is small with high probability. In other words, in the point estimator we try to choose a unique point in the parameter space which can reasonably be considered as the true value of theparameter. On the other hand, in the interval estimation, we choose a subset of the parameter space, say $I\left(\underset{\sim}{x}\right)$, on the basis of a sample $\underset{\sim}{x}$ which reasonably includes the true value of the parameter. More specifically in interval estimation, we choose an interval $I\left(\underset{\sim}{x}\right)$, such that

$$\Pr_\theta\left\{\theta \in I\left(\underset{\sim}{x}\right)\right\} \geq 1 - \alpha \quad \forall \theta.$$

5.3 Construction of Confidence Interval

Method I

A simple procedure for finding a confidence interval

Let T be a statistic and $\Psi(T, \theta)$ be a function of T and θ. Suppose the distribution of $\Psi(T, \theta)$ is free from θ. Then it is always possible to choose two constants K_1 and K_2 $(K_1 \leq K_2)$ such that

$\Pr\{\psi(T,\theta) < K_1\} < \alpha_1$ and $\Pr\{\psi(T,\theta) > K_2\} < \alpha_2$ where $\alpha_1, \alpha_2 > 0$ and $\alpha_1 + \alpha_2 = \alpha$.

Hence $\Pr\{K_1 \le \psi(T,\theta) \le K_2\} \ge 1 - (\alpha_1 + \alpha_2) = 1 - \alpha$.

Suppose it is possible to convert the inequality $K_1 \le \psi(T,\theta) \le K_2$ into the form $\underline{\theta}(T) \le \theta \le \overline{\theta}(T)$.

Then $\Pr\{\underline{\theta}(T) \le \theta \le \overline{\theta}(T)\} \ge 1 - \alpha$. This fact gives us a $(1-\alpha)$ level confidence interval for θ.

Example 5.1 Let $X_1, X_2, \ldots, X_n$ be a random sample form $N(\mu, \sigma^2)$. Find $(1-\alpha)$ level confidence interval for μ when (i) σ^2 is known and (ii) when σ^2 is unknown.

Solution (i) Suppose σ^2 is known.

We take $\psi(T,\theta) = \frac{\sqrt{n}(\bar{x}-\mu)}{\sigma}$ which is an $N(0,1)$ variate. Hence the distribution of $\psi(T,\theta)$ is independent of θ. We can choose k_1 and k_2 from $N(0,1)$ such that

$$P\left[\tau_{1-\alpha_1} \le \frac{\sqrt{n}(\bar{x}-\mu)}{\sigma} \le \tau_{\alpha_2}\right] = 1 - (\alpha_1 + \alpha_2) = 1 - \alpha$$

So, $\left[\bar{x} - \tau_{\alpha_2}\frac{\sigma}{\sqrt{n}}, \bar{x} - \tau_{1-\alpha_1}\frac{\sigma}{\sqrt{n}}\right]$ is a $(1-\alpha)$ level confidence interval for μ if σ is known.

(ii) Suppose σ^2 is unknown:

We take $\psi(T,\theta) = \frac{\sqrt{n}(\bar{x}-\mu)}{s}$ which is student's t statistic with d.f $(n-1)$ where $s^2 = \frac{1}{n-1}\sum(x_i - \bar{x})^2$. The distribution of $\psi(T,\theta)$ is independent of θ. Again we choose k_1 and k_2 using a t-distribution with $(n-1)$ d.f such that

$$P\left[t_{n-1,1-\alpha_1} \le \frac{\sqrt{n}(\bar{x}-\mu)}{s} \le t_{n-1,\alpha_2}\right] = 1 - (\alpha_1 + \alpha_2) = 1 - \alpha$$

$$\Rightarrow P\left[\bar{x} - t_{n-1,\alpha_2}\frac{s}{\sqrt{n}} \le \mu \le \bar{x} - t_{n-1,1-\alpha_1}\frac{s}{\sqrt{n}}\right] = (1-\alpha).$$

So $\left[\bar{x} - t_{n-1,\alpha_2}\frac{s}{\sqrt{n}}, \bar{x} - t_{n-1,1-\alpha_1}\frac{s}{\sqrt{n}}\right]$ is a $(1-\alpha)$ level confidence interval for μ, if σ^2 is unknown.

Example 5.2 Let $X_1, X_2, \ldots, X_n$ be a random sample from $N(\mu, \sigma^2)$. Find $(1-\alpha)$ level confidence interval for σ^2 when (i) μ is known and (ii) μ is unknown.

Solution (i) Suppose μ is known.

We take $\psi(T,\theta) = \frac{\sum(x_i-\mu)^2}{\sigma^2}$ which is distributed as χ^2 with n d.f. Thus its distribution is independent of θ. We can choose k_1 and k_2 from χ^2 distribution with n d.f such that

$$P\left[\chi^2_{n,1-\alpha_1} \le \frac{\sum (x_i-\mu)^2}{\sigma^2} \le \chi^2_{n,\alpha_2}\right] = 1-(\alpha_1+\alpha_2) = 1-\alpha$$

$$\Rightarrow P\left[\frac{\sum (x_i-\mu)^2}{\chi^2_{n,\alpha_2}} \le \sigma^2 \le \frac{\sum (x_i-\mu)^2}{\chi^2_{n,1-\alpha_1}}\right] = 1-\alpha$$

Thus $\left(\frac{\sum (x_i-\mu)^2}{\chi^2_{n,\alpha_2}}, \frac{\sum (x_i-\mu)^2}{\chi^2_{n,1-\alpha_1}}\right)$ is 100(1 − α)% confidence interval of σ^2 when μ is known. (ii) Suppose μ is unknown.

We take the function $\psi(T,\theta) = \frac{\sum (x_i-\bar{x})^2}{\sigma^2}$ which is distributed as χ^2 with (n − 1) d.f. This distribution is independent of θ. Proceeding as in (i), $\left(\frac{\sum (x_i-\bar{x})^2}{\chi^2_{n-1,\alpha_2}}, \frac{\sum (x_i-\bar{x})^2}{\chi^2_{n-1,1-\alpha_1}}\right)$ is 100(1 − α)% confidence interval of σ^2 when μ is unknown.

Example 5.3 Let $X_1, X_2, \ldots, X_n$ be a random sample from density function $f(x|\theta) = \left(\frac{1}{\theta}\right)$, $0 < x < \theta$. Find 100(1 − α)% confidence interval of θ.

Solution The likelihood function is $L = \frac{1}{\theta^n}$. This is maximum when θ is the smallest; but θ cannot be less than $x_{(n)}$, the maximum of sample observations. Thus $\widehat{\theta} = x_{(n)}$.

The p.d.f of $\widehat{\theta}$ is given by

$$h\left(\widehat{\theta}\right) = \frac{n\widehat{\theta}^{\,n-1}}{\theta^n}, 0<\widehat{\theta}<\theta.$$

Let $u = \frac{x_{(n)}}{\theta} = \frac{\widehat{\theta}}{\theta}$. so that $g(u) = nu^{n-1}$, $0 < u < 1$.
Thus the distribution of u is independent of θ.
We find u_1 and u_2 such that

$$P[u_1 < u < u_2] = 1-(\alpha_1+\alpha_2) = 1-\alpha$$

where $\int_0^{u_1} g(u)du = \alpha_1$, $\int_{u_2}^{1} g(u)du = \alpha_2$

i.e. $P\left[u_1 < \frac{\widehat{\theta}}{\theta} < u_2\right] = 1-\alpha. \Rightarrow P\left[\frac{\widehat{\theta}}{u_2} < \theta < \frac{\widehat{\theta}}{u_1}\right] = 1-\alpha$

Thus, $\left(\frac{\max X_i}{u_2}, \frac{\max X_i}{u_1}\right)$ is a 100(1 − α)% confidence interval for θ.

Example 5.4 $X_1, X_2, \ldots, X_n$ is a random sample from a $G\left(\frac{1}{\theta}, 1\right)$ distribution having p.d.f.

$$f(x/\theta) = \frac{1}{\theta} e^{-x/\theta}, x \geq 0.$$

Find $100(1-\alpha)\%$ confidence interval of θ.

Solution Let $t = \frac{\sum_{i=1}^{n} x_i}{\theta} = \frac{n\bar{x}}{\theta}$ which is a $G(1,\ n)$ variate having p.d.f. $g(t) = \frac{1}{\Gamma(n)} e^{-t} t^{n-1}, 0 \leq t < \infty$.

Thus the distribution of t is independent of θ. We find k_1 and k_2 such that

$$P\left[k_1 < t = \frac{n\bar{x}}{\theta} < k_2\right] = 1 - (\alpha_1 + \alpha_2) = 1 - \alpha$$

where

$$\int_0^{k_1} g(t)dt = \alpha_1, \int_{k_2}^{\infty} g(t)dt = \alpha_2$$

i.e.

$$P\left[\frac{n\bar{x}}{k_2} < \theta < \frac{n\bar{x}}{k_1}\right] = 1 - \alpha$$

Method 2: Confidence based methods: A general approach:

Let T be a statistic and $t_1(\theta)$ and $t_2(\theta)$ be two quantities such that $\Pr\{T < t_1(\theta)\} < \alpha_1$ and $\Pr\{T > t_2(\theta)\} < \alpha_2,\ \alpha_1, \alpha_2 > 0,\ \alpha_1 + \alpha_2 = \alpha$. The equation $T = t_1(\theta)$ and $T = t_2(\theta)$ give us two curves as

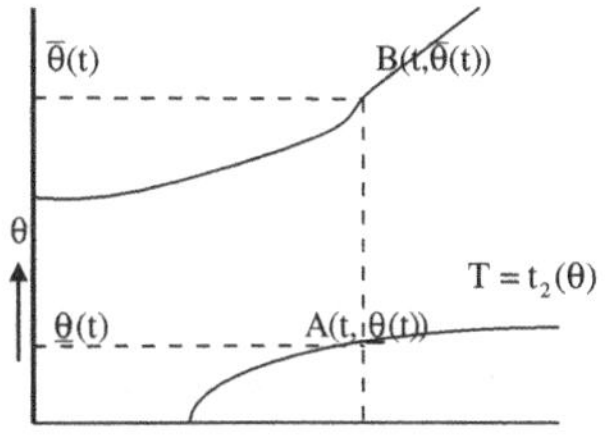

Suppose t be the observed value of the statistic T. Draw a perpendicular at $T = t$. It intersects the curves at A and B. Suppose the co-ordinates of A and B are $(t, \underline{\theta}(t))$ and $(t, \bar{\theta}(t))$ respectively. According to the construction

$$t_1(\theta) \leq T \leq t_2(\theta) \Leftrightarrow \underline{\theta}(t) \leq \theta \leq \bar{\theta}(t).$$

$$\therefore \Pr[t_1(\theta) \leq T \leq t_2(\theta)] = \Pr\{\underline{\theta}(t) \leq \theta \leq \bar{\theta}(T)\} \geq 1 - \alpha.$$

This fact gives us $(1-\alpha)$ level Confidence Interval for θ.

Note 1: To avoid the drawing one may consider inverse interpolation formula.
Note 2: If the L.H.S's of the Eq. (7.1) can be given explicit expression in terms of θ and if the equations can be solved for θ uniquely, then roots are the confidence limits for θ at confidence level $(1-\alpha)$.

Example 5.5 Let $X_1, X_2, \ldots, X_n$ be a random sample from density function $f(x|\theta) = \frac{1}{\theta}, 0<x<\theta$. Find $100(1-\alpha)\%$ confidence interval of θ.

Solution The likelihood function is $L = \frac{1}{\theta^n}$. This is maximum when θ is the smallest; but θ cannot be less than $x_{(n)}$, the maximum of sample observations. Thus $\widehat{\theta} = x_{(n)}$.

The p.d.f of $\widehat{\theta}$ is given by

$$h\left(\widehat{\theta}\right) = \frac{n\widehat{\theta}^{n-1}}{\theta^n}, 0<\widehat{\theta}<\theta.$$

We find $k_1(\theta)$ and $k_2(\theta)$ such that

$$P\left[k_1(\theta)<\widehat{\theta}<k_2(\theta)\right] = 1-(\alpha_1+\alpha_2) = 1-\alpha$$

where

$$\int_0^{k_1(\theta)} h\left(\hat{\theta}\right) d\hat{\theta} = \alpha_1 \tag{7.2}$$

and

$$\int_{k_2(\theta)}^{\theta} h\left(\hat{\theta}\right) d\hat{\theta} = \alpha_2 \tag{7.3}$$

From (7.2), $\left.\frac{\hat{\theta}^n}{\theta^n}\right]_0^{k_1(\theta)} = \alpha_1$ or, $k_1(\theta) = \theta(\alpha_1)^{1/n}$
From (7.3), $\left.\frac{\hat{\theta}^n}{\theta^n}\right]_{k_2(\theta)}^{\theta} = \alpha_2$ or, $1-\frac{[k_2(\theta)]^n}{\theta^n} = \alpha_2$ or, $k_2(\theta) = \theta(1-\alpha_2)^{1/n}$. Therefore, $\mathrm{P}\left[\theta\alpha_1^{1/n}<\widehat{\theta}<\theta(1-\alpha_2)^{1/n}\right] = 1-\alpha$ or, $P\left[\frac{\hat{\theta}}{(1-\alpha_2)^{1/n}}<\theta<\frac{\hat{\theta}}{(\alpha_1)^{1/n}}\right] = 1-\alpha$.

Note We can get the confidence interval of θ by the Method I which is given in Example 5.3.

Large sample confidence interval: Let the asymptotic distribution of a statistic T_n be normal with mean θ and variance $\frac{\sigma^2(\theta)}{n}$, then $\Pr\left\{\tau_{1-\alpha_1} \le \frac{(T_n-\theta)\sqrt{n}}{\sigma(\theta)} \le \tau_{\alpha_2}\right\} \simeq 1-\overline{\alpha_1+\alpha_2} = 1-\alpha$ (say).

This fact gives us a confidence interval for θ at confidence level $(1-\alpha)$ approximately.

Example 5.6 $X_1, X_2, \ldots, X_n$ is a large random sample from $P(\lambda)$. Find the $100(1-\alpha)\%$ confidence interval for λ.

Solution Likelihood function is $L = \frac{e^{-n\lambda}\lambda^{\sum x_i}}{x_1!x_2!.....x_n!}$

MLE of $\lambda = \widehat{\lambda} = \bar{x}$

$$V\left(\widehat{\lambda}\right) = \frac{1}{-E\left(\frac{\partial^2 \log L}{\partial \lambda^2}\right)} = \frac{\lambda}{n}$$

Thus, $\frac{\bar{x}-\lambda}{\sqrt{\lambda/n}} \to N(0,1)$ as $n \to \infty$

Hence $P\left[\tau_{1-\alpha_1} < \frac{\bar{x}-\lambda}{\sqrt{\lambda/n}} < \tau_{\alpha_2}\right] = 1-(\alpha_1+\alpha_2) = 1-\alpha$

$$\Rightarrow P\left[\bar{x} - \tau_{\alpha_2}\sqrt{\bar{x}/n} < \mu < \bar{x} - \tau_{1-\alpha_1}\sqrt{\bar{x}/n}\right] = 1-\alpha$$

using the approximation $\lambda = \hat{\lambda} = \bar{x}$ in the denominator. So $100(1-\alpha)\%$ confidence interval for λ is from $\bar{x} - \tau_{\alpha_2}\sqrt{\bar{x}/n}$ to $\bar{x} - \tau_{1-\alpha_1}\sqrt{\bar{x}/n}$.

Method 3 Method based on Chebysheff's inequality:

By Chebysheff's inequality, $\Pr[|T - E(T)| \leq \varepsilon\sigma_T] > 1 - \frac{1}{\varepsilon^2}$. Now setting $1 - \frac{1}{\varepsilon^2} = 1 - \alpha$, we can construct confidence interval.

Example 5.7 Consider the problem of Example 5.3. Find the $100(1-\alpha)\%$ confidence interval of θ by using the method of Chebysheff's inequality.

Solution

We have $E\left(\widehat{\theta}\right) = \frac{n}{n+1}\theta$ and $E\left(\widehat{\theta}-\theta\right)^2 = \theta^2\frac{2}{(n+1)(n+2)}$

By applying Chebysheff's inequality we get

$$P\left[\frac{\left|\widehat{\theta}-\theta\right|}{\theta}\sqrt{\frac{(n+1)(n+2)}{2}} < \epsilon\right] > 1 - \frac{1}{\epsilon^2}.$$

Since $\widehat{\theta} \xrightarrow{p} \theta$, we replace θ by $\widehat{\theta}$ and for moderately large n,

$$P\left[\frac{\left|\widehat{\theta}-\theta\right|}{\widehat{\theta}}\sqrt{\frac{(n+1)(n+2)}{2}} < \epsilon\right] > 1 - \frac{1}{\epsilon^2}.$$

Choosing $1 - \frac{1}{\epsilon^2} = 1 - \alpha$ or $\epsilon = \frac{1}{\sqrt{\alpha}}$. we have

$$P\left[\widehat{\theta}-\frac{1}{\sqrt{\alpha}}\widehat{\theta}\frac{\sqrt{2}}{\sqrt{(n+1)(n+2)}}<\theta<\widehat{\theta}+\frac{1}{\sqrt{\alpha}}\widehat{\theta}\frac{\sqrt{2}}{\sqrt{(n+1)(n+2)}}\right]>1-\alpha$$

Again $\frac{1}{\sqrt{(n+1)(n+2)}}\simeq\frac{1}{n}$ for large n and the fact that $\widehat{\theta}\leq\theta$, we have $P\left[\widehat{\theta}<\theta<\widehat{\theta}\left(1+\frac{1}{n}\sqrt{\frac{2}{\alpha}}\right)\right]>1-\alpha$. Thus $\left(\widehat{\theta}=\max x_i,\quad \max x_i\left(1+\frac{1}{n}\sqrt{\frac{2}{\alpha}}\right)\right)$ is an approximate $1-\alpha$ level confidence interval for θ.

5.4 Shortest Length Confidence Interval and Neyman's Criterion

From the above discussion, it is clear that $(1-\alpha)$ level C.I is not unique. In fact, infinite number of C.I's can be constructed by simple method [Because the equation $\alpha_1+\alpha_2=\alpha$, $\alpha_1\geq 0$, $\alpha_2\geq 0$ has infinite number of solution for (α_1,α_2)]. Again for different choice of statistic, we get different confidence intervals. For example, in r.s. from

$$f(x,\theta)=\frac{1}{\theta}e^{-\frac{x}{\theta}},0<x<\infty$$

$\left[\frac{2\sum X_i}{\chi^2_{2n,\alpha}}\right]$ is a $(1-\alpha)$ level lower confidence bound for θ

[As $\frac{2X}{\theta}\sim{\chi^2}_2\Rightarrow\frac{2\sum X_i}{\theta}\sim{\chi^2}_{2n}$ since M.g.f. of $X=(1-t\theta)^{-1}\Rightarrow$ M.g.f of $\frac{2X}{\theta}=(1-2t)^{-1}=$ M.g.f. of ${\chi^2}_2$].

On the other hand, $a(1-\alpha)$ level confidence bound for θ based on $X_{(1)}=\min\limits_i X_i$ is $\frac{2nX_{(1)}}{\chi^2_{2,\alpha}}$.

So we need some optimality criteria to choose one of the $(1-\alpha)$ level confidence intervals.

1. Shortest length confidence interval [Wilk's criterion]

A $(1-\alpha)$ level confidence interval $I(\theta)=\left[\underline{\theta}(T),\bar{\theta}(T)\right]$ based on T will be of shortest length if the inequality

$\bar{\theta}(T)-\underline{\theta}(T)\leq\bar{\theta}^*(T)-\underline{\theta}^*(T)$, for all θ holds for every other $(1-\alpha)$ level C.I. $\left[\underline{\theta}^*(T),\bar{\theta}^*(T)\right]$ based on the same statistic T.

Example 5.8 On the basis of an r.s. from $N(\mu,\sigma^2)$, σ^2 being unknown, a $(1-\alpha)$ level C.I. for μ based on $\bar{X}$ is given by

$\left[\bar{X}-\tau_{\alpha_2}\frac{\sigma}{\sqrt{n}},\bar{X}-\tau_{1-\alpha_1}\frac{\sigma}{\sqrt{n}}\right]$, $\alpha_1,\alpha_2\geq 0$ and $\alpha_1+\alpha_2=\alpha$. The length of the interval is $\left(\tau_{\alpha_2}-\tau_{1-\alpha_1}\right)\frac{\sigma}{\sqrt{n}}$.

To find the shortest length confidence interval, we minimize $(\tau_{\alpha 2} - \tau_{1-\alpha_1})$ subject to $\alpha_1 + \alpha_2 = \alpha$; $\alpha_1, \alpha_2 \geq 0$.

Owing to the symmetry of the distribution $\frac{\sqrt{n}(\bar{x}-\mu)}{\sigma}$ about '0', the quantity $\tau_{\alpha 2} - \tau_{1-\alpha_1}$ will be a minimum when $\tau_{\alpha/2} = -\tau_{1-\alpha_1}$, i.e., when $\alpha_1 = \alpha_2 = \alpha/2$. Thus the shortest length $(1-\alpha)$ level C.I. for μ based on $\bar{x}$ is $\left[\bar{x} - \tau_{\alpha/2}\frac{\sigma}{\sqrt{n}}, \bar{x} + \tau_{\alpha/2}\frac{\sigma}{\sqrt{n}}\right]$.

Remarks Occasionally, the length of a C.I is a random quantity. In this case, we minimize its expected length. e.g. In random sampling from $N(\mu, \sigma^2)$, (both μ and σ^2 are unknown), a $(1-\alpha)$ level C.I for μ is given by $\left[\bar{X} - t_{\alpha_2, \overline{n-1}}\frac{s}{\sqrt{n}}, \bar{X} - t_{1-\alpha_1, \overline{n-1}}\frac{s}{\sqrt{n}}\right]$. This length of the C.I is $\left[t_{\alpha_2, \overline{n-1}} - t_{1-\alpha_1, \overline{n-1}}\right]\frac{s}{\sqrt{n}}$. which is a random quantity.

So, to find the shortest (expected) length C.I, we minimize $\left[t_{\alpha_2, \overline{n-1}} - t_{1-\alpha_1, \overline{n-1}}\right]\frac{E(s)}{\sqrt{n}}$ subject to $\alpha_1, \alpha_2 \geq 0$ and $\alpha_1 + \alpha_2 = \alpha$. Owing to the symmetry of t_{n-1} distribution about '0', the minimum is attained at $\alpha_1 = \alpha_2 = \alpha/2$. Therefore the required shortest expected length confidence interval is $\left[\bar{X} - t_{\alpha/2, \overline{n-1}}\frac{s}{\sqrt{n}}, \bar{X} + t_{\alpha/2, \overline{n-1}}\frac{s}{\sqrt{n}}\right]$.

Example 5.9 Consider the problem discussed in Example 5.2. On the basis of a random sample from $N(\mu, \sigma^2)$, μ being known, a $(1-\alpha)$ level CI for σ^2 is given by $\left[\frac{\sum (x_i-\mu)^2}{\chi^2_{n,\alpha_2}}, \frac{\sum (x_i-\mu)^2}{\chi^2_{n,1-\alpha_1}}\right]$, $\alpha_1, \alpha_2 \geq 0$ and $\alpha_1 + \alpha_2 = \alpha$. The length of the interval is $\left[\frac{1}{\chi^2_{n,1-\alpha_1}} - \frac{1}{\chi^2_{n,\alpha_2}}\right]\sum (X_i - \mu)^2$ which has the expected value

$$\left[\frac{1}{\chi^2_{n,1-\alpha_1}} - \frac{1}{\chi^2_{n,\alpha_2}}\right]n\sigma^2.$$

We wish to minimize $\left[\frac{1}{\chi^2_{n,1-\alpha_1}} - \frac{1}{\chi^2_{n,\alpha_2}}\right]$,

subject to $\int\limits_{\chi_1^2}^{\chi_2^2} f(\chi^2)d\chi^2 = 1-\alpha$, where $\chi_1^2 = \chi^2_{n,1-\alpha_1}$, $\chi_2^2 = \chi^2_{n,\alpha_2}$ and $f(\chi^2)$ is the p.d.f. of a chi-square r.v. with n d.f.

Now let $\phi = \frac{1}{\chi_1^2} - \frac{1}{\chi_2^2} + \lambda\left[\int\limits_{\chi_1^2}^{\chi_2^2} f(\chi^2)d\chi^2 - (1-\alpha)\right]$

where λ is a Lagrangian multiplier. We get

$$\frac{\delta\phi}{\delta\chi_1^2} = -\frac{1}{\chi_1^4} - \lambda f\left(\chi_1^2\right) = 0$$

$$\frac{\delta\phi}{\delta\chi_2^2} = \frac{1}{\chi_2^4} + \lambda f\left(\chi_2^2\right) = 0$$

$$\therefore \lambda = \frac{-1}{\chi_1^4 f\left(\chi_1^2\right)} = -\frac{1}{\chi_2^4 f\left(\chi_2^2\right)}$$

Hence χ_1^2 and χ_2^2 are such that the equation

$$\chi_1^4 f\left(\chi_1^2\right) = \chi_2^4 f\left(\chi_2^2\right) \text{ is to be satisfied and } \int_{\chi_1^2}^{\chi_2^2} f(\chi^2)d\chi^2 = 1 - \alpha.$$

It is very difficult to find the actual values of χ_1^2 and χ_2^2. In practice, the equal tails interval, $\left[\frac{\sum (x_i-\mu)^2}{\chi^2_{n,\alpha/2}}, \frac{\sum (x_i-\mu)^2}{\chi^2_{n,1-\alpha/2}}\right]$, is used.

Similarly if μ is unknown, the equal tail confidence interval, $\left[\frac{\sum (x_i-\bar{x})^2}{\chi^2_{n-1,\alpha/2}}, \frac{\sum (x_i-\bar{x})^2}{\chi^2_{n-1,1-\alpha/2}}\right]$, is employed.

Example 5.10 Consider the problem discussed in Example in 5.3. A $(1 - \alpha)$ level C.I. for θ is given by $\left(\frac{\max x_i}{u_2}, \frac{\max x_i}{u_1}\right)$; $\alpha_1, \alpha_2 \geq 0$, $\alpha_1 + \alpha_2 = \alpha$. The length L of the interval is $\left(\frac{1}{u_1} - \frac{1}{u_2}\right)\max x_i$.

We minimize L subject to

$$\int_{u_1}^{u_2} nu^{n-1}du = u_2^n - u_1^n = 1 - \alpha$$

This implies $1 - \alpha < u_2^n$

$$\Rightarrow (1 - \alpha)^{1/n} < u_2 \leq 1$$

and

$$\begin{aligned}\frac{\delta L}{\delta u_2} &= \max x_i\left(\frac{\delta L}{\delta u_1}\frac{\delta u_1}{\delta u_2}+\frac{1}{u_2^2}\right)\\ &= \max x_i\left(-\frac{1}{u_1^2}\frac{nu_2^{n-1}}{nu_1^{n-1}}+\frac{1}{u_2^2}\right)\\ &= \max x_i\frac{u_1^{n+1}-u_2^{n+1}}{u_2^2u_1^{n+1}}<0,\end{aligned}$$

so that the minimum occurs at $u_2 = 1$. When $u_2 = 1$, $u_1 = \alpha^{1/n}$. Thus a $1-\alpha$ level confidence interval is given by $\left(\max x_i, \max x_i \big/ \alpha^{1/n}\right)$. This confidence interval has the smallest length among all confidence intervals for θ based on $\max x_i$

2. Neyman's criterion

Let $I_1(X)$ and $I_2(X)$ be two $(1-\alpha)$ levelconfidence intervals for θ. $I_1(X)$ will be accurate (or shorter) than $I_2(X)$ if

$$P_{\theta'}\{\theta \in I_1(X)\} \le P_{\theta'}\{\theta \in I_2(X)\}\forall\theta,\theta' \in \Theta, \theta \ne \theta'(\theta' = \text{true value})$$

A $(1-\alpha)$ level C.I. $I(X)$ is said to be most accurate (UMA) (or shortest) if $P_{\theta'}\{\theta \in I(X)\} \le P_{\theta'}\{\theta \in I^*(X)\}\forall\theta,\theta' \in \Theta, \theta \ne \theta'$ for any other $(1-\alpha)$ level C.I. $I^*(X)$.

A $(1-\alpha)$ level C.I. $I(X)$ is said to be unbiased if,

$$P_{\theta'}\{\theta \in I(X)\} \le 1-\alpha = P_{\theta'}\{\theta' \in I(X)\}\forall\theta,\theta' \in \Theta, \theta \ne \theta'$$

i.e. Probability (containing wrong value of θ) ≤ Probability (containing true value of θ).

Implication An unbiased confidence interval includes true value more often than it does contain wrong value.

A $(1-\alpha)$ level unbiased C.I. $I(X)$ is said to be most accurate amongst the class of unbiased $(1-\alpha)$ level if $P_{\theta'}\{\theta \in I(X)\} \le P_{\theta'}\{\theta \in I^*(X)\}\forall\theta,\theta' \in \Theta,\theta \ne \theta'$ for any other $(1-\alpha)$ level unbiased C.I. $I^*(X)$

Relation between non randomized test and confidence interval

Theorem 5.1 *Suppose* $A(\theta_0)$ *denoted the acceptance region of a level* α *test for testing* $H_0 : \theta = \theta_0$

Define $S\left(\underset{\sim}{x}\right) = \left\{\theta / \underset{\sim}{x} \in A(\theta)\right\}$

Then $S\left(\underset{\sim}{x}\right)$ *will be a* $(1-\alpha)$ *level confidence interval* for θ.

Proof By the construction of $S\left(\underset{\sim}{x}\right)$, we have

$$\underset{\sim}{x} \in A(\theta) \Leftrightarrow \theta \in S\left(\underset{\sim}{x}\right)$$

$$\therefore P_\theta\left\{\theta \in S\left(\underset{\sim}{x}\right)\right\} = P_\theta\left\{\underset{\sim}{x} \in A(\theta)\right\} \geq 1 - \alpha \forall \theta.$$

Note The implication of this theorem is that for a fixed $\underset{\sim}{x}$, the confidence region $S\left(\underset{\sim}{x}\right)$ is that set of values θ_0 for which the hypothesis $H_0 : \theta = \theta_0$ is accepted when $\underset{\sim}{x}$ is the observed value of $\underset{\sim}{x}$

Theorem 5.2 *Let* $S\left(\underset{\sim}{x}\right)$ *be a* $(1 - \alpha)$ *level confidence interval for* θ. *Define* $A(\theta) = \left\{\underset{\sim}{x}/\theta \in S\left(\underset{\sim}{x}\right)\right\}$. *Then* $A(\theta_0)$ *will be an acceptance region of a level* α *non-randomized test for testing* $H_0 : \theta = \theta_0$.

Proof By the construction of $A(\theta)$, we have

$$\underset{\sim}{x} \in A(\theta) \Leftrightarrow \theta \in S\left(\underset{\sim}{x}\right)$$

$$\therefore P_\theta\left\{\underset{\sim}{x} \in A(\theta)\right\} = P_\theta\left\{\theta \in S\left(\underset{\sim}{x}\right)\right\} \geq 1 - \alpha \forall \theta.$$

Relation between UMP non-randomized test and UMA confidence interval

Theorem 5.3 *Suppose* $A(\theta_0)$ *denoted the acceptance region of an UMP, level-*α *non-randomized test for testing* $H_0 : \theta = \theta_0$. *Define* $S\left(\underset{\sim}{x}\right) = \left\{\theta/\underset{\sim}{x} \in A(\theta)\right\}$. *Then* $S\left(\underset{\sim}{x}\right)$ *will be an UMA* $(1 - \alpha)$ *level confidence interval for* θ.

Proof By Theorem 5.1, it is clear that the level of set $S\left(\underset{\sim}{x}\right)$ is $(1 - \alpha)$.

Consider another acceptance region $A^*(\theta_0)$ of a level α non-randomized test for testing $H_0 : \theta = \theta_0$

Let $S^*\left(\underset{\sim}{x}\right) = \left\{\theta/\underset{\sim}{x} \in A^*(\theta)\right\}$, then the level of $S^*\left(\underset{\sim}{x}\right)$ is also $(1 - \alpha)$.

Since $A(\theta)$ is the acceptance region of a UMP non-randomized test, we can write,

$$P_{\theta_0}\left\{\underset{\sim}{x} \in A(\theta)\right\} \leq P_{\theta_0}\left\{\underset{\sim}{x} \in A^*(\theta)\right\} \quad (\theta \neq \theta_0)$$

$$\therefore P_{\theta_0}\left\{\theta \in S\left(\underset{\sim}{x}\right)\right\} \leq P_{\theta_0}\left\{\theta \in S^*\left(\underset{\sim}{x}\right)\right\} \forall (\theta \neq \theta_0) \theta, \theta_0 \in \Theta$$

Since $S^*\left(\underset{\sim}{x}\right)$ is arbitrary the proof follows immediately.

Theorem 5.4 *Let* $S\left(\underset{\sim}{x}\right)$ *be an UMA* $(1-\alpha)$ *level confidence interval* for θ. *Define* $A(\theta)=\left\{\underset{\sim}{x}/\theta\in S\left(\underset{\sim}{x}\right)\right\}$. *Then* $A(\theta_0)$ *will be an acceptance region of a level-*α *UMP test for testing* $H_0:\theta=\theta_0$.

Proof According to the construction of $A(\theta)$, $A(\theta_0)$ will be the acceptance region of a level-α non-randomized test for testing $H_0:\theta=\theta_0$.

Now corresponding to another $(1-\alpha)$ level C.I. $S^*\left(\underset{\sim}{x}\right)$,

$$\text{let}\, A^*(\theta)=\left\{\underset{\sim}{x}:\theta\in S^*\left(\underset{\sim}{x}\right)\right\}.$$

Then $A^*(\theta_0)$ will be also an acceptance region of a level-α non-randomized test for testing $H_0:\theta=\theta_0$

Now since $S\left(\underset{\sim}{x}\right)$ is an UMA $(1-\alpha)$ level C.I. for θ,

$$P_{\theta_0}\left\{\theta\in S\left(\underset{\sim}{x}\right)\right\}\le P_{\theta_0}\left\{\theta\in S^*\left(\underset{\sim}{x}\right)\right\}\forall(\theta\neq\theta_0)\theta,\theta_0\in\Theta,\ \theta\neq\theta_0$$

$$\Rightarrow P_{\theta_0}\left\{\underset{\sim}{x}\in A(\theta)\right\}\le P_{\theta_0}\left\{\underset{\sim}{x}\in A^*(\theta)\right\}$$

which implies that $A(\theta_0)$ will be the acceptance region of level-α UMP non-randomized test for testing $H_0:\theta=\theta_0$, since $A^*(\theta)$ is arbitrary.

Relation between UMPU non-randomized test and UMAU confidence interval

Theorem 3.5 *Let* $A(\theta_0)$ *be the acceptance region of an UMPU level-*α *non-randomized test for testing* $H_0:\theta=\theta_0$. *Define* $S\left(\underset{\sim}{x}\right)=\left\{\theta/\underset{\sim}{x}\in A(\theta)\right\}$. *Then* $S\left(\underset{\sim}{x}\right)$ *will be an UMAU* $(1-\alpha)$ *level confidence interval* for θ.

Proof According to construction of $S\left(\underset{\sim}{x}\right)$ it will be a $(1-\alpha)$ level Confidence Interval for θ. Let $S^*\left(\underset{\sim}{x}\right)=\left\{\theta/\underset{\sim}{x}\in A^*(\theta)\right\}$ corresponding to any other acceptance region $A^*(\theta_0)$ of a level-α non-randomized test for testing $H_0:\theta=\theta_0$.

Now since $A(\theta_0)$ is the acceptance region of a level-α UMPU non-randomized testfor testing $H_0:\theta=\theta_0$

$$P_{\theta_0}\left\{\underset{\sim}{x}\in A(\theta)\right\}\le P_{\theta_0}\left\{\underset{\sim}{x}\in A^*(\theta_0)\right\}\le 1-\alpha\forall\theta,\theta_0\in\Theta,\ \theta\neq\theta_0$$

$$\Rightarrow P_{\theta_0}\left\{\theta\in S\left(\underset{\sim}{x}\right)\right\}\le P_{\theta_0}\left\{\theta\in S^*\left(\underset{\sim}{x}\right)\right\}\le 1-\alpha$$

i.e., $S\left(\underset{\sim}{x}\right)$ is a UMAU $(1-\alpha)$ level C.I. for θ, since $A^*(\theta_0)$ is arbitrary.

Theorem 5.6 *Let $S\left(\underset{\sim}{x}\right)$ be an UMAU $(1-\alpha)$ level confidence interval for θ. Define $A(\theta)=\left\{\underset{\sim}{x}/\theta \in S\left(\underset{\sim}{x}\right)\right\}$. Then $A(\theta_0)$ will be an acceptance region of a level-α UMPU test for testing $H_0:\theta=\theta_0$.*

Proof According to the construction of $A(\theta)$, $A(\theta_0)$ will be the acceptance region of a level-α non-randomized test for testing $H_0:\theta=\theta_0$.

Now, corresponding to any other $(1-\alpha)$ level C.I. $S^*\left(\underset{\sim}{x}\right)$ for θ,

let $A^*(\theta)=\left\{\underset{\sim}{x}/\theta \in S^*\left(\underset{\sim}{x}\right)\right\}$, then $A^*(\theta)$ will also be an acceptance region of a level-α non-randomized test for testing $H_0:\theta=\theta_0$.

Since $S\left(\underset{\sim}{x}\right)$ is UMAU $(1-\alpha)$ level C.I.

$$\therefore P_{\theta_0}\left\{\theta \in S\left(\underset{\sim}{x}\right)\right\} \le P_{\theta_0}\left\{\theta \in S^*\left(\underset{\sim}{x}\right)\right\} \le 1-\alpha \forall \theta, \theta_0 \in \Theta,\ \theta \ne \theta_0$$

$$\Rightarrow P_{\theta_0}\left\{\underset{\sim}{x} \in A(\theta)\right\} \le P_{\theta_0}\left\{\underset{\sim}{x} \in A^*(\theta_0)\right\} \le 1-\alpha$$

i.e. $A(\theta_0)$ will be an acceptance region of a level-α UMPU test for testing $H_0:\theta=\theta_0$.

Example 5.11 Let $X_1, X_2, \ldots, X_n$ be a r.s. from $R(0,\theta)$. The UMP level-α non-randomized test for testing $H_0:\theta=\theta_0$ against $\theta \ne \theta_0$ is given by the critical region $x_{(n)} > \theta_0$ or $x_{(n)} \le \theta_0 \sqrt[n]{\alpha}$.

$$\text{Let } A(\theta)=\left\{\underset{\sim}{x}\middle|\theta\sqrt[n]{\alpha}<x_{(n)} \le \theta\right\}$$

$$\begin{aligned}\text{Define } S\left(\underset{\sim}{x}\right) &= \left\{\theta \middle| \underset{\sim}{x} \in A(\theta)\right\}\\ &= \left\{\theta|\theta\sqrt[n]{\alpha}<x_{(n)} \le \theta\right\}\\ &= \left\{\theta|x_{(n)} \le \theta < \frac{x_{(n)}}{\sqrt[n]{\alpha}}\right\}\end{aligned}$$

Thus, by Theorem 5.3, $S(x)=\left\{\theta|x_{(n)} \le \theta < \frac{x_{(n)}}{\sqrt[n]{\alpha}}\right\}$ will be a $(1-\alpha)$ level UMA confidence interval for θ.

Chapter 6
Non-parametric Test

6.1 Introduction

In parametric tests we generally assume a particular form of the population distribution (say, normal distribution) from which a random sample is drawn and we try to construct a test criterion (for testing hypothesis regarding parameter of the population) and the distribution of the test criterion depends upon the parent population.

In non-parametric tests the form of the parent population is unknown. We only assume that the population, from which a random sample is drawn, is continuous and try to develop a test criterion whose distribution is independent of the population distribution under the hypothesis under consideration. A non-parametric test is concerned with the form of the population but not with any parametric value.

A test procedure is said to be distribution free if the statistic used has a distribution which does not depend upon the form of the distribution of the parent population from which the sample is drawn. So in such procedure assumptions regarding the population are not necessary.

Note Sometimes the term 'distribution free' is used instead of non-parametric. But we should make some distinction between them.

In fact, the terms 'distribution free' and 'non-parametric' are not synonymous. The term 'distribution free' is used to indicate the nature of the distribution of the test statistic whereas the term 'non-parametric' is used to indicate the type of hypothesis problem investigated.

Advantages and disadvantages of non-parametric method over parametric method

Advantages

(i) Non-parametric methods are readily comprehensible, very simple and easy to apply and do not require complicated sample theory.

P.K. Sahu et al., *Estimation and Inferential Statistics*,
DOI 10.1007/978-81-322-2514-0_6

(ii) No assumption is made about the form of frequency function of the parent population from which the sample is drawn.
(iii) No parametric technique will be applicable to the data which are mere classification (i.e. which are measured in nominal scale), while non-parametric method exists to deal with such data.
(iv) Since the socio-economic data are not, in general, normally distributed, non-parametric tests have found applications in psychometry, sociology and educational statistics.
(v) Non-parametric tests are available to deal with data which are given in ranks or whose seemingly numerical scores have the strength of the ranks. For example, no parametric test can be applied if the scores are given in grades such as A, B, C, D, etc.

Disadvantages

(i) Non-parametric test can be used only if the measurements are nominal and ordinal. Even in that case, if a parametric test exists it is more powerful than the non-parametric test.
In other words, if all the assumptions of a statistical model are satisfied by the data and if the measurements are of required strength, then non-parametric tests are wasteful of time and data.
(ii) No non-parametric method exists for testing interactions in ANOVA model unless special assumptions about the additivity of the model are made.
(iii) Non-parametric tests are designed to test statistical hypothesis only but not for estimating parameters.

6.2 One-Sample Non-parametric Tests

In this section we consider the following one-sample non-parametric tests:

(i) Chi-square test
(ii) Kolmogorov–Smirnov test
(iii) Sign test
(iv) Wilcoxon signed-rank test
(v) Run test

6.2.1 Chi-Square Test (i.e Test for Goodness of Fit)

Let n sample observations are continuous measurements grouped in k class intervals or observations themselves are frequency of k mutually exclusive events

$A_1, A_2, \ldots, A_k$ such that $S = A_1 + A_2 + \cdots + A_k$ is the space of the variable under consideration. The form of the distribution is not known. We want to test $H_o: F(x) = F_0(x)$ against: $H_1: F(x) \neq F_0(x)$. Here $F_o(x)$ is specified with all its parameters.

Under H_0 we can obtain the probability (p_i) of a random observation from F_0 to belong in the ith class $A_i (i = 1, 2, \ldots k)$. The expected frequency in ith class is $e_i = np_i$ for $i = 1, 2, \ldots, k$. These are compared with the observed frequencies x_i. Pearson suggested the statistic.

$$\chi^2 = \sum_{i=1}^{k} \frac{(x_i - np_i)^2}{np_i}.$$

If the agreement between the observed (x_i) and expected frequencies (e_i) is close, then the differences $(x_i - np_i)$ will be small and consequently χ^2 will be small. Otherwise it will be large. The larger the value of χ^2 the more likely is that the observed frequencies did not come from the population under H_0. This means that the test is always right-sided. It can be shown that for large samples the sampling distribution of χ^2 under H_0 follows chi-square distribution with $(k - 1)$ d. f. The approximation holds good if every $e_i \geq 5$. In case there are some $e_i < 5$, we have to combine adjacent classes till the expected frequency in the combined class is at least 5. Then k will be the actual number of classes used in computing χ^2. Thus the null hypothesis H_0 is rejected if Cal $\chi^2 > \chi^2_{\alpha, k-1}$.

6.2.2 *Kolmogrov–Smirnov Test*

Let $X_1, X_2, \ldots, X_n$ be a sample from continuous distribution function $F(x)$. We are to test $H_0: F(x) = F_0(x) \,\forall\, x$ against $H_1: F(x) \neq F_0(x)$ for some x.

Suppose $F_n(x)$ is the sample (empirical) distribution function corresponding to any given x; that is, if the number of observation $\leq x$ is k, then

$$F_n(x) = \frac{k}{n}.$$

Test statistic under H_0 is given by

$$D_n = \operatorname*{Sup}_x |F_n(x) - F_0(x)|$$

which is known as **Kolmogorov–Smirnov statistic**.

The distribution of D_n does not depend on F_0 as long as F_0 is continuous. H_0 is rejected if $D_n > D_{n,\alpha}$.

Similarly, the one-sided KS statistics for one-sided alternatives are the following:

(i) for the alternative $H^+ : F(x) \geq F_0(x)\,\forall x$ the appropriate statistic is

$$D_n^+ = \underset{x}{\text{Sup}}[F_n(x) - F_0(x)]$$

(ii) for the alternative $H^- : F(x) \leq F_0(x)\,\forall x$ the appropriate statistic is

$$D_n^- = \underset{x}{\text{Sup}}[F_0(x) - F_n(x)]$$

The statistics D_n^+ and D_n^- have the same distribution because of symmetry. The test rejects H_0 if $D_n^+ > D_{n,\alpha}^+$ when alternative is $F(x) \geq F_0(x)\,\forall x$ and rejects H_0 if $D_n^- > D_{n,\alpha}^-$ when alternative is $F(x) \leq F_0(x)\,\forall x$ at the level α.

6.2.3 *Sign Test*

$F(x)$ is continuous distribution function of the parent population, which is continuous. $F(x)$ is unknown, from which we draw a random sample $(x_1, x_2, \ldots, x_n)$. We define $\zeta_p = p$th order population quantile.

$$\therefore \Pr\,[X \leq \xi_p] = p \text{ i.e. } \Pr\,[X - \xi_p \leq 0] = p.$$

Assumption $F(x)$ is continuous in the neighbourhood of ζ_p. To test $H_0 : \zeta_p = {\zeta_p}^0$.

Case 1 $H_1 : \xi_p > {\xi_p}^0$

To perform the test we consider the number of positive quantities among $(x_1 - {\xi_p}^0), (x_2 - {\xi_p}^0), \ldots, (x_n - {\xi_p}^0)$. Sample values equal to ${\xi_p}^0$ are ignored. Suppose S = total number of + signs, we note that, under H_0

$$\Pr[X - {\xi_p}^0 \leq 0] = p$$
$$\Rightarrow \Pr\left[X - {\xi_p}^0 > 0\right] = 1 - p = q, \text{ say.}$$

$\therefore$ Under $H_0, S \sim B(n, q)$

Also, under $H_1, \Pr\left[X \leq \xi_p^0\right] < p$, i.e. $\Pr\left[X - {\xi_p}^0 > 0\right] > q$. Suppose, under $H_1, \Pr\left[X - \xi_p^0 > 0\right] = q'$ where $q' > q$.

$\therefore$ Under $H_1,\ S \sim B(n, q')$ where $q' > q$.

Hence a large value of S indicates the rejection of H_0.

$$\text{So the test is } \phi(S) = \begin{cases} 1 & \text{if } \; S > s \\ a & \text{if } \; S = s \\ 0 & \text{if } \; S < s \end{cases}$$

where 's' and 'a' are such that

(I) $\Pr[S > s/H_0] < \alpha \leq \Pr[S \geq s/H_0]$
(II) $E_{H_0}\phi(S) = \alpha$

From (I) we get s and from (II) $\alpha = \Pr[S > s/H_0] + a\Pr[S = s/H_0]$

$$\Rightarrow a = \frac{\alpha - \Pr[S > s/H_0]}{\Pr[S = s/H_0]}.$$

Hence test is given by $S > s \Rightarrow$ Rejection of H_0
$S < s \Rightarrow$ Acceptance of H_0
$S = s \Rightarrow$ To draw a random number with probability of rejection 'a' and probability of acceptance $1 - a$.

Case 2

$$H_2 = \xi_p < \xi_p{}^0 \;\text{ or }\; \xi_p = \xi_p{}' < \xi_p{}^0$$

Under H_2

$$\Pr[X \leq \xi_p{}'] = p$$

$$\therefore \Pr[X \leq \xi_p{}^0] > p$$

or, $\Pr[X - \xi_p{}^0 \leq 0] > p$, i.e. $\Pr[X - \xi_p{}^0 > 0] < 1 - p = q$.

Suppose under $H_2, \Pr[X - \xi_p{}^0 > 0] = q'$ where $q' < q$.

$\therefore$ Under $H_2, S \sim B(n, q')$ where $q' < q$.

So a small value of S indicates the rejection of H_0.

$$\text{So our test is } \phi(S) = \begin{cases} 1 & \text{if } \; S < s \\ a & \text{if } \; S = s \\ 0 & \text{if } \; S > s \end{cases}$$

where 's' and 'a' are such that

$$\begin{aligned}&\Pr\left[S<s/H_0\right]<\alpha\leq \Pr\left[S\leq s/H_0\right] \text{ and } E_{H_0}\phi(S)=\alpha\\&\text{i.e. } \Pr\left[S<s/H_0\right]+a\Pr\left[S=s/H_0\right]=\alpha \text{ or,}\\&a=\frac{\alpha-\Pr\left[S<s/H_0\right]}{\Pr\left[S=s/H_0\right]}\end{aligned}$$

i.e. if $S<s\Rightarrow$ reject H_0

$S>s\Rightarrow$ accept H_0

$S=s\Rightarrow$ draw a random number with probability of rejection 'a' and probability of acceptance $(1-a)$.

Large sample test

Under $H_0, S\sim B(n,q)$

$\therefore$ under H_0 $\tau=\frac{S-nq}{\sqrt{npq}}\sim N(0,1)$

$$\therefore \omega_0:\tau<-\tau_\alpha$$

Case 3 $H_3:\xi_p\neq\xi_p{}^0$

Under $H_3, \Pr[X\leq\xi_p{}^0]\neq p\Rightarrow \Pr[X-\xi_p{}^0>0]\neq q$

Suppose under $H_3, \Pr[X-\xi_p{}^0>0]=q'$ where $q'\neq q$

$\therefore$ Under $H_3, S\sim B(n,q')$ where $q'\neq q$.

So a small or a large value of S indicates the rejection of H_0. Here the test is

$$\phi\,(S)=\begin{cases}1 & \text{if } S<s_1\\ a_1 & \text{if } S=s_1\\ 0 & \text{if } s_1<S<s_2\\ a_2 & \text{if } S=s_2\\ 1 & \text{if } S>s_2\end{cases}$$

where s_1 and s_2 are such that

$$\begin{aligned}&\Pr[S<s_1/H_0]<\alpha_1\leq\Pr[S\geq s_1/H_0],\\&\Pr\left[S>s_2/H_0\right]<\alpha_2\leq\Pr\left[S\geq s_2/H_0\right]\end{aligned}$$

and $\alpha_1+\alpha_2=\alpha$. For simplicity we take $\alpha_1+\alpha_2={}^{\alpha}/_{2}$.

'a_1' and 'a_2' are such that

$${}^{\alpha}/_{2}=\Pr\left[S<s_1/H_0\right]+a_1\Pr\left[S=s_1/H_0\right]$$

$$\Rightarrow a_1=\frac{\frac{\alpha}{2}-\Pr[S<s_1/H_0]}{\Pr[S=s_1]}$$

$$\frac{\alpha}{2} = \Pr\left[S > s_2/H_0\right] + a_2 \Pr\left[S = s_2/H_0\right]$$

$$\Rightarrow a_2 = \frac{\frac{\alpha}{2} - \Pr[S > s_2/H_0]}{\Pr[S = s_2/H_0]}$$

Thus, we reject H_0 if $S < s_1$ or $S > s_2$.
We accept H_0 if $s_1 < S < s_2$ and random or no conclusion if $S = s_1$ or $S = s_2$.
Large sample test: Under $H_0, S \sim B(n, q)$,
$\therefore$ under $H_0, \tau = \frac{S-nq}{\sqrt{npq}} \sim N(0,1)$

$$\omega_0 : |\tau| > \tau_{\frac{\alpha}{2}}.$$

Note $p = \frac{1}{2}, \xi_p = \xi_{\frac{1}{2}} = \text{median}$.

Under $H_0, S \sim B\left(n, \frac{1}{2}\right)$ and then S is symmetric about $\frac{n}{2}$. Therefore for two sided test in case of Case 3,
$\frac{n}{2} - s_1 = s_2 - \frac{n}{2} \Rightarrow s_1 = n - s_2$ and hence $a_1 = a_2$.

6.2.4 *Wilcoxon Signed-Rank Test*

Another similar modification of the sign test is the Wilcoxon signed-rank test. This is used to test the hypothesis that observations have come from symmetrical population with a common specified median, say, μ_0. Thus the problem is to test $H_0 : \mu = \mu_0$. The signed-rank statistic T^+ is computed as follows:

1. Subtract μ_0 from each observation.
2. Rank the resulting differences in order of size, discarding sign.
3. Restore the sign of the original difference to the corresponding rank.
4. Obtain T^+, the sum of the positive ranks.

Similarly, T^- is the sum of the negative ranks. Then under H_0, we expect T^+ and T^- to be the same. We also note that

$$T^+ + T^- = \sum_{i=1}^{n} i = \frac{n(n+1)}{2}.$$

The statistic T^+ (or T^-) is known as the Wilcoxon statistic. A large value of T^+ (or equivalently, a small value of T^-) means that most of the large deviation from μ_0 are positive and therefore we reject H_0 in favour of the alternative $H_1 : \mu > \mu_0$.

Thus the test rejects H_0 at the level α if $T^+ < C_1$ when $H_1 : \mu < \mu_0$
if $T^+ > C_2$ when $H_1 : \mu > \mu_0$
if $T^+ < C_3$ or $T^+ > C_4$ when $H_1 : \mu \neq \mu_0$
where C_1, C_2, C_3 and C_4 are such that

$$P[T^+ < C_1] = \alpha$$

$$P[T^+ > C_2] = \alpha$$

$$P[T^+ < C_3] + P[T^+ > C_4] = \alpha.$$

6.2.5 Run Test

Suppose we have a set of observations $(X_1, X_2 \ldots, X_n)$. We are to test H_0: The set of observations are random against H_1: They are not random.

We replace each observation either by '+' or '−' sign according as it is larger or smaller than the median of the sample observations. Any observation equal to median is simply discarded. A run is defined to be a sequence of values of the same kind bounded by the values of other kind. We compute the total number of runs 'r'. Too many values of 'r' as well as too small values of 'r' give an indication of non-randomness. Thus the test rejects H_0 at the level α if $r < r_1$ or $r > r_2$ where r_1 and r_2 are such that

$$P[r < r_1] = \alpha/2, P[r > r_2] = \alpha/2.$$

The one-sample run test is based on the order or sequence in which the individual scores or observations originally were obtained.

Example 6.1 The theory predicts that the proportion of peas in the four groups A, B, C and D should be 9:3:3:1. In an experiment among 556 peas, the numbers in the four groups were 315, 108, 101 and 32. Does the experimental result support the theory?

Solution If P_1, P_2, P_3 and P_4 be the proportions of peas in the four classes in the whole population of peas, then the null hypothesis to be tested is

$$H_0 : P_1 = \frac{9}{16}, P_2 = \frac{3}{16}, P_3 = \frac{3}{16}, P_4 = \frac{1}{16}$$

The test statistic under H_0 is given by

$$\chi^2 = \sum_{i=1}^{k} \frac{(x_i - np_i^0)^2}{np_i^0} \quad \text{with } (k-1) \text{ d.f}$$

$$= \sum_{i=1}^{k} \frac{x_i^2}{np_i^0} - n$$

The expected frequencies are

$$e_1 = np_1^0 = 556X\frac{9}{16} = 312.75$$

$$e_2 = np_2^0 = 556X\frac{3}{16} = 104.25$$

$$e_3 = np_3^0 = 556X\frac{3}{16} = 104.25$$

$$e_4 = np_4^0 = 556X\frac{1}{16} = 34.75$$

$$\text{So, } \chi^2 = \frac{315^2}{312.75} + \frac{108^2}{104.25} + \frac{101^2}{104.25} + \frac{32^2}{34.75} - 556$$
$$= 556.47 - 556 = 0.47 \text{ with 3 d.f.}$$

From the table we have $\chi^2_{0.05,3} = 7.815$. Since the calculated value of χ^2, i.e. 0.47 is less than the tabulated value, i.e. 7.815, it is not significant. Hence the null hypothesis may be accepted at 5 % level of significance and we may conclude that the experimental result supports the theory.

Example 6.2 Can the following sample be reasonably regarded as coming from a uniform distribution on the interval (35,70): 36, 42, 44, 50, 64, 58, 56, 50, 37, 48, 52, 63, 57, 43, 39, 42, 47, 61, 53, 58? Use Kolmogorov–Smirnov test.

Solution Here we test $H_0 : F(x) = F_0(x)$ for all x, where $F_0(x)$ is the distribution function of the uniform distribution on the interval (35,70). Now

$$F_0(x) = 0 \text{ if } x \leq 35$$
$$= \frac{x-35}{35} \text{ if } 35 < x < 70$$
$$= 1 \text{ if } x \geq 70$$

Rearranging the data in increasing order of magnitude, we have the following results:

x	$F_0(x)$	$F_{20}(x)$	$\lvert F_{20}(x) - F_0(x)\rvert$
36	1/35	1/20	3/140
37	2/35	2/20	6/140
39	4/35	3/20	5/140
42	7/35	4/20	0
42	7/35	5/20	7/140
43	8/35	6/20	10/140
44	9/35	7/20	13/140
47	12/35	8/20	8/140
48	13/35	9/20	11/140
50	15/35	10/20	10/140

(continued)

(continued)

50	15/35	11/20	17/140
52	17/35	12/20	16/140
53	18/35	13/20	19/140
56	21/35	14/20	14/140
57	22/35	15/20	17/140
58	23/35	16/20	20/140
58	23/35	17/20	27/140
61	26/35	18/20	22/140
63	28/35	19/20	21/140
64	29/35	20/20	24/140

$$D_{20} = \operatorname*{Sup}_{x}|F_{20}(x) - F_0(x)| = \frac{27}{140} = 0.1929.$$

Let us take $\alpha = 0.05$. Then from the table $D_{20,0.05} = 0.294$. Since $0.1929 < 0.294$, we accept H_0 at 5 % level of significance. So we can conclude that the given data has come from a uniform distribution on the interval (35,70).

Example 6.3 The following data represent the yields of maize in q/ha recorded from an experiment.

16.4, 19.2, 24.5, 15.4, 17.3, 23.6, 22.7, 20.9, 18.2

Test whether the median yield (M) is 20 q/ha.

Solution We test $H_0 : M = 20$ against $H_1 : M \neq 20$. To test H_0, we find the difference $(X - 20)$ and write their signs

$$- - + - - + + + -$$

Here $n = 9$ and r = number of '+' sign = 4. This r will be binomial variate with parameters $n = 9$ and $p = 0.5$.

To test H_0 against $H_1 : M \neq 20 \equiv H_1 : p \neq 0.5$, the critical region ω will be given by $r \geq r_{\alpha/2}$ and $r \leq r'_{\alpha/2}$, where $r_{\alpha/2}$ is the smallest integer and $r'_{\alpha/2}$ is the largest integer such that

$$P\left[r \geq r_{\alpha/2} \middle| H_0\right] = \sum_{x=r_{\alpha/2}}^{9} \binom{9}{x}\left(\frac{1}{2}\right)^9 \leq \frac{\alpha}{2} = 0.025$$

$$\text{i.e.,} \sum_{x=0}^{r_{\alpha/2}-1} \binom{9}{x}\left(\frac{1}{2}\right)^9 \geq 0.975$$

$$\text{and } P\left[r \leq r'_{\alpha/2} \middle| H_0\right] = \sum_{x=0}^{r'_{\alpha/2}} \binom{9}{x}\left(\frac{1}{2}\right)^9 \leq \frac{\alpha}{2} = 0.025$$

From the table we have $r_{\alpha/2} - 1 = 7$, i.e. $r_{\alpha/2} = 8$ and $r'_{\alpha/2} = 1$. Here $r'_{\alpha/2} = 1 < r = 4 < r_{\alpha/2} = 8$, so H_0 is accepted at 5 % level of significance.

Example 6.4 For the problem given in Example 6.3, test $H_0 : M = 20$ against $H_1 : M \neq 20$ by using Wilcoxon signed-rank test.

Solution The differences $X_i - 20$ are

−3.6, −0.8, 4.5, −4.6, −2.7, 3.6, 2.7, 0.9, −1.8

The order sequence of numbers ignoring the sign and their ranks with original signs are as follows:

0.8	0.9	1.8	2.7	2.7	3.6	3.6	4.5	4.6
−1	2	−3	4.5	−4.5	6.5	−6.5	8	−9

Thus, T^+ = The sum of the positive ranks = 21 and T^- = The sum of negative ranks = 24.

We note that $T^+ + T^- = \frac{n(n+1)}{2} = 45$

To test $H_0 : M = 20$ against $H_1 : M \neq 20$, the critical region ω will be given by $T^+ > C_4$ and $T^+ < C_3$ at the level α. Here we take $\alpha = 0.05$.

From the table we have $P[T^+ > 39] \leq 0.025$ and

$$P[T^+ < 6] \leq 0.025$$

Since $T^+ = 21$ lies between 6 and 39 (table values), we accept H_0. It means that the median yield of maize is 20 q/ha.

Example 6.5 Test whether the observations

21, 19, 22, 18, 20, 24, 15, 32, 35, 28, 30 are random.

Solution We test H_0 : The observation are random against H_1 : The observations are not random.

The sample values are arranged in increasing order.

15, 18, 19, 20, 21, 22, 24, 28, 30, 32, 35

∴ Median = 22

Each original observation is replaced by '+' or '−' sign according as it is larger or smaller than the median, i.e. 22. Any observation equal to median is simply discarded. Thus we have from the original observation

21	19	22	18	20	24	15	32	35	28	30
-	-	X	-	-	+	-	+	+	+	+

Thus number of runs = $r = 4$, number of '+' signs = $n_1 = 5$ and number of '−' signs = $n_2 = 5$. From table for $n_1 = 5$, $n_2 = 5$ any observed r of 2 or less or of 10 or more is in the region of rejection at 5 % level of significance. So H_0 is accepted, i.e. the observations are random.

Example 6.6 The males (M) and females (F) were queued in front of the railway reservation counter in the order below

M F F M M M F M F F M M F M

Test whether the order of males and females in the queue was random.

Solution Here null hypothesis is

H_0 : The order of males and females in the queue was random against

H_1 : The order of males and females in the queue was not random.

For the given sequence,

$$\underline{M}\ \underline{FF}\ \underline{MMM}\ \underline{F}\ \underline{M}\ \underline{FF}\ \underline{MM}\ \underline{F}\ \underline{M}$$

we have,

n_1 = number of males = 8
n_2 = number of females = 6
r = number of runs = 9

Since the observed value of $r = 9$ lies between the critical values 3 and 12, we accept H_0 at 5 % level of significance. It means that the order of males and females in the queue was random.

6.3 Paired Sample Non-parametric Test

In this section we consider the following paired sample non-parametric tests:

(i) Sign test.
(ii) Wilcoxon signed-rank test.

6.3.1 Sign Test (Bivariate Single Sample Problem) or Paired Sample Sign Test

Suppose we have a bivariate population with continuous distribution function $F(x,y)$ which is unknown but continuous. The ordinary sign test for the location parameter of a univariate population is equally applicable to a paired sample problem. This is the non-parametric version of paired 't' test.

We draw a random sample $(x_1, y_1), (x_2, y_2), \ldots, (x_n, y_n)$ from $F(x, y)$. To test $H_0 : \xi_p(x-y) = \xi_p{}^0$ writing $z = x - y \Rightarrow H_0 : \xi_p(z) = \xi_p{}^0$, i.e. $H_0 : \xi_p = \xi_p{}^0$, writing $\xi_p(z) = \xi_p$.

Assumption $z = x - y$ is continuous in the neighbourhood of $\xi_p(z)$. Note that $\Pr[z \leq \xi_p] = p \Rightarrow \Pr[z - \xi_p > 0] = q, q = 1 - p$. We define S = total number of positive signs among $(z_1 - \xi_p{}^0), (z_2 - \xi_p{}^0), \ldots, (z_n - \xi_p{}^0)$.

$\therefore$ Under H_0, $\Pr[z - \xi_p{}^0 > 0] = q$ and $S \sim B(n, q)$. Proceed for Case 1, Case 2 and Case 3 as worked out already in Sect. 6.2

Note Since $\xi_p(x-y)$ is not necessarily equal to $\xi_p(x) - \xi_p(y)$, the paired sample sign test is a test for the quantile difference (but not for the difference of the quantiles), whereas the paired '*t*' test is a test for the mean difference (and also for the difference of the means).

6.3.2 *Wilcoxon Signed-Rank Test*

This is another test used on matched pairs. It is more powerful than the sign test because it gives more weight to large numerical differences between the members of a pair than to small differences. Under matched-paired samples, the differences d within n paired sample values (x_{1i}, x_{2i}) for $i = 1, 2, \ldots, n$ are assumed to have come from continuous and symmetric population differences. If M_d is the median of the population of differences, then the null hypotheses is that $M_d = 0$ and the alternative hypothesis is one of $M_d > 0, M_d < 0$ or $M_d \neq 0$.

The observed differences $d_i = x_{1i} - x_{2i}$ are ranked in increasing order of absolute magnitude and the sum of ranks is computed for all the differences of like sign. The test statistic T is the smaller of these two rank-sums. Paris with $d_i = 0$ are not counted. On the null hypothesis, the expected value of the two ranks-sums would be equal. If the positive rank-sum is the smaller and is equal to or less than the table value, the null hypothesis will be rejected at the corresponding level of significance α in favour of the alternative hypothesis that $M_d > 0$. If the negative rank-sum is the smaller, the alternative will be that $M_d < 0$. If a two-tailed test is required, the alternative being that $M_d \neq 0$, the given levels of significance should be doubled.

Example 6.7 For nine animals, tested under control conditions and experimental conditions, the following values of a measured variable were observed:

Animal	1	2	3	4	5	6	7	8	9
Control (x_1)	21	24	26	32	55	82	46	55	88
Experimental (x_2)	18	9	23	26	82	199	42	30	62

Test whether a significant difference exists between the medians, using (i) the sign test and (ii) the Wilcoxon signed-ranks test.

Solution Let θ be the median of the distribution of differences. Our null hypothesis will be $H_0 : \theta = 0$ against $H_1 : \theta \neq 0$.

(i) Let $d_i = x_{1i} - x_{2i}$ be the difference of the values under control and experimental conditions.

$$d_i : 3,\ 15,\ 3,\ 6,\ -27,\ -117,\ 4,\ 25,\ 26$$

Here we have 7 '+' signs among 9 non-zero values. Under H_o, number(r) of '+' signs will follow a binomial distribution with parameters $n = 9$ and $p = 0.5$. To test $H_0 : \theta = 0 \equiv H_0 : p = 0.5$ against $H_1 : \theta \neq 0 \equiv H_1 : p \neq 0.5$, the critical region ω will be given by $r \geq r_{\alpha/2}$ and $r \leq r'_{\alpha/2}$ where $r_{\alpha/2}$ is the smallest integer and $r'_{\alpha/2}$ is the largest integer such that.

$$P\left[r \geq r_{\alpha/2} \middle| H_0\right] = \sum_{x=r_{\alpha/2}}^{9} \binom{9}{x} \left(\frac{1}{2}\right)^9 \leq \frac{\alpha}{2} = 0.025$$

$$\text{i.e.,} \sum_{x=0}^{r_{\frac{\alpha}{2}}-1} \binom{9}{x} \left(\frac{1}{2}\right)^9 \geq 0.975$$

$$\text{and } P\left[r \leq r'_{\alpha/2} \middle| H_0\right] = \sum_{x=0}^{r'_{\alpha/2}} \binom{9}{x} \left(\frac{1}{2}\right)^9 \leq \frac{\alpha}{2} = 0.025$$

From the table we get $r_{\alpha/2} - 1 = 7 \Rightarrow r_{\alpha/2} = 8$ and $r'_{\alpha/2} = 1$. For our example $r = 7$ which lies between $r_{\alpha/2}(=8)$ and $r'_{\alpha/2}(=1)$. So H_0 is accepted.

(ii) The observed differences $d_i = x_{1i} - x_{2i}$ are ranked in increasing order of absolute magnitude and the sum of the ranks is computed for all the difference of like sign. Thus

d_i	3	15	3	6	−27	−117	4	25	26
Rank	1.5	5	1.5	4	8	9	3	6	7

The test statistic T is the smaller of these two rank-sums (one for positive d_i and one for negative d_i). Here $T = 17$. From the table, we reject H_0 at $\alpha = 0.05$ if either $T > 39$ or $T < 6$. Since $T > 6$ and < 39, we accept H_0.

6.4 Two-Sample Problem

Case 1 The two populations differ in location only:

We take two univariate populations with continuous distribution functions $F_1(x)$ and $F_2(x)$ which are unknown but continuous.

Assumption The two populations differ only in location.

To test $H_0 : F_1(x) = F_2(x)$ against $H_1 : F_2(x)$ is located to the right of $F_1(x) \Leftrightarrow H_0 : F_1(x) = F_2(x)$ against $H_1 : F_1(x) \geq F_2(x)$.

We draw a random sample $(x_1, x_2, \ldots, x_{n_1})$ of size n_1 from the first population and another sample $(x_{n_1+1}, x_{n_1+2}, \ldots, x_{n_1+n_2})$ of size n_2 from the second population. We write, $F_1(x) = F_2\ (x)$ and $F_2(x) = F(x-\delta)$, δ is unknown location parameter. So we are to test $H_0 : \delta = 0$ against $H_1 : \delta > 0$.

A. Wilcoxon–Mann Whitney Rank-Sum Test

We pooled the two samples and give them ranks. Suppose $(R_1, R_2, \ldots, R_{n_1})$ and $(R_{n_1+1}, R_{n_1+2}, \ldots, R_{n_1+n_2})$ be the ranks of the 1st and 2nd sample observations respectively.

[Example (10,7,9,11,3), $n_1 = 5$ is sample 1 and (20,5,17,8), $n_2 = 4$ is the sample 2.

$$\begin{array}{lccccccccc} & 3 < & 5 < & 7 < & 8 < & 9 < & 10 < & 11 < & 17 < & 20 \\ & \downarrow & \downarrow & \downarrow & \downarrow & \downarrow & \downarrow & \downarrow & \downarrow & \downarrow \\ \text{Ranks} & 1 & 2 & 3 & 4 & 5 & 6 & 7 & 8 & 9 \end{array}$$

$\therefore (R_1 = 6, R_2 = 3, R_3 = 5, R_4 = 7, R_5 = 1)$ are the 1st sample ranks and $(R_6 = 9, R_7 = 2, R_8 = 8, R_9 = 4)$ are the 2nd sample ranks.]

If there is any tie then the corresponding observation is ignored. Let $S_1, S_2, \ldots, S_{n_2}$ be the ordered ranks of the 2nd sample observations, i.e. $S_1 < S_1 < \ldots < S_{n_2}$.

[In the example above $2 < 4 < 8 < 9 \therefore R_7 = S_1, R_9 = S_2, R_8 = S_3, R_6 = S_4$]

Define T = sum of the ranks of the 2nd sample observations $= \sum_{j=1}^{n_2} R_{n_1+j} = \sum_{j=1}^{n_2} S_j$

If H_1 is true, then it is expected that the second sample observations are generally of higher ranks and hence T will be large. So a right tail test will be appropriate here.

Hence for testing $H_0 : \delta = 0$ against $H_1 : \delta > 0$, $\omega_0 : T > t_\alpha$ where t_α is such that $\Pr[T > t_\alpha / H_0] \leq \alpha$. Similarly for $H_0 : \delta = 0$ against $H_2 : \delta < 0$, $\omega_0 : T < t_\alpha{}'$ where $t_\alpha{}'$ is such that $\Pr[T < t_\alpha{}' / H_0] \leq \alpha$, and for $H_0 : \delta = 0$ against $H_3 : \delta \neq 0$; $\omega_0 : T < t_1, T > t_2$ where t_1 and t_2 are such that

$$P[T < t_1/H_0] + P[T > t_2/H_0] \leq \alpha.$$

Null distribution of T: Under H_0 all the $n (= n_1 + n_2)$, observations $x_1, x_2, \ldots, x_{n_1}, x_{n_1+1}, x_{n_1+2}, \ldots, x_{n_1+n_2}$ are i.i.d. so that the second sample ranks can be considered as a random sample of size n_2 without replacement from (1, 2,…,n).

$\therefore \mu$ = population mean $= \frac{n+1}{2}$ and σ^2 = Variance $= \frac{n^2-1}{12}$.

$$\therefore E\left(\frac{T}{n_2}/H_0\right) = \mu = \frac{n+1}{2} \Rightarrow E(T/H_0) = \frac{n_2(n+1)}{2}$$

$$V\left(\frac{T}{n_2}/H_0\right) = \frac{n-n_2}{n-1} \cdot \frac{\sigma^2}{n_2} = \frac{n_1}{n-1} \cdot \frac{n^2-1}{12 \cdot n_2} = \frac{n_1(n+1)}{12 \cdot n_2}$$

$$\Rightarrow V(T/H_0) = \frac{n_1 n_2(n+1)}{12}.$$

Hence, if n is large, under H_0

$\tau = \frac{T - \frac{n_2(n+1)}{2}}{\sqrt{n_1 n_2(n+1)/12}}$ asymptotically $\sim N(0,1)$

$\therefore$ For $H_0 : \delta = 0$ against $H_1 : \delta > 0 \Rightarrow \omega_0 : \tau > \tau_\alpha$

$H_0 : \delta = 0$ against $H_2 : \delta < 0 \Rightarrow \omega_0 : \tau < -\tau_\alpha$

and $H_0 : \delta = 0$ against $H_3 : \delta \neq 0 \Rightarrow \omega_0 : |\tau| > \tau_{\alpha/2}$

Mann–Whitney

An alternative description of the test is more convenient.

Let $g(x_i, x_{n_1+j}) = \begin{cases} 1 & \text{if} \quad x_{n_1+j} > x_i \\ 0 & \text{otherwise} \quad i = 1(1)n_1 \\ & \quad j = 1(1)n_2 \end{cases}$

U = no. of pairs in which 2nd sample observation is greater than 1st sample observation

$$= \sum_{j=1}^{n_2} \sum_{i=1}^{n_1} g(x_i, x_{n_1+j})$$

$= \sum_{j=1}^{n_2} \sum_{i=1}^{n_1} g(R_i, R_{n_1+j})$, [no. of pairs in which 2nd sample ranks are greater than 1st sample ranks]

$$= \sum_{j=1}^{n_2} \sum_{i=1}^{n_1} g(R_i, S_j)$$

$= \sum_{j=1}^{n_2} \left\{ \sum_{i=1}^{n_1} g(R_i, S_j) \right\}$, [$\sum_{i=1}^{n_1} g(R_i, S_j)$ = no. of 1st sample ranks which are less than S_j]

$$= \sum_{j=1}^{n_2} \{(S_j - 1) - (j-1)\} = \sum_{1}^{n_2} (S_j - j) = T - \frac{n_2(n_2+1)}{2}$$

$$\therefore E(U/H_0) = E(T/H_0) - \frac{n_2(n_2+1)}{2} = \frac{n_1 n_2}{2}.$$

$$V(U/H_0) = V(T/H_0) = \frac{n_1 n_2(n+1)}{12}$$

Hence, for large n, under H_0

$$\tau = \frac{U - \frac{n_1 n_2}{2}}{\sqrt{\frac{n_1 n_2(n+1)}{12}}} \overset{a}{\sim} N(0,1)$$

Therefore

(1) For $H_0 : \delta = 0$ against $H_1 : \delta > 0, \omega_0 : \tau > \tau_\alpha$
(2) For $H_0 : \delta = 0$ against $H_2 : \delta < 0, \omega_0 : \tau < -\tau_\alpha$
(3) For $H_0 : \delta = 0$ against $H_3 : \delta \neq 0, \omega_0 : |\tau| > \tau_{\alpha/2}$

B. Mood's Median Test

Here we test $H_0 : F_1(x) = F_2(x)$ against $H_1 : F_1(x) \geq F_2(x)$, i.e. $H_0 : \delta = 0$ against $H_1 : \delta > 0$.

We draw a sample $(x_1, x_2, \ldots, x_{n_1})$ of size n_1 from the 1st population and another sample $(x_{n_1+1}, x_{n_1+2}, \ldots, x_{n_1+n_2})$ of size n_2 from the 2nd population.

We mix the two samples and arrange them in ascending order of magnitude. Say $x_{(1)} < x_{(2)} < \cdots < x_{(n)}$ & $x_{(m)}$ = combined sample median.

$$\begin{aligned} \text{Define } T &= \text{total no. of 2nd sample size} > x_{(m)} \\ &= \text{total no. of 2nd sample ranks} > m \end{aligned}$$

Here T is the test statistic.

Under H_1, T would be too large and hence a right tail test is appropriate.

So for $H_1 : \delta > 0 \Rightarrow \omega_0 : T > t_\alpha$ where, t_α is such that $P_{H_0}[T \geq t_\alpha] \leq \alpha$

for $H_2 : \delta < 0 \Rightarrow \omega_0 : T < t_\alpha{}'$ where $P_{H_0}[T \leq t_\alpha] \leq \alpha$ and

for $H_3 : \delta \neq 0 \Rightarrow \omega_0 : T \leq t_1$ and $T \geq t_2$ where t_1, t_2 are such that $P_{H_0}[T \leq t_1] + P_{H_0}[T \geq t_2] \leq \alpha$.

Null distribution of T: We want to get $P(T = t/H_0)$.

Note that the totality of the pooled ranks (1, 2,.., n) is comprised of two subsets: $\{1, 2, \ldots, m\}$ and $\{m+1, m+2, \ldots, n\}$. Under H_0, the second sample ranks represent a random sample without replacement of size n_2 from the entire set. Since T = no. of 2nd sample ranks exceeding m, the probability that there will be just t number of members from 2nd subset in the random sample of size n_2 is given by the hypergeometric law:

$$\therefore P(T = t/H_0) = \frac{\binom{n-m}{t}\binom{m}{n_2 - t}}{\binom{n}{n_2}}$$

$$\therefore E(T/H_0) = \frac{n_2(n-m)}{n} \text{ and } V(T/H_0) = \frac{n_1 n_2 m(n-m)}{n^2(n-1)}.$$

As $n \to \infty, \frac{m}{n} \simeq \frac{1}{2}$ and then $E(T/H_0) \simeq \frac{n_2}{2}$ and $V(T/H_0) \simeq \frac{n_1 n_2}{4n}$.
$\therefore$ For large n, under H_0

$$\tau = \frac{T - n_2/2}{\sqrt{\frac{n_1 n_2}{4n}}} \underset{\sim}{a} N(0,1)$$

$\therefore$ for $H_1 : \delta > 0 \Rightarrow \omega_0 : \tau > \tau_\alpha$
for $H_1 : \delta < 0 \Rightarrow \omega_0 : \tau < -\tau_\alpha$
and for $H_3 : \delta \neq 0 \Rightarrow \omega_0 : |\tau| > \tau_{\alpha/2}$.

Case II The two populations differ in every respect, i.e. with respect to location, dispersion, skewness, kurtosis, etc.

C. Wald–Wolfowitz Run test

$H_0 : F_1(x) = F_2(x)$ against $H_1 : F_1(x) \neq F_2(x)$
Here also we arrange the combined sample in ascending order $x_{(1)} < x_{(2)} < \ldots < x_{(n)}$.

Suppose $(R_1, \ldots, R_{n_1})$ be the ranks of the 1st sample observation and $(R_{n_1+1}, \ldots, R_{n_1+n_2})$ be the ranks of the 2nd sample observation. According to the ordered arrangement,

we write $z_\alpha = 0$ if $x_{(\alpha)}$ comes from 1st sample
$= 1$ if $x_{(\alpha)}$ comes from 2nd sample.

We note that, 1st sample can be written as $\left\{x_{(R_1)}, x_{(R_2)}, \ldots, x_{(R_{n1})}\right\}$ and the 2nd sample can be written as $\left\{x_{(R_{n_1}+1)}, x_{(R_{n_1}+2)}, \ldots, x_{(R_{n_1}+n2)}\right\}$.

$$\begin{aligned} \therefore z_\alpha &= 0 \text{ if } \alpha \in (R_1, R_2, \ldots R_{n_1}) \\ &= 1 \text{ if } \alpha \in (R_{n_1+1}, R_{n_2+2}, \ldots R_{n_1+n_2}). \end{aligned}$$

So $z_1, z_2, \ldots, z_n$ is a sequence of 0's and 1's and are determined by $(R_1, R_2, \ldots, R_n)$. Let U = number of '0' runs and V = number of '1' runs and $W = U + V$ = total number of runs.

Here W is our test statistic.

The idea is that if the populations are identical, then the 1st sample and 2nd sample ranks would get thoroughly mixed up, i.e. the runs of '0' and '1' would be mixed up thoroughly, i.e. W would be too large. On the other hand, if the two populations are not identical, i.e. if H_0 is not true, then the arrangement of runs will be patching. So ω would be too small. Hence a left tail test would be appropriate.

Hence $\omega_0 : W \leq \omega_\alpha$ where ω_α is such that $P_{H_0}[W \leq \omega_\alpha] \leq \alpha$. It can be shown that under H_0

$$\Pr[U = u, V = v] = \begin{cases} 0 \text{ if } |u - v| \geq 2 \\ \dfrac{\binom{n_1-1}{u-1}\binom{n_2-1}{v-1}}{\binom{n}{n_1}} \text{ if } |u - v| = 1 \\ \dfrac{2\binom{n_1-1}{u-1}\binom{n_2-1}{v-1}}{\binom{n}{n_1}} \text{ if } u - v = 0 \end{cases}$$

$$\therefore P_{H_0}[W = 2m] = P_{H_0}\{u = m, v = m\} = \frac{2\binom{n_1-1}{m-1}\binom{n_2-1}{m-1}}{\binom{n}{n_1}} \text{ and}$$

$$P_{H_0}[W = 2m+1] = P_{H_0}\{u = m, v = m+1\} + P_{H_0}\{u = m+1, v = m\} = \frac{\binom{n_1-1}{m-1}\binom{n_2-1}{m} + \binom{n_1-1}{m}\binom{n_2-1}{m-1}}{\binom{n}{n_1}}$$

It can be shown that $E(W/H_0) = \frac{2n_1n_2}{n} + 1$;

$$V(W/H_0) = \frac{2n_1n_2}{n(n-1)}\left(\frac{2n_1n_2}{n} - 1\right).$$

For large n_1 and n_2, under H_0

$$\tau = \frac{W - E_{H_0}(W)}{\sqrt{V_{H_0}(W)}} \overset{a}{\sim} N(0,1). \tag{6.1}$$

(**Note:** Since U and V are not independent, so the traditional CLT for $W = U + V$ is not applicable here. Still (6.1) is true here as shown by Wald and Wolfowitz using Strilings' approximation). We write $\lambda_1 = \frac{n_1}{n}$ and $\lambda_2 = \frac{n_2}{n} \therefore \lambda_1 + \lambda_2 = 1$

$$\therefore E(W/H_0) = 2n\lambda_1\lambda_2 + 1 \simeq 2n\lambda_1\lambda_2 \text{ and } V(W/H_0) \simeq 4n\lambda_1^2\lambda_2^2.$$

Then $\tau = \frac{W - 2n\lambda_1\lambda_2}{\sqrt{4n\lambda_1{}^2\lambda_2{}^2}} \underset{\sim}{a} N(0,1)$

$$\omega_0 : \tau \leq -\tau_\alpha.$$

D. Kolmogorov–Smirnov test

Let $X_1, X_2, \ldots, X_{n_1}$ be from F_1 and $X_{n_1+1}, X_{n_1+2}, \ldots, X_n$ be from F_2. We are to test $H_0 : F_1(x) = F_2(x) \forall x$ against

$H_1: F_1(x) \geq F_2(x) \forall x, F_1(x) > F_2(x)$ for some x
Or, $H_2: F_1(x) \leq F_2(x) \forall x, F_1(x) < F_2(x)$ for some x
Or, $H_3: F_1(x) \neq F_2(x) \forall x$, for some x.
Let '#' symbol implies the number of cases satisfying a stated condition.

$$F_{1n_1}(x) = \frac{\# x_\alpha \leq x, \alpha = 1, 2, \ldots, n_1}{n_1}$$

$$F_{2n_2}(x) = \frac{\# x_\beta \leq x, \beta = n_1 + 1, n_1 + 2, .., n_2}{n_2}$$

Test statistic

$$D^+_{n_1,n_2} = \underset{x}{\text{Sup}}\{F_{1n_1}(x) - F_{2n_2}(x)\} \text{ for } H_1$$

$$D^-_{n_1,n_2} = \underset{x}{\text{Sup}}\{F_{2n_2}(x) - F_{1n_1}(x)\} \text{ for } H_2$$

$$D_{n_1,n_2} = \underset{x}{\text{Sup}}\,|F_{1n_1}(x) - F_{2n_2}(x)|$$

$$= \max\left\{D^+_{n_1,n_2}, D^-_{n_1,n_2}\right\} \text{ for } H_3$$

Let 2nd sample ranks be $R_{n_1+1}, \ldots, R_n$ and ordered ranks be $S_1 < S_2 < .. < S_{n_2}$. Similarly for 1st sample ranks are $R_1, R_2, \ldots, R_{n_1}$ and ordered ranks are $S'_1 < S'_2 .. < S'_{n_1}$. Then $D^+_{n_1,n_2} = \underset{x}{\text{Sup}}\{F_{1n_1}(x) - F_{2n_2}(x)\} = \max\limits_{i=0,1,..,n_1} \underset{X_{S'_i} \leq x < S'_{i+1}}{\text{Sup}} \{F_{1n_1}(x) - F_{2n_2}(x)\}$

$$= \max\left\{\max_{i=1,..,n_1}\left(\frac{i}{n_1} - \frac{S'_i - i}{n_2}\right), 0\right\}.$$

Similarly, $D^-_{n_1,n_2} = \max\left\{0, \max\limits_{j=1,..,n_2}\left(\frac{j}{n_2} - \frac{S_j - j}{n_1}\right)\right\}.$

$$D_{n_1,n_2} = \max\left\{D^+_{n_1,n_2}, D^-_{n_1,n_2}\right\}.$$

Under H_0, D is uniform and D^+, D^- and D are distribution free. [Under H_0, distribution of $\left\{(s_1, s_2, \ldots s_{n_2}), (s'_1, s'_2, s'_3, \ldots s'_{n_1})\right\}$ is independent of $(F_1 = F_2)$]. Critical region: under H_0, we expect that D^+, D^- and D are very small. Hence right tailed test based on D's would be appropriate.

Asymptotic distribution

For one-sided test $P_{H_0}\left[\sqrt{\frac{n_1 n_2}{n_1 + n_2}} D^+_{n_1,n_2} \leq z\right] \to 1 - e^{-2z^2}$ as $\min(n_1, n_2) \to \infty, z > 0$

Practically we find a z such that $e^{-2z^2} = \alpha$ and reject H_0 if $\sqrt{\frac{n_1 n_2}{n_1 + n_2}}$ (observed $D^+_{n_1,n_2}) \geq z$.

For two sided test $P_{H_0}\left[\sqrt{\frac{n_1 n_2}{n_1+n_2}}D_{n_1,n_2} \leq z\right] \to 1 - 2\sum_{i=1}^{\infty}(-1)^{i-1}e^{-2i^2z^2}$ as min $(n_1, n_2) \to \infty$.

Advantages of K–S test over Homogeneity χ^2 test are as follows

1. K–S test is applicable to ungrouped data, while χ^2 is applicable to grouped data only.
2. Under H_0 K–S is exactly distribution free, while χ^2 is asymptotically distribution free.
3. K–S test is consistent against any alternative, while χ^2 is so for specific alternative only.

Example 6.8 Twelve 4-year-old boys and twelve 4-year-old girls were observed during two 15 min play sessions and each child's play during these two periods was scored as follows for incidence and degree of aggression:

$$\text{Boys} : 86, 69, 72, 65, 113, 65, 118, 45, 141, 104, 41, 50$$
$$\text{Girls} : 55, 40, 22, 58, 16, 7, 9, 16, 26, 36, 20, 15$$

Test the hypothesis that there were sex differences in the amount of aggression shown, using (a) the Wald-Wolfowitz runs test, (b) the Mann–Whitney–Wilcoxon test and (c) the Kolmogorov–Smirnov test.

Solution We want to test H_0 : incidence and degree of aggression are the same in four-year olds of both sexes against H_1 : four-year-old boys and four-year-old girls display differences in incidence and degree of aggression.

(a) Wald–Wolfowitz runs test

We combine the scores of boys (B's) and girls (G's) in a single-ordered series, we may determine the number of runs of G's and B's. The ordered series is given below.

Score	7	9	15	16	16	20	22	26	36	40	41	45	50	55	58
Groups	G	G	G	G	G	G	G	G	G	G	B	B	B	G	G
Runs					1							2		3	
Score	65	65	69	72	86	104	113	118	141						
Groups	B	B	B	B	B	B	B	B	B						
Runs					4										

Each run is underlined and we observe that $r = 4$.

From the table for $n_1 = 12$, $n_2 = 12$, we reject H_0 at $\alpha = 0.05$ if $r \leq 7$. Since our value of r is smaller than 7, we may reject H_0. So we can conclude that boys and girls display differences in aggression.

	7	9	15	16	16	20	22	26	36	40	41	45	50	55	58	65	65	69	72	86	104	113	118	141
	G	G	G	G	G	G	G	G	G	G	B	B	B	G	G	B	B	B	B	B	B	B	B	B
Rank	1	2	3	4.5	4.5	6	7	8	9	10	11	12	13	14	15	16.5	16.5	18	19	20	21	22	23	24

(b) Mann–Whitney–Wilcoxon test

The pooled sample and the ranks are given below:
The sum of the ranks for the observations corresponding to the boys is

$$R_1 = 11 + 12 + 13 + 16.5 + 16.5 + 18 + 19 + 20 + 21 + 22 + 23 + 24 = 216$$

and that for girls is

$$R_2 = 1 + 2 + 3 + 4.5 + 4.5 + 6 + 7 + 8 + 9 + 10 + 14 + 15 = 84$$

The smaller rank-sum is 84. This corresponds to girls.
Hence

$$\begin{aligned} U &= n_1 n_2 + \frac{n_2(n_2+1)}{2} - R_2 \\ &= 144 + 78 - 84 = 138 \end{aligned}$$

Or, equivalently,

$$\begin{aligned} U &= n_1 n_2 + \frac{n_1(n_1+1)}{2} - R_1 \\ &= 144 + 78 - 216 = 6 \end{aligned}$$

The test statistic is given by the smaller of the two quantities. Here $U = 6$. The other value of U can be obtained from the relation $U' = n_1 n_2 - \mathrm{U} = 144 - 6 = 138$. The critical value of U for a two-tailed test at $\alpha = 0.05$ and $n_1 = n_2 = 12$ is 37. The observed $U = 6$ is less than the table value. Hence it is significant at 5 % level. Hence H_0 is rejected.

(c) Kolmogorov–Smirnov test

The scores of the boys and girls are presented in two frequency distributions shown below:

Score (x)	No. of boys	No. of girls	$F_{12}(x)$	$G_{12}(x)$	$\lvert F_{12}(x) - G_{12}(x) \rvert$
7–20	0	6	0	6/12	6/12
21–34	0	2	0	8/12	8/12
35–48	2	2	2/12	10/12	8/12
49–62	1	2	3/12	12/12	9/12
63–76	4	0	7/12	12/12	5/12
77–90	1	0	8/12	12/12	4/12
91–104	1	0	9/12	12/12	3/12
105–118	2	0	11/12	12/12	1/12
119–132	0	0	11/12	12/12	1/12
133–146	1	0	12/12	12/12	0

$D_{12,12} = \text{Sup}|F_{12}(x) - G_{12}(x)| = 9/12$. From the table, the critical value for $n_1 = n_2 = 12$ at level $\alpha = 0.05$ is $D_{12,12;05} = 6/12$. Since $D_{12,12} > D_{12,12;0.5}$, we reject H_0.

6.5 Non-parametric Tolerance Limits

We draw a random sample $(X_1, X_2, \ldots, X_n)$ from a distribution with distribution function $F(x)$ which is continuous. We define functions of sample observations $L = L(x_1, x_2, \ldots, x_n)$ and $U = U(x_1, x_2, \ldots, x_n)$ such that $L < U$.

$$\text{If } \Pr[\Pr(L \le X \le U) \ge \beta] = \gamma \tag{6.2}$$

then the interval (L,U) is called 100 β% tolerance interval with tolerance coefficient γ. L and U are called lower and upper tolerance limits respectively. If the determination of γ does not depend upon F then the limit (L,U) are called non-parametric (distribution free) tolerance limits. We note that, (6.2) can be written as,

$$\Pr\{F(U) - F(L) \ge \beta\} = \gamma \tag{6.3}$$

that is a tolerance interval (L,U) for a continuous distribution having c.d.f. $F(x)$ with tolerance coefficient γ is a random interval such that the probability is γ that the area between the endpoints of the interval (L,U) is at least a certain pre-assigned quantity 'β'.

If L and U are two-order statistics say $x_{(r)}$ and $x_{(s)}$, $(r < s)$, then (6.3) is equivalent to $\Pr\{F(x_{(s)}) - F(x_{(r)}) \ge \beta\} = \gamma$.

Wilks has shown that the order statistics provide non-parametric tolerance limits, while it is Robbins who has shown that it is only the order statistics which provide distribution free tolerance limits.

Determination of Tolerance Limits

Joint distribution of $x_{(r)}, x_{(s)}$ is

$$g\{x_{(r)}, x_{(s)}\} = \frac{n!}{(r-1)!(s-r-1)!(n-s)!}\left[F(x_{(r)})\right]^{r-1}$$
$$\left[F(x_{(s)}) - F(x_{(r)})\right]^{s-r-1}\left[1 - F(x_{(s)})\right]^{n-s} f(x_{(r)})f(x_{(s)}); x_{(r)} < x_{(s)}$$

Putting $U = F(x_{(r)})$ and $V = F(x_{(s)})$ we get,

$$g(u,v) = \frac{n!}{(r-1)!(s-r-1)!(n-s)!}u^{r-1}(v-u)^{s-r-1}(1-v)^{n-s}; 0<u<v<1.$$

Again we put $\begin{matrix} U = W \\ V - U = Y \end{matrix} \Rightarrow \begin{matrix} U = W & 0<y<1 \\ V = W + Y, & 0<W<1-y. \end{matrix}$

$$\therefore g(w,y) = \frac{n!}{(r-1)!(s-r-1)!(n-s)!} w^{r-1} y^{s-r-1} (1-w-y)^{n-s}$$

$$\therefore g(y) = \frac{n!}{(r-1)!(s-r-1)!(n-s)!} y^{s-r-1} \int_0^{1-y} w^{r-1}(1-w-y)^{n-s} dw$$

$$= \frac{n!}{(r-1)!(s-r-1)!(n-s)!} y^{s-r-1} \int_0^1 (1-y)^{r-1} t^{r-1} (1-y)^{n-s} (1-t)^{n-s} (1-y) dt$$

$$= \frac{n!}{(r-1)!(s-r-1)!(n-s)!} y^{s-r-1} (1-y)^{n+r-s} \int_0^1 t^{r-1}(1-t)^{n-s} dt$$

$$= \frac{\Gamma(n+1)}{\Gamma(s-r)\Gamma(n+r-s+1)} y^{s-r-1}(1-y)^{n+r-s}$$

$$= \frac{1}{\beta(s-r, n+r-s+1)} y^{s-r-1}(1-y)^{n+r-s}, 0<y<1.$$

$$\therefore \Pr\left[F(x_{(s)}) - F(x_{(r)}) \geq \beta\right] = \gamma$$

$$\Leftrightarrow \Pr[y \geq \beta] = \gamma \Leftrightarrow \Pr[y \leq \beta] = 1 - \gamma$$

$$\text{i.e. } \int_0^\beta g(y) dy = 1 - \gamma$$

$$\text{i.e. } \frac{\int_0^\beta y^{s-r-1}(1-y)^{n+r-s} dy}{\beta(s-r, n+r-s+1)} = 1 - \gamma$$

$$\text{i.e. } I_\beta(s-r, n+r-s+1) = 1 - \gamma \tag{6.4}$$

For given β, γ and n we choose r and s satisfying (6.4) such that $r + s = n + 1$ that is $x_{(r)}$ and $x_{(s)}$ are symmetrically placed.

Particular case: $r = 1$, $s = n$; Then (6.4) $\Rightarrow I_\beta(n-1, 2) = 1 - \gamma$

$$\text{i.e. } 1 - \gamma = \frac{\int_0^\beta t^{n-2}(1-t) dt}{\beta((n-1), 2)}$$

$$\text{i.e. } 1 - \gamma = \left(\frac{\beta^{n-1}}{n-1} - \frac{\beta^n}{n}\right) \Big/ \frac{\Gamma(n-1)\Gamma(2)}{\Gamma(n+1)}$$

$$= \frac{n\beta^{n-1} - (n-1)\beta^n}{n(n-1)} n(n-1)$$

$$\Rightarrow 1 - \gamma = n\beta^{n-1}(1-\beta) + \beta^n$$

that is $1-\gamma \simeq n\beta^{n-1}(1-\beta)$ as $0<\beta<1$ and $n\to\infty$. So for large 'n', $1-\gamma \simeq n\beta^{n-1}(1-\beta)$.

For given β and γ, one can find n from this relationship.

Alternative

For Bin(n,p), we know

$$\sum_{x=0}^{c}\binom{n}{x}p^x q^{n-x} = I_q(n-c, c+1)$$
$$= 1 - I_p(c+1, n-c)$$

$$\text{Then } (6.4) \Rightarrow \gamma = 1 - I_\beta(s-r, n+r-s+1)$$
$$= \sum_{x=0}^{s-r-1}\binom{n}{x}\beta^x(1-\beta)^{n-x}.$$

So for given n, β and γ we can find s and r such that $x_{(r)}$ and $x_{(s)}$ are symmetrically placed.

6.6 Non-parametric Confidence Interval for ξ_p

Suppose $F(x)$ is continuous and a random sample $(x_1, x_2, \ldots, x_n)$ is drawn from it. ξ_p is the p-th order quantile. So $P[X \le \xi_p] = p$. Define $X_{(r)}$ and $X_{(s)}$ as the rth and sth order statistics, $r < s$. Then $\left(X_{(r)}, X_{(s)}\right)$ is said to be $100(1-\alpha)\%$ confidence interval for ξ_p if

$$\Pr\left[X_{(r)} \le \xi_p \le X_{(s)}\right] = 1 - \alpha \tag{6.5}$$

$$\begin{aligned}
\text{Now, } \Pr\left[X_{(r)} \le \xi_p \le X_{(s)}\right] &= \Pr\left[\xi_p \le X_{(s)}\right] - \Pr\left[\xi_p \le X_{(r)}\right] \\
&= \Pr\left[X_{(s)} \ge \xi_p\right] - \Pr\left[X_{(r)} \ge \xi_p\right] \\
&= 1 - \Pr\left[X_{(s)} < \xi_p\right] - 1 + \Pr\left[X_{(r)} < \xi_p\right] \\
&= \Pr\left[X_{(r)} < \xi_p\right] - \Pr\left[X_{(s)} < \xi_p\right] \\
&= \Pr\left[\text{at least } r \text{ of the observations } < \xi_p\right] \\
&\quad - \Pr\left[\text{at least } s \text{ of the observations } < \xi_p\right]
\end{aligned}$$

$$= \sum_{x=r}^{s-1} \binom{n}{x} p^x (1-p)^{n-x} \tag{6.6}$$

$$= \sum_{x=0}^{s-1} \binom{n}{x} p^x (1-p)^{n-x} - \sum_{x=0}^{r-1} \binom{n}{x} p^x (1-p)^{n-x}$$
$$= 1 - I_p(s, n-s+1) - 1 + I_p(r, n-r+1)$$
$$= I_p(r, n-r+1) - I_p(s, n-s+1)$$

Since, $\Pr\left[X_{(r)} \le \xi_p \le X_{(s)}\right] = 1 - \alpha$, so r and s are such that

$$1 - \alpha = I_p(r, n-r+1) - I_p(s, n-s+1) \tag{6.7}$$

Given α and n, the selection of r and s satisfying (6.7) is not unique. We select that pair of r and s for which $(s - r)$ is minimum.

For symmetrically placed order statistics $x_{(r)}$ and $x_{(s)}$, we select that pair of (r, s) such that $r + s = n + 1 \Rightarrow s - 1 = n - r$.

$$\therefore \text{ From (6.7) } 1 - \alpha = \sum_{r}^{n-r} \binom{n}{x} p^x (1-p)^{n-x}.$$

From this relation one can find r and hence $s = n + 1 - r$.

Note If in (6.7) the exact probability $(1 - \alpha)$ is not attained then we choose that pair of r and s such that

$$\Pr\left[X_{(r)} \le \xi_p \le X_{(s)}\right] \ge 1 - \alpha \text{ i.e. } I_p(r, n-r+1) - I_p(s, n-s+1) \ge 1 - \alpha.$$

Non-parametric confidence interval for $\xi_{1/2}$ (=median) using sign test

The sign test technique can be applied to obtain a class interval estimate for the unknown population median $\xi_{1/2}$. Suppose $X_{(1)}, X_{(2)}, \ldots, X_{(n)}$ be the order statistics. We consider the testing problem $H_0 : \xi_{1/2} = \xi^0$ against $H_1 : \xi_{1/2} \neq \xi^0$.

Define, S = total no. of +ve signs among $\left(X_{(i)} - \xi^0\right) \forall i = 1(1)n$

The ordinary sign test is

$$\phi(s) = \begin{cases} 1 & \text{if } s < s_1 \\ a_1 & \text{if } s = s_1 \\ 0 & \text{if } s_1 < s < s_2 \\ a_2 & \text{if } s = s_2 \\ 1 & \text{if } s > s_2 \end{cases}$$

where s_1 and s_2 are such that

$$\left.\begin{aligned} \Pr\cdot[s < s_1/H_0] < \frac{\alpha}{2} \le \Pr\cdot[s \le s_1/H_0] \\ \Pr\cdot[s > s_2/H_0] < \frac{\alpha}{2} \le \Pr\cdot[s \ge s_2/H_0] \end{aligned}\right\} \tag{6.8}$$

Also a_1 and a_2 are such that $a_1 = \frac{\frac{\alpha}{2} - \Pr[s < s_1/H_0]}{P[s = s_1/H_0]}$ and $a_2 = \frac{\frac{\alpha}{2} - \Pr[s > s_2/H_0]}{P[s = s_2/H_0]}$
We accept H_0 if $s_1 < s < s_2$ and so

$$\Pr[s_1 < s < s_2] = 1 - \alpha$$

$$\text{i.e., } \Pr[s_1 + 1 \le s \le s_2 - 1] = 1 - \alpha \tag{6.9}$$

In order to obtain a confidence interval for $\xi_{1/2}$ we need only to translate the inequality in the LHS of (6.9) to an equivalent statement involving the order statistics and $\xi_{1/2}$. We have seen earlier that $1 - \alpha = \Pr\left[X_{(r)} \le \xi_p \le X_{(s)}\right]$ $= \sum_{x=r}^{s-1} \binom{n}{x} p^x (1-p)^{n-x}$.

Now, for

$$p = \frac{1}{2},\ 1 - \alpha = \Pr\left[X_{(r)} \le \xi_{1/2} \le X_{(s)}\right] = \sum_{x=r}^{s-1} \binom{n}{x} \left(\frac{1}{2}\right)^n$$

$$= \Pr[r \le S \le s - 1] \text{ as } S \sim B\left(n, \frac{1}{2}\right) \text{ under } H_0.$$

$$\therefore \Pr\left[X_{(r)} \le \xi_{1/2} \le X_{(s)}\right] = \Pr[r \le S \le s - 1] = 1 - \alpha \tag{6.10}$$

Comparing (6.9) and (6.10), we can write

$$\Pr\left[X_{(s_1+1)} \le \xi_{\frac{1}{2}} \le X_{(s_2)}\right] = 1 - \alpha$$

$\therefore$ 100$(1 - \alpha)$% C.I. for $\xi_{1/2}$ using sign test is $\left[X_{(s_1+1)}, X_{(s_2)}\right] = \left[X_{(s_1+1)}, X_{(n-s_1)}\right]$ {since S is symmetric about $n/2, \frac{n}{2} - s_1 = s_2 - n/2$}
For large samples, (6.9) is equivalent to

$$\Pr\left[\frac{s_1+1-{}^n\!/_2}{\sqrt{{}^n\!/_4}} \le \frac{S-\frac{n}{2}}{\sqrt{{}^n\!/_4}} \le \frac{s_2-1-\frac{n}{2}}{\sqrt{{}^n\!/_4}}\right] = 1-\alpha$$

$$\text{or, } \Pr\left[\frac{s_1+1-{}^n\!/_2-0.5}{\sqrt{{}^n\!/_4}} \le \tau \le \frac{s_2-1-\frac{n}{2}+0.5}{\sqrt{{}^n\!/_4}}\right] = 1-\alpha$$

$$\therefore \frac{s_1+1-{}^n\!/_2-0.5}{\sqrt{{}^n\!/_4}} = -\tau_{\alpha/2} \text{ and } \frac{s_2-1-\frac{n}{2}+0.5}{\sqrt{{}^n\!/_4}} = \tau_{\alpha/2}$$

$$\text{i.e. } s_1 = {}^n\!/_2 - 0.5 - \sqrt{{}^n\!/_4}\tau_{\alpha/2} \ \&\ s_2 = {}^n\!/_2 + 0.5 + \sqrt{{}^n\!/_4}\tau_{\alpha/2} \qquad (6.11)$$

So, $100(1-\alpha)\%$ C.I. for $\xi_{1/2}$ using sign test is

$\left[X_{(s_1+1)}, X_{(s_2)}\right] = \left[X_{(s_1+1)}, X_{(n-s_1)}\right]$ where s_1 and s_2 are given by (6.11).

6.7 Combination of Tests

When several tests of the same hypothesis H_0 are made on the basis of independent sets of data, it is quite likely that some of the tests will dictate rejection of the hypothesis (at the chosen level of significance) while the others will dictate its acceptance. In such a case, one would naturally like to have a means of combining the results of the individual tests to reach a firm, overall decision. While one may well apply the same test to the combined set of data, what we are envisaging is a situation where only the values of the test statistics used are available.

Let us denote by T_i the statistic used in making the ith test (say, for $i = 1, 2, \ldots, k$). Commonly $T_1, T_2, \ldots, T_k$ will be statistics defined in the same way (like χ^2 statistics or t-statistics), but with varying sampling distributions simply because they are based on varying sample sizes. To fix ideas, let us assume that in each case the test requires that H_0 be rejected if, and only if, the observed value of the corresponding statistic be too large. Consider, in this situation, the probabilities $y_i = \Pr[T_i > t_i/H_0]$, for $i = 1, 2, \ldots, k$.

Provided T_i has a continuous distribution under H_0, say with probability density function $g_i(t)$, so that $y_i = \int_{t_i}^{\infty} g_i(t)\mathrm{d}t$, where t_i is a randomly taken value of T_i, y_i has the rectangular distribution over the interval [0,1] under H_0 and hence $-2\log_e y_i$ has the χ^2 distribution with df = 2. Consequently $P_\lambda = -2\sum_{i=1}^{k}\log_e y_i$ has, under H_0, the χ^2 distribution with $2k$ degrees of freedom. This statistic is used as the test statistic for making the combined test. One would reject H_0 if, and only if, the observed value of P_λ exceeds $\chi^2_{\alpha,2k}$.

The case where each individual test requires rejection of H_0 if, and only if, the observed value of the corresponding test statistic is too small, or the case where each individual test requires rejection of H_0 if, and only if, the observed value of the test statistic is either too large or too small, is to be similarly dealt with. The reason is that, if T_i have continuous distributions under H_0, then $u_i = \Pr[T_i < t_i/H_0]$ and $v_i = \Pr[|T_i| > |t_i|/H_0]$ are also rectangularly distributed over (0,1). This implies that the statistic P_λ to be appropriate to these situations, viz., $P_\lambda = -2\sum_{i=1}^{k} \log_e u_i$ and $P_\lambda = -2\sum_{i=1}^{k} \log_e v_i$, are also distributed as χ^2 statistics with df = 2k under H_0. In each of these cases also, the overall decision will be to reject H_0 if, and only if, the observed value of the respective P_λ exceeds $\chi^2_{\alpha,2K}$.

Example 6.9 In order to test whether the mean height (μ) of a variety of paddy plants, when fully grown, is 60 cm, or less than 60 cm, five experimenters made independent (student's) t-tests with their respective data. The probabilities of the t-statistics (with the appropriate df in each case) to be less than their respective observed values are 0.023, 0.061, 0.07, 0.105 and 0.007. If the tests are made at 5 % level, then the hypothesis $H_0 : \mu = 60$ cm, has to be accepted in three cases out of the five.

In order to combine the results of the 5 tests, we note that log y_i, for i = 1, 2, 3, 4 and 5, are $\bar{2}.36173, \bar{2}.78533, \bar{2}.23045, \bar{1}.02119$ and $\bar{3}.84510$, respectively. Hence for the data, $\sum_{i=1}^{5} \log_e u_i = -10 + 2.24380 = -7.75620$, so that $P_\lambda = -\sum_{1}^{5} 2\log_e u_i = 2.30259 \times 15.5124 = 35.719$.

This is to be compared with $\chi^2_{.05,10} = 18.307$ and $\chi^2_{.01,10} = 23.205$. Since the observed value of P_λ exceeds the tabulated values, the combined result of the experimenter's tests leads to the rejection of H_0 at both 5 % and the 1 % level. In other words, in the light of all 5 experimenters' data, we may conclude that the mean height at the variety of paddy plant is less than 60 cm.

6.8 Measures of Association for Bivariate Samples

A. Spearman's rank correlation coefficient

In many situations, the individuals are ranked by two judges or the measurements taken for two variables are assigned ranks within the samples independently. Now it is desired to know the extent of association between the ranks. The method of calculating the association between ranks was given by Charles Edward Spearman in 1906 and is known as Spearman's rank correlation.

Let $(X_1, Y_1), (X_2, Y_2), \ldots, (X_n, Y_n)$. be a sample from a bivariate population. If the sample values $X_1, X_2, \ldots, X_n$ and $Y_1, Y_2, \ldots, Y_n$ are each ranked from 1 to n in increasing order of magnitude separately and if the X's and Y's have continuous distribution functions, we get a unique set of rankings. The data will then reduce to n pairs of ranking. Let us write

$$R_{1\alpha} = \text{Rank of } X_\alpha, \ \alpha = 1, 2, \ldots, n.$$
$$R_{2\alpha} = \text{Rank of } Y_\alpha, \ \alpha = 1, 2, \ldots, n.$$

Pearsonian coefficient of correlation between the ranks $R_{1\alpha}$'s and $R_{2\alpha}$'s is called the Spearman's rank correlation coefficient r_s which is given by

$$r_s = \frac{\sum_{\alpha=1}^{n} (R_{1\alpha} - \bar{R}_1)(R_{2\alpha} - \bar{R}_2)}{\left\{\sum_{\alpha=1}^{n} (R_{1\alpha} - \bar{R}_1)^2 \sum_{\alpha=1}^{n} (R_{2\alpha} - \bar{R}_2)^2\right\}^{1/2}}$$
$$= \frac{12 \sum_{\alpha=1}^{n} \left(R_{1\alpha} - \frac{n+1}{2}\right)\left(R_{2\alpha} - \frac{n+1}{2}\right)}{n(n^2 - 1)}$$

If for n individuals, $D_\alpha = R_{1\alpha} - R_{2\alpha}$, is the difference between ranks of the αth individual for $\alpha = 1, 2, \ldots, n$, the formula for Spearman's rank correlation is

$$r_s = 1 - \frac{6 \sum_{i=1}^{n} D_\alpha^2}{n(n^2 - 1)}.$$

The value of r_s lies between −1 and +1. If X, Y are independent then $E(r_s) = 0$. Also Population Spearman's rank correlation coefficient, i.e. $\rho_s = 0 \Rightarrow E(r_s) = 0$. Kendall in 1962 derived the frequency function of r_s and gave exact critical value r_s. But the approximate test of r_s which is the same as t-test for Pearsonian correlation coefficient is good enough for all practical purposes. Here we test $H_0 : \rho_s = 0$ against $H_1 : \rho_s \neq 0$. The test statistic

$t = \frac{r_s\sqrt{n-2}}{\sqrt{1-r_s^2}}$ has $(n - 2)$ d.f. The decision about H_0 is taken in the usual way. For large samples under H_0, the random variable $Z = r_s\sqrt{n-1}$ has approximately a standard normal distribution. The approximation is good for $n \geq 10$.

B. Kendall's rank correlation coefficient

Kendall's rank correlation coefficient τ is suitable for the paired ranks as in case of Spearman's rank correlation. Let $(X_1, Y_1), (X_2, Y_2), \ldots, (X_n, Y_n)$ be a sample from a bivariate population.

For any two pairs (X_i, Y_i) and (X_j, Y_j) we say that the relation is perfect concordance if

$X_i < X_j$ whenever $Y_i < Y_j$ or $X_i > X_j$ whenever $Y_i > Y_j$ and that the relation is perfect discordance if $X_i > X_j$ whenever $Y_i < Y_j$ or $X_i < X_j$ whenever $Y_i > Y_j$.

Let π_c and π_d be the probability of perfect concordance and of perfect discordance respectively defined by

$$\pi_c = P\left[(X_j - X_i)(Y_j - Y_i) > 0\right]$$
$$\text{and } \pi_d = P\left[(X_j - X_i)(Y_j - Y_i) < 0\right].$$

The measure of association between the random variables X and Y defined by

$$\tau = \pi_c - \pi_d$$

is known as Kendall's tau (τ)

It is noted that

$\tau = 0$ if X and Y are independent.
$= +1$ if X and Y be in prefect concordance.
$= -1$ if X and Y be in prefect discordance.

We now need to find an estimate of τ from the sample.

Using sample observations, Kendall's measure of association becomes

$$T = \frac{1}{\binom{n}{2}} \sum_{1 \le i < j \le n}^{n} \sum s(x_j - x_i)s(y_j - y_i) \tag{6.12}$$

where $s(r) = 1$ if $r > 0$
$= 0$ if $r = 0$
$= -1$ if $r < 0$

Naturally $E\left[s(x_j - x_i)s(y_j - y_i)\right] = \pi_c - \pi_d = \tau$

The statistic T defined in (6.12) is known as Kendall's sample tau (τ) coefficient. The procedure for calculating T consists of the following steps:

Step 1: Arrange the rank of the first set (X) in ascending order and rearrange the ranks of the second set (Y) in such a way that n pairs of rank remain the same.
Step 2: After operating Step 1, the ranks of X are in natural order. Now we are left to determine how many pairs of ranks on the set Y are in their natural order and how many are not. A number is said to be in natural order if it is smaller than the succeeding number and is coded as +1 and also if it is greater than its succeeding number then it will not be taken in natural order and will be coded as −1. In this way all $\binom{n}{2}$ pairs of the set (Y) will be considered and assigned the values +1 and −1.

Step 3: Find the sum 'S' of all the coded values.
Step 4: The formula for Kendall's rank correlation coefficient-T is

$$T = \frac{S}{\binom{n}{2}} = \frac{\text{Actual value}}{\text{Maximum possible value}} = \frac{2S}{n(n-1)}$$

Here we test $H_0 : \tau = 0$ against $H_1 : \tau \neq 0$. Thus we reject H_0 if the observed value of $|T| > t_{\alpha/2}$ where $P\left[|T > t_{\alpha/2}|H_0\right] = \alpha$. The values of t_α are given in the table for selected values of n and α. Values for $4 \leq n \leq 10$ are tabulated by Kendall.

It can be shown that $E(T) = \tau$ and $V(T) = \frac{4(n-2)}{9n(n-1)} + \frac{1-\tau^2}{\binom{n}{2}}$. If $n \to \infty$ under $H_0 : \tau = 0$, $\frac{3\sqrt{n}}{2} T \sim N(0,1)$ and we can test the independence of x and y.

Remark An important difference between T and r_s is that T provides an unbiased estimate of τ, whereas r_s is not an unbiased estimate of ρ_s.

Example 6.10 Following are the ranks awarded to seven debators in a competition by two judges.

Debators	A	B	C	D	E	F	G
Ranks by judge I (x)	3	2	1	6	7	4	5
Ranks by judge II (y)	5	6	3	7	4	2	1

Compute (i) Spearmen's rank correlation coefficient (r_s) and Kendall's sample tau coefficient (T) and test their significance.

Solution (i) First we find $d_i = x_i - y_i \forall i$ which are
$d : -2\ -4\ -2\ -1\ 3\ 2\ 4$
Also, $\sum_{i=1}^{7} d_i^2 = 54$
thus $r_s = 1 - \frac{6\sum d_i^2}{n(n^2-1)} = 1 - \frac{6\times54}{7\times48} = 0.036$
To test $H_0 : \rho_s = 0$ against $H_1 : \rho_s \neq 0$, the statistic

$$t_5 = \frac{r_s\sqrt{n-2}}{\sqrt{1-r_s^2}} = \frac{0.036\sqrt{7-2}}{\sqrt{1-(0.036)^2}} = 0.080$$

From the table, $t_{0.025,5} = 2.571$. Calculated value of $|t| = 0.080 < 2.571$, hence we accept H_0. It means there is a dissociation between the ranks awarded by two judges.

(ii) We write below ranks of x in natural order and ranks of y correspondingly

x	1	2	3	4	5	6	7
y	3	6	5	2	1	7	4

For this problem, $n = 7$

For S, take the rank 3 and give +1 or −1 value for all pairs with subsequent ranks of y. $3 < 6$, give a number +1; $3 < 5$, again +1; $3 > 2$, give a number −1 and so on. Then choose 6 and take the pairs (6,5), (6,2), (6,1), (6,7) and (6,4) and continue the process till we reach the last pair (7,4). Proceeding in this manner,

S = (+1 +1 −1 −1 +1 +1) + (−1 −1 −1 +1 −1) + (−1 −1 +1 −1) + (−1 +1 +1) + (+1 +1) + (−1)

= 2 − 3 − 2 + 1 + 2 − 1 = −1

Thus $T = \frac{S}{\binom{n}{2}} = \frac{-1 \times 2}{7 \times 6} = -0.048$

To test the significance of T, we test

$H_0 : \tau = 0$ against $H_1 : \tau \neq 0$.

From the table, for $n = 7$ we have $t_{0.025} = 0.62$. Since $|T| = 0.048 < 0.62$, we accept H_0. It reveals that there is no association between the ranks awarded by two judges.

Example 6.11 A random sample of 12 couples showed the following distribution of heights (in inches):

Couple no.	1	2	3	4	5	6	7	8	9	10	11	12
Husband height	80	70	73	72	62	65	74	71	63	64	68	67
Wife height	72	60	76	62	63	46	68	71	61	65	66	67

(a) Compute r_s and T.

(b) Test the hypothesis that the heights of husband and wife are independent using r_s as well as T. In each case use the normal approximation.

Solution (a) The heights of husband and wife are each ranked from 1 to 12 in increasing order of magnitude separately and let us denote their ranks by x_i and y_i respectively ($i = 1,2, \ldots, 12$).

x_i	: 12	7	10	9	1	4	11	8	2	3	6	5
y_i	: 11	2	12	4	5	1	9	10	3	6	7	8
$d_i = x_i - y_i$	: 1	5	−2	5	−4	3	2	−2	−1	−3	−1	−3

$$\sum d_i^2 = 108.$$

Thus $r_s = 1 - \frac{6\sum d_i^2}{n(n^2-1)} = 1 - \frac{6 \times 108}{12 \times 143} = 0.6224$

We write below the ranks of x in natural order and ranks of y correspondingly

x_i	:	1	2	3	4	5	6	7	8	9	10	11	12
y_i	:	5	3	6	1	8	7	2	10	4	12	9	11

Total number of scores = $\binom{n}{2} = \frac{12 \times 11}{2} = 66$

Actual score = S = 3 + 6 + 3 + 8 + 1 + 2 + 5 + 0 + 3 – 2 + 1 = 30 (procedure for calculations of S is explained in Example 6.10 (ii))

Thus, $T = \frac{30}{60} = 0.4545$

(b) To test $H_0 : \rho_s = 0$ against $H_1 : \rho_s \neq 0$, the approximate test statistic is

$$Z = r_s\sqrt{n-1}$$

$$= 0.6224 \times \sqrt{11} = 2.06 \sim N(0,1)$$

Since Cal $|Z|$, i.e., 2.06 > $Z_{0.025}$ = 1.96, hence we reject H_0.

It means that the heights of husband and wife are not independent.

To test $H_0 : \tau = 0$ against $H_1 : \tau \neq 0$, the approximate test statistic is

$$Z = \frac{3}{2}(\sqrt{n})T = \frac{3}{2}\left(\sqrt{12}\right)0.4545 = 2.36 \sim N(0,1)$$

Since Cal $|Z|$, i.e., 2.36 > $Z_{0.025}$ = 1.96, hence we reject H_0. Hence we can conclude that there is an association between the heights of husband and wife.

[illegible] $= 0.622$

[illegible] the ranks of [illegible] and [illegible] of [illegible]

[illegible]

Total number of [illegible] $= \binom{8}{2} = [illegible]$

Actual score = [illegible] $= 30$ [illegible]

calculation of [illegible] Example 6.10 [illegible]

$= 0.854$

[illegible] test statistic is

[illegible]

[illegible] means that the [illegible] of [illegible]

[illegible]

$Z = [illegible]$

[illegible] conclude that there is an association [illegible]

Chapter 7
Statistical Decision Theory

7.1 Introduction

In this chapter we discuss the problems of point estimation, hypothesis testing and interval estimation of a parameter from a different standpoint.

Before we start the discussion, let us first define certain terms commonly used in statistical inerence problem and decision theory. Let $X_1, X_2, \ldots, X_n$ denote a random sample of size n from a distribution that has the p.d.f. $f(x, \theta)$, where θ is an unknown state of nature or an unknown parameter and Θ is the set of all possible values of θ, i.e. parameter space (known).

To make some inference about θ, i.e. to take some decisions or action about θ, the statistician takes an action on the basis of the sample point $(x_1, x_2, \ldots, x_n)$.

Let us define

$$\begin{aligned} Œ &= \text{the set of all possible actions for statistician (action space)} \\ &\equiv \text{to choose an action a from Œ.} \end{aligned}$$

So, θ = true state of nature and a = action taken by the statistician.

The value $L(\theta, a)$ is the loss incurred by taking action 'a' when θ is true. Equivalently, it is a measure of the degree of undesirability of choosing an action 'a' when θ is true and this gives a preference pattern over œ for given θ, i.e. the smaller the loss the better the action under θ. $L(\theta, a)$ is a real-valued function on Θ x œ = Loss function. Thus (Θ, œ, L) is the basic element in our discussion.

Example 7.1 Let θ = average life length of electric bulbs produced in a factory and $\Theta = (0, \infty)$.

Point estimation of θ

To estimate the value of $\theta \equiv$ to choose one value from $(0, \infty)$; so $a = (0, \infty)$.

Observe life lengths of some randomly selected bulbs.

Define $L(\theta, a) = (\theta - a)^2$ = squared error loss function

P.K. Sahu et al., *Estimation and Inferential Statistics*,
DOI 10.1007/978-81-322-2514-0_7

(or) = $|\theta - a|$ = absolute error loss function
(or) = $w(\theta)(\theta - a)^2$ = weighted squared error loss function where
$w(\theta)$ = a known function of θ.

Desired nature of (L, θ) graph should be a convex function with minimum at θ and increasing in $|\theta - a|$.

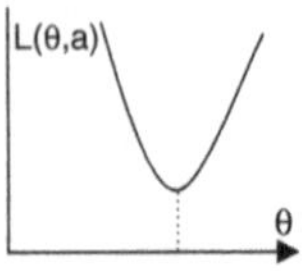

Testing of hypothesis of θ

To test $H_0 : \theta \le \theta_0$ (a given value of θ) against

$$H_1 : \theta > \theta_0$$

$Œ = \{a_0, a_1\}$ where a_0 = accept H_0 and a_1 = accept H_1. Here, simple (0–1) loss function is as

	a_0	a_1
$\theta \le \theta_0$	0	1
$\theta > \theta_0$	1	0

or, assigned value loss function is as

$$\begin{array}{c|cc} & a_0 & a_1 \\ \theta \le \theta_0 & l_{00} & l_{01} \\ \theta > \theta_0 & l_{10} & l_{11} \end{array} \left.\right\} \begin{array}{l} l_{00} < l_{01} \\ l_{11} < l_{10} \end{array}$$

or, a $(0 - \omega)$ type loss function is as

$$\begin{array}{c|cc} & a_0 & a_1 \\ \theta \le \theta_0 & 0 & \omega_1(\theta) \\ \theta > \theta_0 & \omega_2(\theta) & 0 \end{array} \left.\right\} \begin{array}{l} w_1(\theta) \uparrow \text{ in } \theta_0 - \theta \\ w_2(\theta) \uparrow \text{ in } \theta - \theta_0 \end{array}$$

Interval estimation

Here, we are to choose one interval from $(0, \infty)$.

$$\begin{aligned} \text{So, } Œ &= \text{The set of all possible intervals of } (0, \infty) \\ &= (a_1, a_2). \end{aligned}$$

$$L(\theta, a) = \begin{cases} 1 \text{ if } \theta \notin a \\ 0 \text{ if } \theta \in a \end{cases}$$ or, may be $L(\theta, a) = a_2 - a_1$ = length of the interval.

Let $R =$ A random experiment performed

$X =$ Random outcomes of the experiment $=$ Random variable or vector

$x =$ Observed value of X

$\mathcal{X} =$ Sample space

The probability distribution of X depends on θ, (say)

$$P_\theta : P_\theta[X \in A] \text{ or, } \quad F_\theta(x) = P_\theta[X \leq x]$$
$$\text{or, } f_\theta(x) = \text{p.d.f or p.m.f of } X.$$

The statistician observes the value x of X to take his decision. If $X = x$ is observed the statistician takes an action $d(x) \in \mathcal{Œ}$, $d(x): \mathcal{X} \rightarrow \mathcal{Œ}$ where

$$d(x) = \text{A decision rule in its simplest form}$$
$$= \text{A non-randomized decision rule.}$$

If $d(x)$ = action taken; loss incurred under $\theta = L(\theta, d(x))$. If $d(x)$ = decision rule, then loss incurred (under θ) $= L(\theta, d(x))$ (random quantity) = a real-valued random variable. Expected loss (under θ) $= E_\theta L(\theta, d(x)) = R_d(\theta)$ = risk of $d(x)$ under θ.

$$\therefore R_d(\theta) : \theta \in \Theta \rightarrow \text{Risk function of } d(x).$$

Let us restrict to rule $d(x)$ for which $R_d(\theta) < \infty \forall \theta$ and let D = the set of all such $d(x)$'s. $R_d(\theta)$ gives a preference pattern D for given θ. The smaller the risk the better is the decision rule $d(x)$.

Thus, $(\Theta, \mathcal{Œ}, L) \xrightarrow{X} (\Theta, D, R)$

Example 7.2 Point estimation of real $\theta : \mathcal{Œ} = \Theta$

$d(x)$: $\mathcal{X} \rightarrow \mathcal{Œ}(\Theta)$; $d(x)$ = point estimator of θ.

For squared error loss $R_d(\theta) = E_\theta(d(x) - \theta)^2 =$ MSE of $d(x)$ under θ.

Example 7.3 $\mathcal{Œ} = \{a_0, a_1\}$; $a_i =$ accept H_i, i = 0, 1,

$$d(x) : \mathcal{X} \rightarrow \{a_0, a_1\}$$
$$\mathcal{X}_0 = \{x : d(x) = a_0\} = \text{acceptance region}$$
$$\mathcal{X}_1 = \{x : d(x) = a_1\} = \text{rejection region}$$

$$\therefore d(x) = a_0 \text{ if } x \in \mathcal{X}_0$$
$$a_1 \text{ if } x \in \mathcal{X}_1$$

$\mathcal{X}_0$ and $\mathcal{X}_1$ are disjoint and $\mathcal{X}_0 + \mathcal{X}_1 = \mathcal{X}$

For (0–1) loss if $\theta \in \Theta_0, R_d(\theta) = P_\theta\{d(x) = a_1\}$
$= P_\theta\{X \in \mathcal{X}_1\}$
$=$ Probability of first kind of error.

If $\theta \in \Theta_1, R_d(\theta) = P_\theta\{d(x) = a_0\} = P_\theta\{X \in \mathcal{X}_0\}$
$= 1 - P_\theta\{X \in \mathcal{X}_1\} =$ Probability of type 2 error.

Interval estimation of real θ

Œ = set of all possible intervals of Θ.

$$d(x) : \mathcal{X} \to \text{Œ}$$

$$d(x) = (d_1(x), d_2(x))$$

$$L(\theta, a) = \begin{cases} 1 \text{ if } \theta \notin a \\ 0 \text{ if } \theta \in a \end{cases}$$

Then $R_d(\theta) = P_\theta\{\theta \notin d(x)\} = 1 - P_\theta\{\theta \in d(x)\}$
If $L(\theta, a) = a_2 - a_1$
then $R_d(\theta) = E_\theta[d_2(x) - d_1(x)]$ = Expected length of $d(x)$.
Thus, (Θ, Œ, L) = Basic element of a statistical decision problem.
X = observable random variable; for each x, $d(x) \in$ Œ, i.e. $d : \mathcal{X} \to$ Œ
$d(x)$ = a non-randomized decision rule.

$$R_d(\theta) = E_\theta(L(\theta, d(x))) = \text{ Risk of } d(x)$$

D = the set of all non-randomized decision rules (with finite risks $\forall\theta$)

Randomized Decision Rules

Randomized action

Example 7.4 Let $\Theta = \{\theta_1, \theta_2\}$, Œ $= \{a_1, a_2, a_3\}$ and

Loss function as		a_1	a_2	a_3
	θ_1	1	4	3
	θ_2	4	1	3

Neither a_1 nor a_2 is better than a_3 for every value of θ. Now define an action

$a^* : a^* = a_1$ with probability $\frac{1}{2}$

$= a_2$ with probability $\frac{1}{2}$

The expected loss for a^* is

$$L(\theta_1, a^*) = \frac{1}{2}L(\theta_1, a_1) + \frac{1}{2}L(\theta_1, a_2) = 2.5$$

$$L(\theta_2, a^*) = \frac{1}{2}L(\theta_2, a_1) + \frac{1}{2}L(\theta_2, a_2) = 2.5$$

Thus a^* is to be preferred to a_3 both under θ_1 and θ_2. Such an a^* is called randomized action.

Generally, by randomized action a^* we mean actually a probability distribution over Œ and loss due to a randomized action a^* is

$L(\theta, a^*) = EL(\theta, z)$ where z is a random variable with probability distribution a^* over Œ.

Advantages of considering randomized actions

1. Extends the class of actions, i.e. allows more flexibility for the statistician.
2. The set of all randomized actions is convex, i.e. if a_1^*, a_2^* are two randomized actions, then for every $0 \le \alpha \le 1$; $\alpha a_1^* + (1-\alpha)a_2^*$ is also a randomized action with $L(\theta, \alpha a_1^* + (1-\alpha)a_2^*) = \alpha L(\theta, a_1^*) + (1-\alpha)L(\theta, a_2^*)$.

We shall consider only randomized actions a^* for which $L(\theta, a^*)$ is finite $\forall\theta$ and shall denote by Œ* the set of all such randomized actions.

Note Clearly Œ $\subseteq$ Œ* because a non-randomized action 'a' ≡ A probability distribution over Œ degenerate at the point 'a'.

First definition of randomized decision rule

Let X = observable random variable
x = observed value of X
For each x, let $\delta(x) \in$ Œ*, i.e. $\delta : \mathcal{X} \to$ Œ*
$\delta = \delta(x)$ = a (behavioural) randomized decision rule.
$R_\delta(\theta)$ = Risk of δ at $\theta = E_\theta L(\theta, \delta(x))$
We shall consider only behavioural rules δ for which $R_\delta(\theta)$ is finite $\forall\theta$ and shall denote by $\mathcal{D}$ as the class of all such behavioural rules. Clearly, $D \subseteq \mathcal{D}$.

Example 7.5 Test of hypothesis problem $H_0 : \theta \in \Theta_0$ against $H_1 : \theta \in \Theta_1$.

$$\text{Œ} = \{a_0, a_1\}, a_i = \text{ accept } H_i, i = 0, 1, \ldots$$

A typical randomized action $a^* = \phi$
where ϕ = probability of accepting H_1
$1 - \phi$ = probability of accepting $H_0, 0 \le \phi \le 1$.

A typical behavioural decision rule: $\delta = \delta(x) = \phi(x)$
where $\phi(x) =$ probability of accepting H_1 for $X = x$

$$1-\phi(x) = \text{ probability of accepting } H_0 \text{ for } X = x$$

$0 \leq \phi(x) \leq 1$. For 0–1 loss, $L(\theta, a^*) = \phi \cdot 1 + (1-\phi) \cdot 0 = \phi$ for $\theta \in \Theta_0$

$$L(\theta, a^*) = \phi \cdot 0 + (1-\phi) \cdot 1 = 1-\phi \text{ for } \theta \in \Theta_1$$

$$\begin{aligned} R_\phi(\theta) &= E_\theta \phi(x) \text{ for } \theta \in \Theta_0 \\ &= E_\theta[1-\phi(x)] \text{ for } \theta \in \Theta_1 \end{aligned}$$

Second definition of randomized decision rule

Let X = observable random variable; x = observed value of X.
D = the set of all non-randomized decision rules.

δ = A probability distribution over D
= A randomized (mixed) decision rule with $R_\delta(\theta) = ER_z(\theta)$ = Risk of δ at θ where
Z = A random variable with probability distribution δ over D.

Example 7.6 $Œ = \{a_1, a_2\}$ $\mathfrak{X} = \{x_1, x_2\}$

$$D = \{d_1, d_2, d_3, d_4\}$$

$$\begin{aligned} d_1 &: d_1(x_1) = a_1, d_1(x_2) = a_1 \\ d_2 &: d_2(x_1) = a_2, d_2(x_2) = a_2 \\ d_3 &: d_3(x_1) = a_1, d_3(x_2) = a_2 \\ d_4 &: d_4(x_1) = a_2, d_4(x_2) = a_1 \end{aligned}$$

A typical mixed decision rule is $\delta = (p_1, p_2, p_3, p_4)$
$p_i \geq 0 \ \forall \ i = 1(1)4$, $\sum_1^4 p_i = 1$ where

$$p_i = \text{ probability of choosing non-randomized rule } d_i$$

$$R_\delta(\theta) = \sum_{i=1}^{4} p_i R_{d_i}(\theta).$$

We shall consider only mixed rules δ for which $R_\delta(\theta)$ is finite $\forall \theta$ and shall denote by D^* as the class of all such mixed decision rules. Clearly, $D \subseteq D^*$ since a non-randomized rule d = a probability distribution over D degenerate at d.

First mode of randomization:

$$(\Theta, Œ, L) \rightarrow (\Theta, Œ^*, L) \xrightarrow{X} (\Theta, \mathscr{D}, R)$$

Second mode of randomization:

$$(\Theta, Œ, L) \xrightarrow{X} (\Theta, D, L) \rightarrow (\Theta, D^*, R)$$

Note The two modes of randomization can be considered to be equivalent in the sense that given any $\delta \in D^*$ one can find a $\delta^* \in \mathscr{D}$ with $R_\delta(\theta) = R_{\delta^*}(\theta)\ \forall\theta$ and conversely.

Example 7.7 $Œ = \{a_1, a_2\}$, $\mathscr{X} = \{x_1, x_2\}$
$D = \{d_1, d_2, d_3, d_4\}$ as defined earlier.

A typical $\delta \in D^*$ is $\delta = (p_1, p_2, p_3, p_4)$, $p_i \geq 0$ for i = 1(1)4, $\sum_1^4 p_i = 1$, where $p_i =$ probability of choosing d_i.

$$D^* = \left\{(p_1, p_2, p_3, p_4)\big/ p_i \geq 0 \forall i, \sum p_i = 1\right\}$$

A typical $\delta^* \in \mathscr{D}$ is $\delta^* = (\phi_1, \phi_2), 0 \leq \phi_1, \phi_2 \leq 1$, where $\phi_i = \phi(x_i)$ = probability of taking action a_1 if $X = x_i$,

$$1 - \phi_i = \text{ probability of taking action } a_2 \text{ if } X = x_i.$$

$$\mathscr{D} = \{(\phi_1, \phi_2)/0 \leq \phi_1, \phi_2 \leq 1\}$$

If one chooses a $\delta \in D^*$,

$$\left.\begin{array}{l} a_1 \text{ is chosen with probability } p_1 + p_3 \\ a_2 \text{ is chosen with probability } 1 - (p_1 + p_3) = p_2 + p_4 \end{array}\right\} \quad \text{for } X = x_1$$

$$\left.\begin{array}{l} a_1 \text{ is chosen with probability } p_1 + p_4 \\ a_2 \text{ is chosen with probability } 1 - (p_1 + p_4) = p_2 + p_3 \end{array}\right\} \quad \text{for } X = x_2$$

Thus, δ can be considered to be equivalent to a $\delta^* \in \mathscr{D}$ with $\phi_1 = p_1 + p_3$, $\phi_2 = p_1 + p_4$.

Similarly, a $\delta^* \in \mathscr{D}$ can be considered to be equivalent to a $\delta = D^*$ with $p_1 + p_3 = \phi_1$, $p_1 + p_4 = \phi_2$.

Advantages of considering randomized rules

1. Extends the class of decision rules, i.e. allows more flexibility to the statistician
2. The set of all randomized rules is convex, i.e. if $\delta_1, \delta_2 \in D$ (or D^*) then $\alpha\delta_1 + (1-\alpha)\delta_2 \in D$ (or D^*).

For every $0 \leq \alpha \leq 1$ and $R_{\alpha\delta_1 + (1-\alpha)\delta_2}(\theta) = \alpha R_{\delta_1}(\theta) + (1-\alpha)R_{\delta_2}(\theta)\forall\theta$.
Thus, $\theta \in \Theta$, $a \in Œ$; $L(\theta, a)$; $(\Theta, Œ, L)$
X = observable random variable
$P = \{P_\theta/\theta \in \Theta\} =$ family of probability distribution of X

$d(x)$ = a non-randomized decision rule
D = the class of all non-randomized decision rules
$\delta(X)$ = a behavioural or randomized decision rule
$\mathscr{D}$ = the class of all behavioural rules
D^* = the class of all randomized rules
$\mathscr{D}$ and D^* are equivalent classes.
We shall hereafter denote both $\mathscr{D}$ and D^* as $\mathscr{D}$.

Note $D \subset \mathscr{D}$
Let $\delta \in \mathscr{D}$, $R_\delta(\theta)$ = risk function of δ; $\theta \in \Theta$.
Goodness of a δ is measured by risk function.

A natural ordering of decision rules
Let $\delta_1, \delta_2 \in \mathscr{D}$

1. δ_1 is said to be equivalent to $\delta_2 (\delta_1 \equiv \delta_2)$ if $R_{\delta_1}(\theta) = R_{\delta_2}(\theta)\ \forall \theta \in \Theta$
2. δ_1 is at least as good as $\delta_2 (\delta_1 \geq \delta_2)$ if $R_{\delta_1}(\theta) \leq R_{\delta_2}(\theta)\ \forall \theta \in \Theta$
3. δ_1 is said to be better than $\delta_2 (\delta_1 > \delta_2)$ if $R_{\delta_1}(\theta) \leq R_{\delta_2}(\theta)\ \forall \theta \in \Theta$ with strict inequality for at least one θ.

Note

1. $\delta_1 \geq \delta_2 \Rightarrow$ either $\delta_1 > \delta_2$, or $\delta_1 \equiv \delta_2$
   $\delta_1 > \delta_2 \Rightarrow \delta_1 \geq \delta_2$
2. $\delta_1 > \delta_2, \delta_2 > \delta_3 \Rightarrow \delta_1 > \delta_3$, similarly for $\geq$ case
3. It may so happen that neither $\delta_1 > (\text{or} \geq) \delta_2$ nor $\delta_2 > (\text{or} \geq) \delta_1$. In such case δ_1 and δ_2 are non-comparable. Thus $> (\text{or} \geq)$ gives a partial ordering of rules $\in \mathscr{D}$

Example 7.8 $X \sim N(\theta, 1)$
To estimate $\theta, \Theta = \text{Œ} = (-\infty, \infty)$.
$L(\theta, a) = (\theta - a)^2 =$ squared error loss. For any real constant C, let $d_c(X) = CX = A$ non-randomized rule (Fig. 7.1).

$$\begin{aligned} R_{dc}(X) &= E_\theta[CX - \theta]^2 = E_\theta[C(X - \theta) - \theta(1 - C)]^2 \\ &= C^2 E_\theta (X - \theta)^2 + \theta^2 (1 - C)^2 - 2C(1 - C)\theta \cdot E_\theta (X - \theta) \\ &= C^2 + \theta^2 (1 - C)^2 \end{aligned}$$

Fig. 7.1

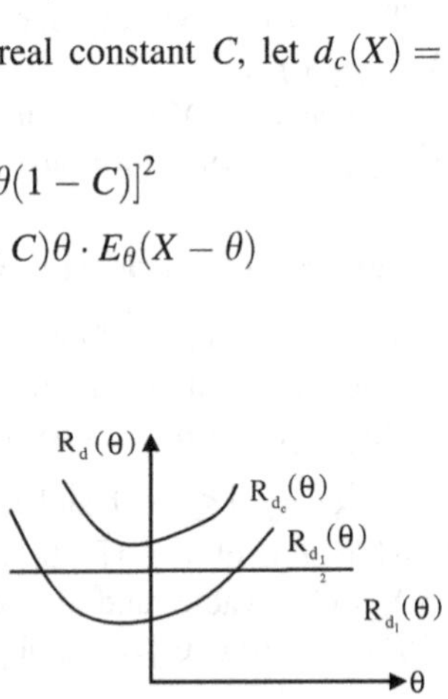

For $C = 1$, $R_{d_1}(\theta) = 1\ \forall\theta$.
For $C > 1$, $R_{d_c}(\theta) > 1 = R_{d_1}(\theta)\ \forall\theta \Rightarrow d_1 > d_c$
If $C = \frac{1}{2}$, $R_{d_{1/2}}(\theta) = \frac{1}{4} + \frac{\theta^2}{4}$
Here neither $d_1 > d_{1/2}$, nor $d_{1/2} > d_1$
Hence d_1 and $d_{1/2}$ are non-comparable.

Admissibility of Decision Rules

Definition A $\delta \in \mathscr{D}$ is said to be an admissible decision rule if there does not exist any $\delta' \in \mathscr{D}$ such that $\delta' > \delta$. Otherwise δ is said to be inadmissible, i.e. δ is said to be an inadmissible rule if there exists a $\delta' \in \mathscr{D}$ such that $\delta' > \delta$.

In the above example, for any $C > 1$, d_c is inadmissible as $d_1 > d_c$.

Note Admissibility is the minimum requirement for any reasonably good decision rule though the criterion is of negative nature.

7.2 Complete and Minimal Complete Class of Decision Rules

Definition Let $C(\subseteq\mathscr{D})$ be a class of decision rules. C is said to be a complete class of decision rule if given any $\delta \notin C$ such that a $\delta' \in C$ exists such that $\delta' > \delta$ (Fig. 7.2).
C is said to be minimal complete if

Fig. 7.2

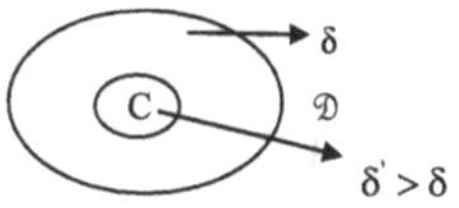

(i) C is complete and
(ii) No proper sub-class of C is complete.

Significance

If a complete class of C is available one can restrict to this class only for finding a reasonable decision rule and thus reduce the problem.

A minimal complete class, if exists, provides maximal reduction to this extent.

Note A minimal complete class does not necessarily exist.

Some relationship between a complete (or a minimal complete) class and the class of all admissible rules

Let A = the class of all admissible rules.

Result 1 For any complete class C, $A \subseteq C$, i.e. any complete class C contains all admissible rules.

Proof Let $\delta \in A$. If possible let $\delta \notin C$. So there exists a $\delta' \in C$ such that $\delta' > \delta \Rightarrow$ δ is inadmissible, which is a contradiction as we have assumed δ is an admissible rule. So $\delta \in A \Rightarrow \delta \in C$, i.e. $A \subseteq C$. □

Result 2 If A is complete, then A is minimal complete.

Proof Assume A is complete. Result 1 $\Rightarrow$ No proper sub-class of A can be complete. Hence A is minimal complete. □

Result 3 If a minimal complete class C exists, then $C \equiv A$.

Proof Let C be a minimal complete class. Then C is complete. By Result 1, $A \subseteq C$. So it is enough to prove that $C \subseteq A$. Suppose this is not true. Then there exists a δ_0 such that $\delta_0 \in C$ but

$$\delta_0 \notin A \tag{7.1}$$

This will imply that there exists a $\delta_1 \in C$ such that

$$\delta_1 > \delta_0 \tag{7.2}$$

(Since $\delta_0 \notin A$, i.e. δ_0 is inadmissible. Hence, there exists a δ such that $\delta > \delta_0$. If $\delta \in C$, take $\delta = \delta_1$. If $\delta \notin C$, there exists a $\delta_1 \in C$ such that $\delta_1 > \delta > \delta_0$. Thus, in all cases there exists a $\delta_1 \in C$ such that $\delta_1 > \delta_0$).

Let us define $C_1 = C - \{\delta_0\}$.

$$\text{Let us define } C_1 = C - \{\delta_0\}. \text{ Then it follows that } C_1 \text{ is also complete} \tag{7.3}$$

(Let $\delta \notin C_1$ □

Case 1 $\delta = \delta_0$. By (7.2), there exists a $\delta_1 \in C$ and hence $\delta_1 \in C_1$ such that $\delta_1 > \delta_0$.

Case 2 $\delta \neq \delta_0$. Then $\delta \notin C$, so there exists a $\delta' \in C$ such that $\delta' > \delta$.

A: $\delta' = \delta_0$. By (7.2), there exists a $\delta_1 \in C$ and hence $\in C_1$ such that $\delta_1 > \delta_0 > \delta$.

B: $\delta' \neq \delta_0$. $\delta' \in C_1$. Hence, there exists a $\delta' \in C_1$ such that $\delta' > \delta$.

Thus, given any $\delta \notin C_1$ in all cases there will exist a $\delta' \in C_1$ such that $\delta' > \delta \Rightarrow$ C_1 is complete)

Now (7.3) contradicts that C is minimal complete and hence (7.1) must be false $\Rightarrow C \subseteq A$. So $C \equiv A$.

Result 2 + Result 3 gives us $\Rightarrow$ A minimal complete class exists iff A is complete and in this case $C \equiv A$.

Corollary 1 *A minimal complete class, if it exists, is unique.*

Proof Let C = a minimal complete class. $C \equiv A$ which is unique. □

Corollary 2 *Let C be a minimal complete class and let $\delta \in C$. Then if $\delta' \sim \delta$, δ' also $\in C$.*

Proof $C \equiv A$, $\delta \in C \Leftrightarrow \delta \in A$. $\delta' \sim \delta \Rightarrow \delta'$ also $\in A$ and hence $\in C$. □

Corollary 3 *If δ is admissible and $\delta' \sim \delta$ then δ' is also admissible.*

Essential complete class and minimal essential complete class

Definition Let $C(\subseteq \mathscr{D})$ be a class of decision rules. Then C is said to be an essential complete class if given any $\delta \notin C$ there exists a $\delta' \in C$ such that $\delta' \geq \delta$.

C is said to be minimal essential complete class if

(i) C is essential complete; and (ii) No proper sub-class of C is essential complete.

Note A complete class C is also essential complete since $\delta' > \delta \Rightarrow \delta' \geq \delta$.

Result 1 Let A = the class of all admissible rules and C = an essential complete class.

If $\delta \in A$ but $\notin C$, then there exists a $\delta' \sim \delta$ such that $\delta' \in C$ (and hence $\in A$).

Proof Let $\delta \in A$ but $\notin C$. Then there exists a $\delta' \in C$ such that $\delta' \geq \delta$. But as $\delta \in A$, it is impossible that $\delta' > \delta$. So, $\delta' \sim \delta$. □

Result 2 Let C be minimal essential complete and let $\delta \in C$. If $\delta' \sim \delta$, then $\delta' \notin C$.

Proof If possible, let $\delta' \in C$. Define $C' = C - \{\delta'\}$ then C' will be also essential complete. This contradicts that C is minimal essential complete. Hence $\delta' \notin C$. □

Note Let $\mathscr{D}_1(\subseteq \mathscr{D})$ be a class of decision rules. D_1 is said to be an equivalent class if all rules $\in \mathscr{D}_1$ are equivalent to each other, but no rule $\in \mathscr{D} - \mathscr{D}_1$ is equivalent to a rule $\in \mathscr{D}_1$. Then $\mathscr{D}$ can be considered as the disjoint union of some equivalent classes.

Then,

(i) If C = a min. complete class then C does or does not entirely contain an equivalent class (by Corollary 2)
(ii) If C = a minimal essential complete class then C contains at most one rule from each equivalent class (by Result 2)

Further if $\delta \in C$ and in C, δ is replaced by $\delta' \sim \delta$, then resultant class is also minimal essential complete.

So,

(a) A minimal complete class $\supseteq$ A minimal essential complete class (by (i) and (ii) above)
(b) A min. essential complete class is not necessarily unique. (by 2nd part of (ii) above).

If C be a complete class such that C contains no proper essentially complete sub-class, then C is minimal complete and is also minimal essential complete.

Example 7.9 Examples of complete and essential complete class

(1) Essential completeness of the class of rules based on a sufficient statistic:

Let $\delta \equiv \delta(x) \in D$. For such x, $\delta(x)$ is a probability distribution over Œ. $T = t(x)$ = a statistic. δ is said to be based on T if $\delta(x)$ is a function of $t(x)$, i.e. $\delta(x) = \delta(x')$ whenever $t(x) = t(x')$.

Such a rule can be denoted by $\delta(T)$. T is said to be a sufficient statistic if the conditional probability distribution of X given T is the same $\forall\theta$.

Let T = a sufficient statistic and $\mathscr{D}_0$ = the class of rules based on T.

Lemma 1 *For any $\delta \in \mathscr{D}$, there exists a $\delta_0 \in \mathscr{D}_0$ such that $\delta_0 \sim \delta$. [Cor. $\mathscr{D}_0$ is an essential complete class]*

Proof Let $\delta \in \mathscr{D}$

For each given value t of T we define a probability distribution $\delta_0(t)$ over Œ as follows:

Observe the value of a random variable X' having the probability distribution the same as the conditional probability distribution of X given $T = t$ (which is independent of θ) and then if $X' = x'$ choose an action $a \in$ Œ according to the probability distribution $\delta(x')$. □

Clearly, $\delta_0(T) = a$ decision rule based on T, i.e. $\in \mathscr{D}_0$.

Also, $L(\theta, \delta_0(t)) = E\{L(\theta, \delta(x))/T = t\}$

$$\Rightarrow R_{\delta_0}(\theta) = E_\theta L(\theta, \delta(T)) = E_\theta E\{L(\theta, \delta_0(x))/T\}$$

$$= E_\theta L(\theta, \delta(x)) = R_\delta(\theta) \text{ i.e., } \delta_0 \sim \delta$$

Thus, given any $\delta \in \mathscr{D}$ we can find a $\delta_0 \in \mathscr{D}_0$ D_0 such that $\delta_0 \sim \delta$.

(2) Essential completeness of the class of non-randomized rules for convex (strictly convex) loss. Let R_k = k-dimensional real space. $S \subseteq R_k$.

S is said to be a convex subset if for any two $\underset{\sim}{x}, \underset{\sim}{y} \in S$ and for any $0 \le \alpha \le 1$, $\alpha \underset{\sim}{x} + (1 - \alpha) \underset{\sim}{y}$ also $\in S$ (Fig. 7.3).

Fig. 7.3

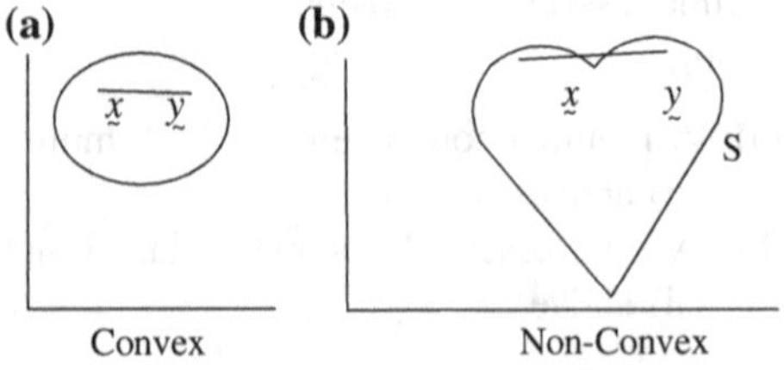

Let S = a convex subset of R_k.
$f\left(\underset{\sim}{x}\right) \doteq$ a real-valued function defined on S (Fig. 7.4).

Fig. 7.4

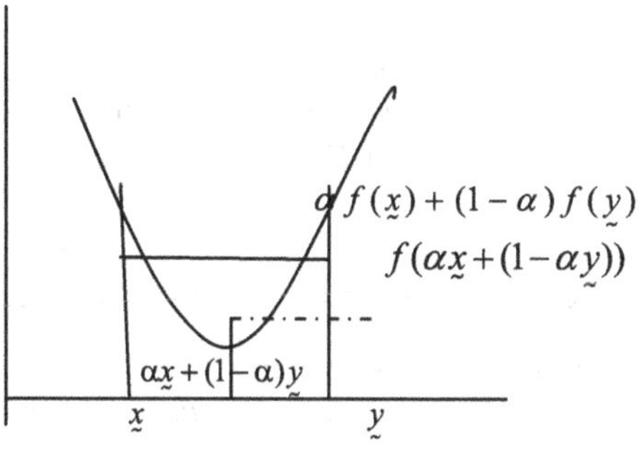

$f\left(\underset{\sim}{x}\right)$ is said to be a convex function if for any two $\underset{\sim}{x}, \underset{\sim}{y} \in S$ and for any $0 \leq \alpha \leq 1$,

$$f\left(\alpha \underset{\sim}{x} + (1-\alpha) \underset{\sim}{y}\right) \leq \alpha f\left(\underset{\sim}{x}\right) + (1-\alpha) f\left(\underset{\sim}{y}\right) \tag{7.4}$$

If strict inequality holds in (7.4) whenever $\underset{\sim}{x} \neq \underset{\sim}{y}$, $f\left(\underset{\sim}{x}\right)$ is said to be strictly convex.

Examples 7.10 $f(x) = \underbrace{x^2, e^x,}_{\text{Strictly convex}} \quad \underset{\text{convex}}{|x|,} \quad x \in R_1$

Lemma 2 (Jensen's inequality) *Let S = a convex subset of R_k; $f\left(\underset{\sim}{x}\right) = a$ real-valued convex function defined on S. Let $\underset{\sim}{Z} = a$ random variable, such that $P\left[\underset{\sim}{Z} \in S\right] = 1$ and $E\left(\underset{\sim}{Z}\right)$ exists. Then (i) $E\left(\underset{\sim}{Z}\right) \in S$; (ii) $Ef\left(\underset{\sim}{Z}\right) \geq f\left(E\,\underset{\sim}{Z}\right)$*

If f is strictly convex, then strict inequality holds in (ii) unless the distribution of $\underset{\sim}{Z}$ is degenerate.

Let Œ = a convex subset of R_k. The loss function $L(\theta, a)$ is said to be convex (or strictly convex) if for each given θ, $L(\theta, a)$ is a convex (or strictly convex) function of a.

Example 7.11

$$\text{Œ} = R_1,\ L(\theta, a) = \underset{\text{Strictly convex}}{\underset{\downarrow}{(\theta - a)^2}} \text{ or } \underset{\text{convex}}{\underset{\downarrow}{|\theta - a|}}$$

Let $\delta \in \mathscr{D}$. For each x, $\delta(x)$ is a probability distribution over Œ. Let $Z_x = a$ random variable with probability distribution $\delta(x)$ over Œ.

We assume that Ez_x exists for each

$$x \in \mathscr{X} \tag{7.5}$$

Let D = the class of all non-randomized rules $D \subseteq D$.

Lemma 3 *Let Œ = a convex subset of R_k and the loss function be convex. Then for each $\delta \in \mathscr{D}$ satisfying (7.5) there exists a $d_0 \in D$, viz, $d_0(x) = EZ_x$ such that $d_0 \geq \delta$. If the loss function is strictly convex, then $d_0 > \delta$ unless δ itself $\in \mathscr{D}$.*

Corollary 1 *Let Œ = a convex subset of R_k, the loss function be strictly convex and every $\delta \in \mathscr{D}$ satisfying (7.5), then D (=the class of all non-randomized rules) is essential complete.*

Proof of Lemma 3 Let $\delta \in \mathscr{D}$

$\delta(x)$ = a probability distribution over Œ. For each x, Z_x = a random variable with probability distribution $\delta(x)$. Define $d_0(x) = EZ_x$. By (i) of Lemma 2, $d_0(x) \in$ Œ $\forall x$, i.e. $d_0 = d_0(x) \in D$. Also, by (ii) of Lemma 2 $L(\theta, d_0(x)) = L(\theta, EZ_x) \leq EL(\theta, Z_x) = L(\theta, \delta(x))$.

$$\begin{aligned} &\Rightarrow R_{d_0}(\theta) = E_\theta L(\theta, d_0(x)) \leq E_\theta(L, \theta, \delta(x)) = R_\delta(\theta) \forall \theta \\ &\Rightarrow d_0 \geq \delta \end{aligned} \tag{7.6}$$

If the loss function is strictly convex, strict inequality holds in (7.6) for at least one θ unless Z_x-distribution is degenerate, i.e. $\forall x$ except possibly for $x \in A$ such that $P_\theta[x \in A] = 0\ \forall \theta$, in which case it means that δ itself $\in D \Rightarrow d_0 > \delta$ unless δ itself $\in D$ □

Corollary 2 *Let Œ = a convex subset of R_k, the loss function is strictly convex and every $\delta \in \mathscr{D}$ satisfying (7.5). Let T be a sufficient statistic and D_0 = the class of non-randomized rules based on T, $D_0 \subseteq D$. Then D_0 is essential complete (complete).*

Proof Let $\delta \in \mathscr{D}$.

$\mathscr{D}_0$ = the class of all randomized decision rules based on T. By Lemma 1, there exists a $\delta_0 = \delta_0(T) \in \mathscr{D}_0$ such that $\delta_0 \sim \delta$. For each t, $\delta_0(T)$ is a probability distribution over Œ. Define $Z_t = a$ random variable with probability distribution $\delta_0(t)$ and $d_0(t) = EZ_t$. As in proof of Lemma 3, $d_0(t) \in$ Œ, i.e. $d_0 = d_0(T) \in D_0$ and $d_0 \geq \delta_0(> \delta_0$ for strictly convex loss function unless $\delta_0 \in D, \sim \delta)$. Thus, given any $\delta \in D$, there exists a $d_0 \in D_0$ such that $d_0 \geq \delta$ ($> \delta$ for strictly convex loss function unless $\delta \in D_0$).

$\therefore D_0$ is essential complete (complete). □

Note On the condition stated by (7.5)

Let $\delta \in \mathscr{D}$, $Z_x =$ a random variable with probability distribution $\delta(x)$ over Œ. $L(\theta, \delta(x)) = EL(\theta, Z_x)$ which exists for each x and θ. This in many cases implies (7.5) holds.

Example 7.12 $k = 1,\ L(\theta, a) = (\theta - a)^2$ Œ $= R_1$

$EL(\theta, Z_x) = E(\theta - Z_x)^2$ exists $\forall x$ and $\forall \theta$

$\Rightarrow EZ_x$ exists $\forall x$.

$$L(\theta, a) = |\theta - a|$$

$$EL(\theta, Z_x) = E|Z_x - \theta| \geq E|Z_x| - \theta$$

i.e. $E|Z_x| \leq \theta + E|Z_x - \theta|$.

Thus $E|Z_x - \theta|$ exists $\forall x$ and $\forall \theta \Rightarrow$ (7.5) holds.

For $K \geq 2$, Œ $= = R_k = \Omega$

$$L\left(\underset{\sim}{\theta}, \underset{\sim}{a}\right) = \sum_{i=1}^{k} |a_i - \theta_i|^2 = \left\| \underset{\sim}{a} - \underset{\sim}{\theta} \right\|^2$$

$EL\left(\underset{\sim}{\theta}, \underset{\sim}{Z_x}\right) = E\left\| \underset{\sim}{Z_x} - \underset{\sim}{\theta} \right\|$ which exists $\forall x$ and $\forall \theta \Rightarrow$ (7.5) holds.

Proposition *Suppose for some* θ

$L(\theta, a) \geq C_1|a| + C_2$ *for some* $C_1(>0), C_2$. *Then* $EL(\theta, Z_x)$ *exists* $\forall x \Rightarrow$ *(7.5) holds.*

This fact gives a sufficient condition on loss function for (7.5) to hold (Fig. 7.5).

Fig. 7.5

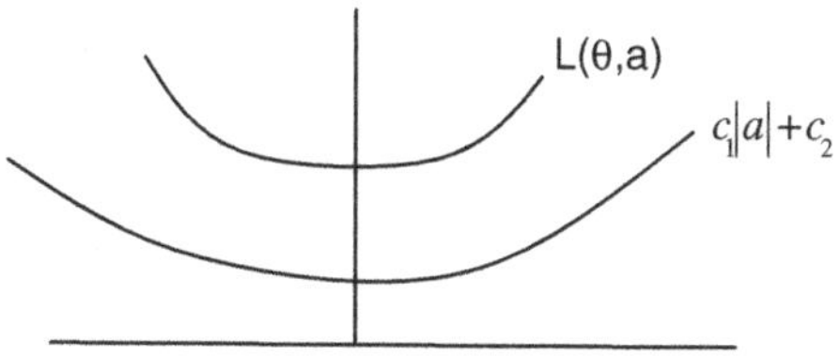

Rao-Blackwell Theorem

Let $T =$ a sufficient statistic.

$\mathscr{D} =$ the class of random values.

$\mathscr{D}_0 =$ the class of random vales based on T.

$D =$ the class of non-random values.

D_0 = the class of non-random values based on T.

$$\text{Let } d \in D \text{ satisfy } E(d(x)/T = t) \text{ exists} \tag{7.7}$$

Lemma 4 (Rao-Blackwell Theorem) *Let* æ *be a convex subset of* R_k *and let the loss function be convex. For any* $d \in D$ *satisfying (7.7), there exists a* $d_0 \in D_0$*, viz,* $d_0(t) = E(d(x)/T = t)$*. If the loss function be strictly convex* $d_0 > d$ *unless d itself* $\in D_0$.

Proof $d_0(t) = E(d(x)/T = t)$ is independent of θ.

$$\begin{aligned}
&L(\theta, d_0(t)) = L(\theta, E(d(x)/T = t)) \\
&\leq E\{L(\theta, d(x)/T = t)\} \text{ by Lemma 2.} \\
&\Rightarrow R_{d_0}(\theta) = E_\theta L(\theta, d_0(T)) \leq E_\theta E\{L(\theta, d(x)/T = t)\} \\
&= E_\theta L(\theta, d(x)) = R_d(\theta) \quad \forall\theta \\
&\Rightarrow d_0 \geq d
\end{aligned}$$

If L is strictly convex, '=' in the above inequality $\forall\theta$
iff d is a function of t, i.e. d itself $\in D_0$ implying that $d_0 > d$ unless d itself $\in D_0$. □

Corollary *Let* æ *be a convex subset of* R_k *and the loss function be convex. Let every* $d \in \mathscr{D}$ *satisfy (7.6) and every* $d \in D$ *satisfy (7.7), then* D_0 *is essential complete. If the loss function be strictly convex,* D_0 *is complete.*

Proof Let $\delta \in D$
By Lemma 3, there exists a $d \in \mathscr{D}$ such that $d \geq \delta$. Also, by Lemma 4 there exists a $d_0 \in \mathscr{D}$ such that $d_0 \geq d \geq \delta$. Thus given any $d \in \mathscr{D}$, there exists a $d_0 \in D_0$ such that $d_0 \geq \delta \Rightarrow D_0$ is essentially complete. If the loss function is strictly convex $d_0 > \delta$ unless δ itself $\in D_0 \Rightarrow D_0$ is complete. □

Note on condition (7.7) For every $d \in D$, $R_d(\theta) = E_\theta L(\theta, d(x))$ exists $\forall\theta$.
This generally implies that $E_\theta(d(x))$ exists $\forall\theta$.
$\Rightarrow E(d(x)/T = t)$ exists, i.e. (7.7) holds.

Example 7.13 To estimate a real parameter $\theta, \Omega = \text{Œ} = (-\infty, \infty)$

$$L(\theta, a) = (\theta - a)^2$$

$R_d(\theta) = E_\theta(d(x) - \theta)^2$ exists $\forall\theta \Rightarrow E_\theta(d(x))$ exists $\forall\theta \Rightarrow$ (7.7) holds.
Similarly, it can be shown for absolute error loss $L(\theta, a) = |\theta - a|$

Proposition *Let for some* θ, $L(\theta, a) \geq C_1|a| + C_2$ *for some constant* $C_1(>0)$ and C_2.

Then $R_d(\theta)$ exists $\forall\theta \Rightarrow E_\theta(d(x))$ exists $\Rightarrow$ (7.7) holds. Thus the proposition gives a sufficient condition on loss function for (7.7) to hold.

7.3 Optimal Decision Rule

$\delta_1 \geq \delta_2$ if $R_{\delta_1}(\theta) \leq R_{\delta_2}(\theta)$ $\forall\theta$ and it is a natural partial ordering of decision rules. $\delta_0 \in \mathscr{D}$ is said to be best or optimal if $\delta_0 \geq \delta \; \forall \; \delta \in \mathscr{D}$, but generally such an optimal rule does not exist.

Example To estimate a real parameter θ, $\Omega = Œ \; = (-\infty, \infty)$. Let $L(\theta, a) = (\theta - a)^2$. If possible, suppose there exists a best rule, say δ_0. Consider any given value of θ, say θ_0 and define $d_0(x) = \theta_0 \; \forall x$. Clearly, $R_{d_0}(\theta_0) = 0 \Rightarrow R_{\delta_0}(\theta_0) = 0$ where $\delta_0 \geq d_0$. Since θ_0 is arbitrary we must have $R_{\delta_0}(\theta) = 0, \forall\theta$ which is generally impossible.

$\Rightarrow$ generally there does not exist a best rule.

So to find a reasonably good decision rule we need some additional principles. Two such principles are generally followed:

(i) Restriction principle
(ii) Linear ordering principle

Restriction principle Put some reasonable restrictions on decision rules, i.e. consider a reasonable restricted sub-class of decision rules having good overall performances and then try to find a best in this restricted sub-class.

Two restriction criteria often used are

(i) Unbiasedness and
(ii) Invariance

Linear ordering principle

For every δ replace the risk function by a representative number and then compare the rules in terms of these representative numbers.

If representative number of $\delta_1 \leq$ representative number of δ_2, then we prefer δ_1 to δ_2. δ_0 is considered to be optimal if representative number of $\delta_0 \leq$ representative number of $\delta \; \forall \; \delta \in \mathscr{D}$.

Thus a linear ordering principle $\equiv$ is a way of specifying representative number

Note Any linear ordering principle should not disagree with partial ordering principle, i.e. if $\delta_1 \geq \delta_2$ we must have representative number of $\delta_1 \leq$ as representative number of δ_2.

Two linear ordering principles that are used in general are

(i) Bayes principle
(ii) Minimax principle

Bayes Principle Let Ω may be finite or countable

$\tau(\theta) : \theta \in \Omega \to$ *a* suitable weight function over Ω. $\tau(\theta) \geq 0 \; \forall \theta$ and $\sum_{\theta \in \Omega} \tau(\theta) = 1$.

Take representative number as weighted average risk

$$= \sum_{\theta \in \Omega} \tau(\theta) R_\delta(\theta) = r(\tau, \delta)$$

$$\begin{aligned} \tau(\theta) &= \text{a p.m.f of a (discrete) distribution over } \Omega \\ &= \text{prior p.m.f of } \theta. \\ r(\tau, \delta) &= \text{Bayes risk of } \delta \text{ with respect to } \tau. \end{aligned}$$

If $\Omega =$ a non-degenerate interval of R_k,
$\tau(\theta) =$ p.d.f of a (continuous) distribution over Ω.
Bayes risk of $\delta = \mathrm{r}(\tau, \delta) = \int_\Omega R_\delta(\theta)\tau(\theta)\mathrm{d}\theta$.

$\delta' S$ are compared with respect to $\mathrm{r}(\tau, \delta)$, i.e. if $\mathrm{r}(\tau, \delta_1) \leq \mathrm{r}(\tau, \delta_2)$, then δ_1 is preferred to δ_2. A $\delta_0 \in \mathscr{D}$ is considered to be optimum if it minimizes $\mathrm{r}(\tau, \delta)$ with respect to $\delta \in \mathscr{D}$. Such a δ_0 is called a Bayes rule with respect to prior τ.

Definition A rule $\delta_0 \in \mathscr{D}$ is said to be a Bayes rule with respect to a prior τ if it minimizes Bayes risk (w.r.t. τ) $\mathrm{r}(\tau, \delta)$ w.r.t. $\delta \in \mathscr{D}$, i.e. if $\mathrm{r}(\tau, \delta_0) = \inf_{\delta \in \infty} \mathrm{r}(\tau, \delta)$.

Note

1. A Bayes rule may or may not exist. If it exists, inf $\equiv$ min.
2. A Bayes rule depends on prior τ.
3. A Bayes rule, even if exists, may not be unique.
4. Bayes principle does not disagree with partial ordering principle, i.e. $R_{\delta_1}(\theta) \leq R_{\delta_2}(\theta) \; \forall \theta \Rightarrow \mathrm{r}(\tau, \delta_1) \leq \mathrm{r}(\tau, \delta_2)$ whatever be τ.

Minimax principle

For a $\delta \in \mathscr{D}$, representative number is taken as

$\operatorname{Sup}_{\theta \in \Omega} R_\delta(\theta) =$ Max. Risk that may be incurred due to choice of δ. δ_1 is preferred to δ_2 if $\operatorname{Sup}_{\theta \in \Omega} R_{\delta_1}(\theta) \leq \operatorname{Sup}_{\theta \in \Omega} R_{\delta_2}(\theta)$.

δ_0 is considered to be optimum if it minimizes $\operatorname{Sup}_{\theta \in \Omega} R_\delta(\theta)$ with respect to $\delta \in \mathscr{D}$.

Such a δ_0 is called a "Minimax Rule".

Definition A rule $\delta_0 \in \mathscr{D}$ is said to be a minimax rule if it minimizes $\operatorname{Sup}_{\theta \in \Omega} R_\delta(\theta)$ with respect to $\delta \in \mathscr{D}$, i.e. if

$\operatorname{Sup}_{\theta \in \Omega} R_{\delta_0}\theta = \inf_{\delta \in \mathscr{D}} \operatorname{Sup}_{\theta \in \Omega} R_\delta \theta$.

Notes

1. A minimax rule may or may not exist.
2. A minimax rule does not involve any prior τ.
3. A minimax rule, even if exists, may not be unique.
4. Minimax principle doesn't disagree with partial ordering principle

$$\text{i.e.}\, R_{\delta_1}(\theta) \leq R_{\delta_2}(\theta) \quad \forall \theta$$
$$\Rightarrow \underset{\theta \in \Omega}{\text{Sup}}\; R_{\delta_1}(\theta) \leq \underset{\theta \in \Omega}{\text{Sup}}\; R_{\delta_2}(\theta)$$

7.4 Method of Finding a Bayes Rule

τ = a given prior.

To find a Bayes rule δ_0 with respect to $\tau \equiv$ to find a rule δ_0 that minimizes Bayes risk $\mathrm{r}(\tau, \delta)$ with respect to δ.

Proposition *If a Bayes rule δ_0 with respect to a given prior τ exists, then there exists a non-randomized rule d_0 which is Bayes with respect to τ.*

Implication For finding a Bayes rule, we can without any loss of generality consider non-randomized rules only.

Proof Let δ_0 be a Bayes rule with respect to τ. δ_0 may be considered as a probability distribution over D (=the class of non-randomized rules).

Let Z = a random variable with probability distribution δ_0 over D. Then

$$\mathrm{r}(\tau, \delta_0) = E_z \mathrm{r}(\tau, z) \tag{7.8}$$

[Let Ω be finite or countable. $r(\tau, \delta_0) = \sum_{\theta \in \Omega} \tau(\theta) R_{\delta_0}(\theta) = \sum_{\theta \in \Omega} \tau(\theta) E_z R_z(\theta)$

$$= E_z \sum_{\theta \in \Omega} \tau(\theta) R_z(\theta) (\text{assuming that it is permissible})$$
$$= E_z r(\tau, z)$$

Similarly, we can show if when $\Omega = a$ non-degenerate interval of R_k].

$$\begin{aligned}
&\text{Now } \delta_0 \text{ is Bayes } \Rightarrow r(\tau, \delta_0) \leq r(\tau, \delta)\, \forall\, \delta \in \mathscr{D} \\
&\Rightarrow r(\tau, \delta_0) \leq r(\tau, d)\; \forall d \in D \text{ as } D \subseteq \mathscr{D} \\
&\Rightarrow r(\tau, \delta_0) \leq r(\tau, z)\, \forall \text{ values of } z. \\
&\Rightarrow r(\tau, \delta_0) \leq E_z r(\tau, z) = r(\tau, \delta_0)
\end{aligned} \tag{7.9}$$

by (7.8).

We must have equality in (7.9), and consequently Z must $\in D_0$ with probability 1, where $D_0 = \{d/d \in D, r(\tau, d) = r(\tau, \delta_0)\}$. □

Consider any $d_0 \in D_0$,

then $r(\tau, d_0) = r(\tau, \delta_0) = \inf_{\delta \in D} r(\tau, \delta)$ (since δ_0 is Bayes)

$\Rightarrow d_0$ is also Bayes. This proves the Proposition.

Note It is clear from the proof that

(1) A randomized Bayes rule = A probability distribution over D_0, i.e. the class of non-randomized Bayes rules.
(2) If a non-randomized Bayes rule is unique, i.e. D_0 consists of a single d_0, then a Bayes rule is unique and is d_0.

Method of finding Bayes rule

$\tau(\theta) = a$ prior distribution of θ.

To minimize $r(\tau, \delta)$ with respect to $\delta \in D$,

Without any loss of generality we may restrict to non-randomized rules only. So we are to minimize $r(\tau, d)$ with respect to $d \in D$.

Let Ω be countable and $\mathcal{X}$ be also countable (If $\mathcal{X}$ is an open interval of R_k, replace Σ by $\int$).

Then for any $d \in D$

$$\begin{aligned} r(\tau, d) &= \sum_{\theta \in \Omega} \tau(\theta) R_d(\theta) = \sum_{\theta \in \Omega} \tau(\theta) \sum_{x \in \mathcal{X}} p(x/\theta) L(\theta, d(x)) \\ &= \sum_{x \in \mathcal{X}} \sum_{\theta \in \Omega} \tau(\theta) p(x/\theta) L(\theta, d(x)) \end{aligned} \tag{7.10}$$

assuming it is permissible.

Suppose there exists a $d_0 = d_0(x)$ such that for each x, $d_0(x)$ minimizes $\sum_{\theta \in \Omega} \tau(\theta) p(x/\theta) L(\theta, d(x))$ with respect to $d(x) \in \mathcal{A}$.

Then clearly, d_0 minimizes (7.10) w.r.t. $d \in D \Rightarrow d_0$ is Bayes rule with respect to τ.

$p(x/\theta) =$ conditional p.m.f of X given θ.
$\tau(\theta) =$ marginal p.m.f of θ.
$p(x/\theta)\tau(\theta) =$ Joint p.m.f of X and θ.

$$\bar{p}(x) = \sum_{\theta \in \Omega} p(x/\theta)\tau(\theta) = \text{ marginal p.m.f of } X.$$

$$q(\theta/x) = \frac{p(x/\theta)\tau(\theta)}{\bar{p}(x)} = \text{ conditional (Posterior) p.m.f. of } \theta \text{ given } X = x$$

if $\bar{p}(x) > 0$ $[p(x) = 0 \Leftrightarrow \tau(\theta)p(x/\theta) = 0 \forall \theta \in \Omega]$.

To minimize $\sum_{\theta\in\Omega} \tau(\theta)p(x/\theta)L(\theta, \mathrm{d}(x))$ with respect to $d(x) \in$ Œ

$\Leftrightarrow$ to min. $\overline{p}(x) \sum_{\theta\in\Omega} q(\theta/x)L(\theta, \mathrm{d}(x))$ with respect to $d(x) \in$ Œ.

$\Leftrightarrow$ min $\sum_{\theta\in\Omega} q(\theta/x)L(\theta, \mathrm{d}(x))$ w.r.t. $d(x) \in$ Œ.

(It is conditional (posterior) loss given $X = x$), i.e. $E\{L(\theta, d(x))/X = x\}$.

Thus if there exists a $d_0 \equiv d_0(x)$ such that for each x, $d_0(x)$ gives min $E\{L(\theta, d(x))/X = x\} =$ Conditional (posterior) loss given $X = x$ w.r.t. $d(x) \in$ Œ.

Then d_0 is a Bayes rule.

If the minimizing $d_0(x)$ is unique for each x, then d_0 is the unique Bayes rule.

[Let Ω be an open interval of R_k and ¥ be also an open interval of R_k

(If ¥ is countable, replace Σ by $\int$)

Then for any $d \in D$

$$
\begin{aligned}
r(\tau, d) &= \int_{\Omega} \tau(\theta)R_d(\theta)d(\theta) \\
&= \int_{\Omega} \tau(\theta)\left[\int_{¥} p(x/\theta)L(\theta, d(x))\mathrm{d}x\right]\mathrm{d}\theta \qquad (7.11) \\
&= \int_{¥}\int_{\Omega} \tau(\theta)p(x/\theta)L(\theta, d(x))\mathrm{d}\theta\mathrm{d}x
\end{aligned}
$$

(assuming this to be permissible)

Suppose there exists a $d_0 \equiv d_0(x)$ such that for each x, $d_0(x)$ minimize $\int_{\Omega} \tau(\theta)p(x/\theta)L(\theta, d(x))\mathrm{d}\theta$ with respect to $d(x) \in$ Œ.

Then clearly, d_0 minimizes (7.11) with respect to $d \in D \Rightarrow d_0$ is Bayes rule with respect to τ.

$p(x/\theta) =$ conditional p.d.f of X given θ.

$\tau(\theta) =$ marginal p.d.f of θ

$p(x/\theta)\tau(\theta) =$ Joint p.d.f of X and θ.

$\overline{p}(x) = \int_{\Omega} \tau(\theta)p(x/\theta)\mathrm{d}\theta =$ marginal p.d.f of X.

$q(\theta/x) = \frac{p(x/\theta)\tau(\theta)}{\overline{p}(x)} =$ conditional (posterior) p.d.f of θ given $X = x$, if $\overline{p}(x) > 0$.

To minimize $\int_{\Omega} \tau(\theta)p(x/\theta)L(\theta, d(x))\mathrm{d}\theta$ with respect to $d(x) \in$ Œ

$\Leftrightarrow$ min. $\overline{p}(x) \int_{\Omega} q(\theta/x)L(\theta, d(x))\mathrm{d}\theta$ with respect to $d(x) \in$ Œ

$\Leftrightarrow$ min. $\int_{\Omega} q(\theta/x)L(\theta, d(x))\mathrm{d}\theta$ with respect to $d(x) \in$ Œ

which is to min conditional (posterior) loss given $X = x$.

i.e. $E(L(\theta, d(x))/X = x)$.

Thus if there exists a $d_0 \equiv d_0(X)$ such that for each x, $d_0(x)$ min $E\{L(\theta, d(x))/X = x\}$ = conditional (posterior) loss given $X = x$ with respect to $d(x) \in \text{œ}$ then d_0 is a Bayes rule.

If the minimizing $d_0(x)$ is unique for each x, then d_0 is unique Bayes rule]

Summary To min $r(\tau, d)$ with respect to $d \in D$

$$\begin{aligned} r(\tau, d) &= E_\theta R_d(\theta) \\ &= E_\theta E_{X/\theta} L(\theta, d(x)) \qquad \left[\because R_d(\theta) E_{X/\theta} L(\theta, d(x))\right] \\ &= E_X E_{\theta/X} L(\theta, d(x)) \text{ min for each } X = x \text{ with respect to } d(x) \in \text{Œ} \end{aligned}$$

If $d_0(x)$ is the minimizing, then $d_0 = d_0(x)$ is Bayes rule.

Applications

1 Estimation of a real parameter θ for squared error loss. To estimate a real parameter θ where $\Omega = \text{œ} = R_1$ or an open interval of it.

$L(\theta, a) = (\theta - a)^2$, $\tau(\theta) = a$ prior p.d.f of θ

To min. $E\{L(\theta, d(x))/X = x\} = \int_\Omega (\theta - d(x))^2 q(\theta/x) \mathrm{d}\theta$ w.r.t. $d(x) \in \text{Œ}$.

Clearly, minimizing $d_0(x)$ is given by

$$d_0(x) = E\left(\theta/X = x\right) = \int_\Omega \theta q(\theta/x) \mathrm{d}\theta = \frac{\int_\Omega \theta p(\theta/x) \tau(\theta) \mathrm{d}\theta}{\int_\Omega \tau(\theta) p(\theta/x) \mathrm{d}\theta}$$

Thus, here unique Bayes rule is d_0 where

$$d_0(x) = \text{ Mean of the posterior distribution of } \theta \text{ given } X = x.$$

Example 7.14

$$X \sim R(0, \theta), 0 < \theta < \infty$$

To estimate θ under squared error loss

Let $\tau(\theta) =$ prior p.d.f of $\theta = \theta e^{-\theta}, \theta > 0$

$$p(x/\theta) = \frac{1}{\theta}, 0 < x < \theta$$

$$q(\theta/x) = \text{conditional P.d.f of } \theta \text{ given } X = x$$
$$= \frac{e^{-\theta}}{\int_x^{\infty} e^{-\theta} d\theta}, x < \theta < \infty$$
$$= e^{-\theta}/e^{-x}$$

Mean of the posterior distribution of θ given $(X = x)$ $= \dfrac{\int_x^{\infty} \theta e^{-\theta} d\theta}{e^{-x}}$

$$= \frac{-\theta e^{-\theta}\big|_x^{\infty} + \int_x^{\infty} e^{-\theta} d\theta}{e^{-x}} = \frac{xe^{-x} + e^{-x}}{e^{-x}} = x + 1.$$

Thus unique Bayes estimator of θ w.r.t. τ is $d_0(x) = X + 1$.

Example 7.15 $X \sim \text{Bin}(n, \theta)$, n given, $0 < \theta < 1$

To estimate θ under squared error loss.

$$p(x/\theta) = \binom{n}{x} \theta^x (1-\theta)^{n-x}, x = 0, 1, \ldots, n$$

Let $\tau(\theta) =$ prior p.d.f of θ

$$= \frac{1}{B(\alpha, \beta)} \theta^{\alpha-1} (1-\theta)^{\beta-1}, \alpha, \beta > 0$$
$$= \text{Beta prior}$$

$$q(\theta/x) = \text{posterior distribution of } \theta \text{ given } X = x$$
$$= \frac{\binom{n}{x} \frac{1}{B(\alpha,\beta)} \theta^{x+\alpha-1} (1-\theta)^{n-x+\beta-1}}{\binom{n}{x} \frac{1}{B(\alpha,\beta)} \int_0^1 \theta^{x+\alpha-1} (1-\theta)^{n-x+\beta-1} d\theta}$$
$$= \frac{1}{B(x+\alpha, n-x+\beta)} \theta^{x+\alpha-1} (1-\theta)^{n-x+\beta-1}, 0 < \theta < 1.$$

$$d_0(x) = \text{mean of posterior distribution of } \theta \text{ given } (X = x)$$
$$= \frac{1}{B(x+\alpha, n-x+\beta)} \int_0^1 \theta^{x+\alpha} (1-\theta)^{n-x+\beta-1} d\theta$$
$$= \frac{B(x+\alpha+1, n-x+\beta)}{B(x+\alpha, n-x+\beta)} = \frac{x+\alpha}{\alpha+\beta+n}.$$

Thus the unique Bayes estimator of θ w.r.t. Beta (α, β) prior is $d_0(x) = \frac{X+\alpha}{n+\alpha+\beta}$.

Particular case if $\alpha = 1, \beta = 1$ $\tau(\theta) = 1$ $\forall 0 < \theta < 1$, i.e. uniform prior.
Unique Bayes estimator is $\frac{X+1}{n+2}$.

Example 7.16 Let $X \sim$ Poisson (θ), $0 < \theta < \infty$
To estimate θ under squared error loss.
To find Bayes estimator w.r.t. Γ prior.
i.e. $\tau(\theta) \propto e^{-\alpha\theta}\theta^{\beta-1}, \theta \geq 0$
Let $\tau(\theta) = Ke^{-\alpha\theta}\theta^{\beta-1}, \theta \geq 0$
as $\int_0^\infty \tau(\theta) d\theta = 1 \Rightarrow K\frac{\Gamma\beta}{\alpha^\beta} = 1 \Rightarrow K = \frac{\alpha^\beta}{\Gamma\beta}$

$$p(x/\theta) = e^{-\theta}\frac{\theta^x}{x!}, x = 0, 1, \ldots$$

$$q(\theta/x) = \frac{\frac{e^{-\theta}\theta^x}{x!}\frac{\alpha^\beta}{\Gamma(\beta)}e^{-\alpha\theta}\theta^{\beta-1}}{\frac{\alpha^\beta}{\Gamma(\beta)} \cdot \frac{1}{x!}\int_0^\infty e^{-(1+\alpha)\theta}\theta^{x+\beta-1} d\theta}$$

$$= \frac{e^{-(1+\alpha)\theta}.\theta^{x+\beta-1}}{\Gamma(x+\beta)}(1+\alpha)^{x+\beta}$$

$$d_0(x) = \frac{(1+\alpha)^{x+\beta}}{\Gamma(x+\beta)}\int_0^\infty e^{-(1+\alpha)\theta}\theta^{x+\beta} d\theta$$

$$= \frac{(1+\alpha)^{x+\beta}}{\Gamma(x+\beta)} \cdot \frac{\Gamma(x+\beta+1)}{(1+\alpha)^{x+\beta+1}} = \frac{x+\beta}{1+\alpha}$$

$\therefore$ Unique Bayes estimator of θ w.r.t. Γ prior is

$$d_0(x) = \frac{x+\beta}{1+\alpha}.$$

Notes

1. $d_0(x)$ is also (unique) Bayes if $L(\theta, a) = c(\theta - a)^2 \propto (\theta - a)^2$, c = a given constant
2. If a sufficient statistic T exists we may consider rules based on T only (because of essential completeness of rules based on T) and then may find Bayes rule based on T.

Example 7.17 $X = (X_1, X_2, .., X_n)$, $X_1, X_2, .., X_n$ i.i.d. $\sim N(\theta, 1)$ $-\infty < \theta < \infty$
To estimate θ under squared error loss.

$T = \overline{X} =$ min. Sufficient statistic $\sim N\left(\theta, \frac{1}{n}\right)$.

$\tau(\theta) := \theta \sim N(0, \sigma^2)$, $\sigma^2 (> 0)$ is known.

$$p(t/\theta)\tau(\theta) = \text{Cont.}\, e^{-\frac{n}{2}(t-\theta)^2} \cdot e^{-\theta^2/2\sigma^2}$$

$$= \text{Cont.}\, e^{-\frac{n}{2}t^2} \cdot e^{-\frac{\theta^2}{2}\left(n+\frac{1}{\sigma^2}\right) + n\theta t}$$

$$= \text{cont.}\, e^{-\frac{n}{2}t^2 + \frac{n^2\sigma^2 t^2}{2(n\sigma^2+1)}} \cdot e^{-\frac{n\sigma^2+1}{2\sigma^2}\left(\theta - \frac{n\sigma^2}{n\sigma^2+1}t\right)^2}$$

$$q(\theta/t) = \text{Posterior p.d.f of } \theta \text{ given } t$$

$$= \frac{\text{Const.e}^{-\frac{n}{2}t^2 + \frac{n^2\sigma^2 t^2}{2(n\sigma^2+1)}} \cdot e^{-\frac{n\sigma^2+1}{2\sigma^2}\left(\theta - \frac{n\sigma^2}{n\sigma^2+1}t\right)^2}}{\text{Const.e}^{-\frac{n}{2}t^2 + \frac{n^2\sigma^2 t^2}{2(n\sigma^2+1)}} \int e^{-\frac{n\sigma^2+1}{2\sigma^2}\left(\theta - \frac{n\sigma^2}{n\sigma^2+1}t\right)^2}}$$

$$= \text{Const.e}^{-\frac{n\sigma^2+1}{2\sigma^2}\left(\theta - \frac{n\sigma^2}{n\sigma^2+1}t\right)^2}$$

$$\Rightarrow \text{given } t,\ \theta \sim N\left(\frac{n\sigma^2}{n\sigma^2+1}t, \frac{\sigma^2}{n\sigma^2+1}\right)$$

Posterior mean $= K\overline{x}$, $K = \frac{n\sigma^2}{n\sigma^2+1}$.
$\therefore$ (Unique) Bayes estimator of $\theta = K\overline{x} = d_0(\overline{x})$
Also, Min. Bayes risk = Bayes risk of $d_0 = E_\theta E_{\overline{x}/\theta}(d_0 - \theta)^2$

$$= E_{\overline{x}} E_{\theta/\overline{x}}(d_0 - \theta)^2 = E_{\overline{x}} \frac{\sigma^2}{n\sigma^2+1} = \frac{\sigma^2}{n\sigma^2+1}$$

Applications

2. Estimation of a real θ under weighted squared error loss: $\theta =$ a real parameter. To estimate θ, $\Omega = Œ =$ some interval of R_1

Let $L(\theta, a) = w(\theta)(\theta - a)^2$, $w(\theta) > 0$
d_0 be Bayes if for each x, $d_0(x)$ minimizes

$$E_{\theta/X=x} w(\theta)(\theta - d(x))^2 = \int w(\theta)(\theta - d(x))^2 q(\theta/x) \mathrm{d}\theta$$

with respect to $d(x) \in$ æ
Clearly, $d_0(x) = \frac{\int \theta w(\theta) q(\theta/x) \mathrm{d}\theta}{\int w(\theta) q(\theta/x) \mathrm{d}\theta}$.

Example 7.18 $X \sim \text{Bin}(n, \theta)$, n known, $0<\theta<1$

To estimate θ with $L(\theta, a) = \frac{(\theta-a)^2}{\theta(1-\theta)} = w(\theta)(\theta - a)^2$

where $w(\theta) = \frac{1}{\theta(1-\theta)}$

Let $\tau(\theta) = 1\ \forall 0<\theta<1$; i.e. uniform prior.

$$q(\theta/x) = \frac{\binom{n}{x}\theta^x(1-\theta)^{n-x}}{\binom{n}{x}\int\theta^x(1-\theta)^{n-x}\mathrm{d}\theta} = \frac{\theta^x(1-\theta)^{n-x}}{B(x+1, n-x+1)},\quad 0<\theta<1$$

$$d_0(x) = \frac{\int\theta w(\theta)q(\theta/x)\mathrm{d}\theta}{\int w(\theta)q(\theta/x)\mathrm{d}\theta} = \frac{\int_0^1 \theta\frac{1}{\theta(1-\theta)}\cdot\frac{\theta^x(1-\theta)^{n-x}}{B(x+1,n-x+1)}\mathrm{d}\theta}{\int_0^1\frac{1}{\theta(1-\theta)}\cdot\frac{\theta^x(1-\theta)^{n-x}}{B(x+1,n-x+1)}\mathrm{d}\theta}$$

$$= \frac{\int_0^1\theta^x(1-\theta)^{n-x-1}\mathrm{d}\theta}{\int_0^1\theta^{x-1}(1-\theta)^{n-x-1}\mathrm{d}\theta} = \frac{B(x+1, n-x)}{B(x, n-x)}$$

$$= \frac{x}{n},\ \text{for}\ x = 1, 2, .., \overline{n-1}$$

$$\text{For}\ x = 0, \int w(\theta)(\theta - d_0(0))^2\, q(\theta/x=0)\mathrm{d}\theta \propto \int_0^1 (\theta - c)^2\theta^{-1}(1-\theta)^{n-1}\mathrm{d}\theta$$

$= \text{finite if}\ c = 0 \qquad [\text{by taking}\ d_0(0) = c]$

$= \infty\ \text{if} \qquad c \neq 0$

$$\Rightarrow \int w(\theta)(\theta - d_0(0))^2\, q(\theta/x=0)\mathrm{d}\theta\ \text{is min for}\ d_0(0) = 0 = \frac{x}{n}.$$

Similarly, for $x = n$, $\int w(\theta)(\theta - d_0(0))^2 q(\theta/x = n)d\theta$ is min for $d_0(n) = 1 = \frac{x}{n}$

Thus for every $x = 0, 1, 2, \ldots, n$; $d_0(x) = \frac{x}{n}$ minimizes

$\int w(\theta)(\theta - d_0(x))^2 q(\theta/x)\mathrm{d}\theta$ with respect to $d(x) \in æ$

$\Rightarrow d_0(x) = \frac{x}{n}$ (= minimum variance unbiased estimator or maximum likelihood estimator of θ) is unique Bayes rule.

Application

3. Estimation of a real θ under absolute error loss. To estimate $\theta =$ a real parameter, $\Omega = æ$ some interval of R_1

Let $L(\theta, a) = |\theta - a|$

$d_0 = d_0(X)$ be Bayes if for each x $d_0(x)$ minimizes $E_{\theta/X=x}|\theta - d(x)|$ with respect to $d(x) \in æ$

Clearly, $d_0(x)$ = median of the posterior distribution of θ given $X = x$. If the median of the posterior distribution is unique, then d_0 is the unique Bayes rule.

Example 7.19 $X = (X_1, X_2, \ldots, X_n)$, $X_1, X_2, \ldots, X_n$ i.i.d. $\sim N(\theta, 1)$; $-\alpha < \theta < \alpha$

To estimate θ under absolute error loss, without loss of any generality we restrict to rules based on $T = \overline{X}$. Let $\tau(\theta) : \theta \sim N(0, \sigma^2)$, $\sigma^2(>0)$ known.

Median of posterior distribution of θ given $t = k\bar{x}$, $k = \frac{n\sigma^2}{n\sigma^2 + 1}$

$\Rightarrow$ (Unique) Bayes estimator of θ is $k\bar{x}$.

Application

4. Estimation of function of θ:

To estimate $g(\theta)$ = a real-value function of θ.

$$æ = \Omega^* = \text{ the set of possible values of } g(\theta)$$

Let $L(\theta, a) = (g(\theta) - a)^2 \rightarrow$ squared error loss.

d_0 be Bayes if it minimizes $E_{\theta/X=x}\{g(\theta) - d(x)\}^2$ with respect to $d(x) \in$ æ for each given x. Clearly, $d_0(x) = E_{\theta/x=x}\{g(\theta)\}$

$\Rightarrow d_0(x) = E_{\theta/x}\{g(\theta)\}$ is (unique) Bayes.

Similarly, we can find it for weighted squared error loss or for absolute error loss.

Example 7.20 $X = (X_1, X_2)$; X_i's independent and $X_i \sim \text{Bin}(n_i, \theta_i)$, where n_1, n_2 known, $0 < \theta_1, \theta_2 < 1$; $\theta = (\theta_1, \theta_2)$

To estimate $g(\theta) = \theta_1 - \theta_2$ under squared error loss.

$\tau(\theta) : \theta_1, \theta_2$ independent, $\theta_i \sim R(0, 1), i = 1, 2$

$$q(\theta/x) = \frac{\binom{n_1}{x_1}\theta_1^{x_1}(1-\theta_1)^{n_1-x_1}\binom{n_2}{x_2}\theta_2^{x_2}(1-\theta_2)^{n_2-x_2}}{\int_0^1\int_0^1 \binom{n_1}{x_1}\theta_1^{x_1}(1-\theta_1)^{n_1-x_1}\binom{n_2}{x_2}\theta_2^{x_2}(1-\theta_2)^{n_2-x_2}d\theta_1 d\theta_2}$$
$$= \frac{\theta_1^{x_1}(1-\theta_1)^{n_1-x_1}\theta_2^{x_2}(1-\theta_2)^{n_2-x_2}}{B(x_1+1, n_1-x_1+1)B(x_2+1, n_2-x_2+1)}, 0 < \theta_1, \theta_2 < 1.$$

i.e. posterior distribution of θ is, θ_1, θ_2 independent and $\theta_i \sim B(x_i + 1, n_i - x_i + 1), i = 1, 2$

$$d_0(x) = E_{\theta/x}(\theta_1 - \theta_2) = E_{\theta_1/x}(\theta_1) - E_{\theta_2/x}(\theta_2)$$
$$= \frac{x_1+1}{n_1+2} - \frac{x_2+1}{n_2+2}$$

Thus (unique) Bayes estimator of $\theta_1 - \theta_2$ is

$$d_0(X) = \frac{X_1+1}{n_1+2} - \frac{X_2+1}{n_2+2}.$$

7.5 Methods for Finding Minimax Rule

I. Geometric or Direct Method

We find geometrically or directly a rule δ_0 such that

$$\operatorname*{Sup}_{\theta\in\Omega} R_{\delta_0}(\theta) = \inf_{\delta\in\mathscr{D}} \operatorname*{Sup}_{\theta\in\Omega} R_\delta(\theta).$$

Let $\Omega = \{\theta_1, \theta_2, \ldots, \theta_k\}, \delta \in \mathscr{D}$, S = risk set

$$\underset{\sim}{y} = \text{risk point of } \delta$$

$$\operatorname*{Sup}_{\theta\in\Omega} R_\delta(\theta) = \max_{1\le j\le k} y_j$$

Two risk points $\underset{\sim}{y}^{(1)}, \underset{\sim}{y}^{(2)}$ may be considered to be equivalent if

$$\max_{1\le j\le k} y_j^{(1)} = \max_{1\le j\le k} y_j^{(2)}.$$

A risk point $\underset{\sim}{y_0}$ is said to be a minimax point if $\max_{1\le j\le k} y_{j0} = \inf_{\underset{\sim}{y}\in S}\max_{1\le j\le k} y_j$.

If $\underset{\sim}{y_0}$ is a minimax point and δ_0 is a rule with risk point $\underset{\sim}{y_0}$, then δ_0 is minimax.

For any real C, let $Q_c = Q_{(c,c,..,c)} = \left\{\underset{\sim}{y} \Big/ y_j \le c \forall j = 1, 2, ..k\right\}$.

All risk points lying on the boundary of a Q_c are equivalent points (Figs. 7.6 and 7.7).

Fig. 7.6

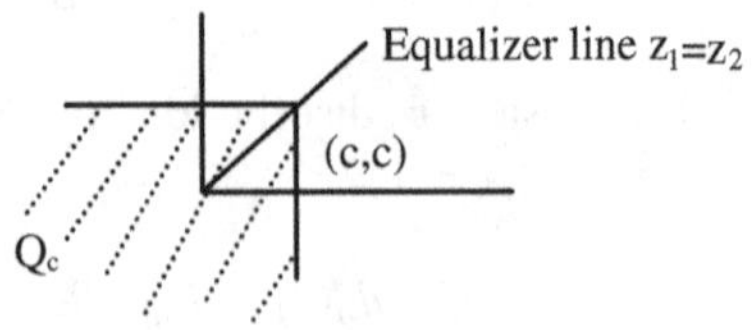

Fig. 7.7

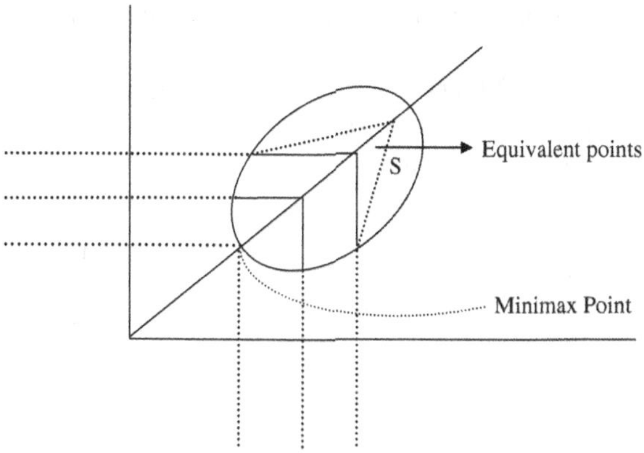

(For any such point $\underset{\sim}{y}$, max $y_j = c$)

Let $C_0 = \inf\{C/Q_c \cap S \neq \phi\}$.

Any risk point $\in$ boundary of Q_{c_0} is a minimax point. Any rule δ_0 with risk point $\underset{\sim}{y_0}$ is minimax.

Notes

1. If S does not contain its boundary points, a minimax rule may not exist.
2. A minimax point may not be unique

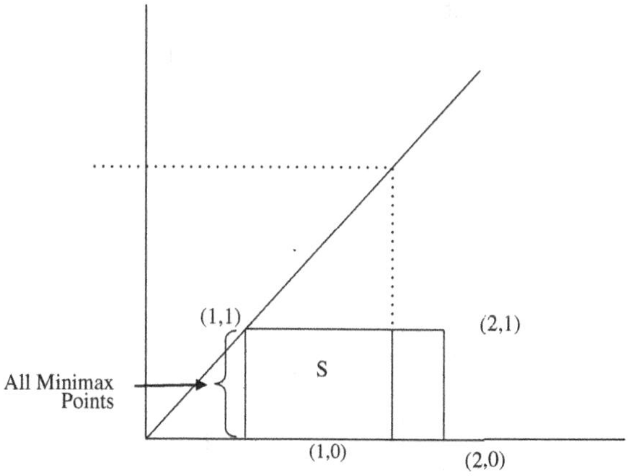

3. A minimax point does not necessarily lie on the equalizer line (Figs. 7.8 and 7.9).

Example 7.20 Let $\Omega = \{\theta_1, \theta_2\}$ æ $= \{a_1, a_2\}$
Loss is (0–1). $\mathcal{X} = \{0, 1, 2, \ldots\}$
$P_{\theta_1}[X = x] = 0$ if $x = 0$

$$= \frac{1}{2^x} \text{ if } x \geq 1$$

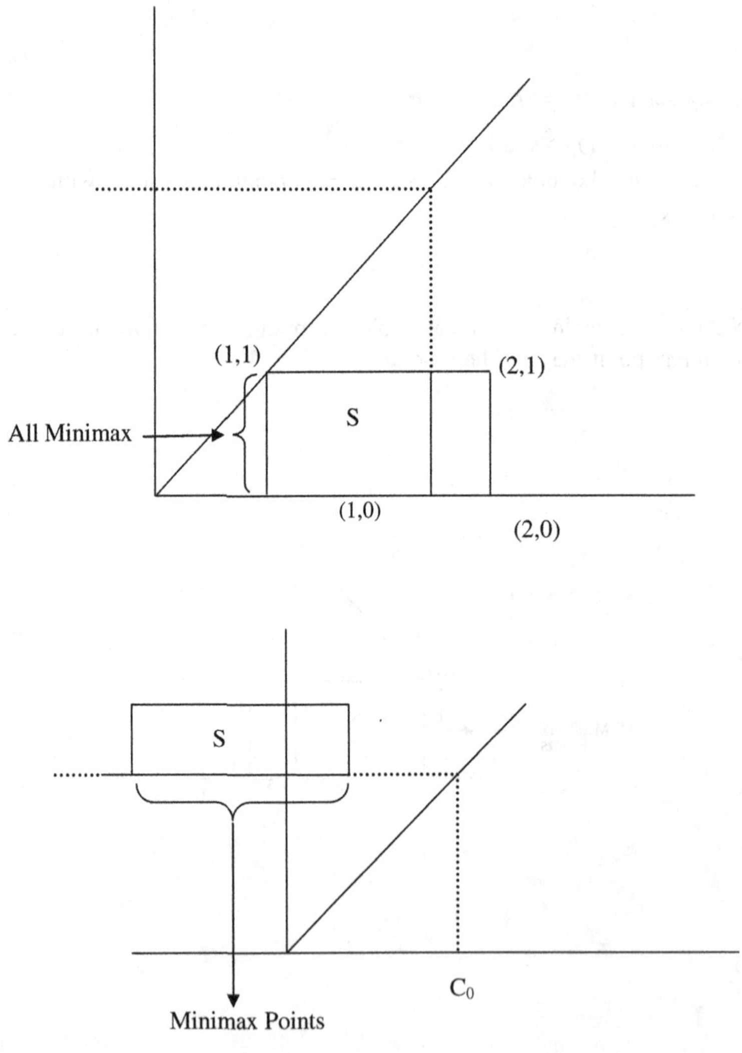

Fig. 7.8

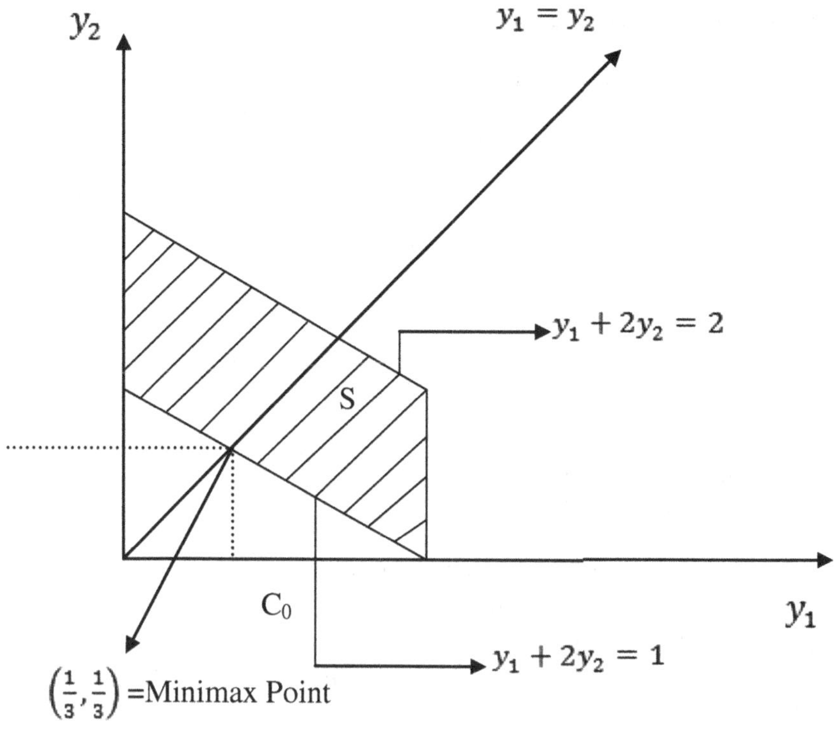

Fig. 7.9

$$P_{\theta_2}[X = x] = \frac{1}{2^{x+1}}, x = 0, 1, \ldots$$

Let $\delta \in \mathscr{D}$. $\delta(a_2/x) = \delta(x)$ $\delta(a_1/x) = 1 - \delta(x)$
$0 \leq \delta(x) \leq 1$

$$y_1 = R_\delta(\theta_1) = \sum_{x=1}^{\infty} \delta(x) \cdot P_{\theta_1}(X = x)$$

$$y_2 = R_\delta(\theta_2) = \sum_{x=0}^{\infty} \{1 - \delta(x)\} \cdot P_{\theta_2}(X = x)$$
$$= 1 - \delta(0) \cdot \frac{1}{2} - \frac{1}{2} \sum_{x=1}^{\infty} \delta(x) \frac{1}{2^x}$$

To find $\delta(x)$ such that $y_1 = y_2 = \frac{1}{3}$ we take

$$\delta(x) = \frac{1}{3} \; \forall x \geq 1, \quad \delta(0) = 1$$

Thus, a minimax rule is given as

$$\delta(a_2/0) = 1 \quad \delta(a_1/0) = 0$$
$$\delta(a_2/x) = \frac{1}{3} \quad \delta(a_1/x) = \frac{2}{3};\ x = 1, 2, \ldots$$

Example 7.21

$$\Omega = \left\{\theta_1 = \frac{1}{4}, \theta_2 = \frac{1}{2}\right\}$$

$$æ = \left\{a_1 = \frac{1}{4}, a_2 = \frac{1}{2}\right\}$$

Loss matrix:

	a_1	a_2
θ_1	1	4
θ_2	3	2

$$\left.\begin{aligned}\text{Let } X &= 0 \text{ with probability } \theta\\ &= 1 \text{ with probability } (1-\theta)\end{aligned}\right\} \theta = \theta_1, \theta_2$$

Then $D = \{d_1, d_2, d_3, d_4\}$

$d_1(0) = d_1(1) = a_1$; $d_2(0) = d_2(1) = a_2$; $d_3(0) = a_1$ but $d_3(1) = a_2$ and $d_4(0) = a_2$ but $d_4(1) = a_1$

$R_{d_1}(\theta_1) = 1, R_{d_1}(\theta_2) = 3$; $R_{d_2}(\theta_1) = 4, R_{d_2}(\theta_2) = 2$

$$R_{d_3}(\theta_1) = \frac{1}{4}\cdot 1 + \frac{3}{4}\cdot 4 = 3\frac{1}{4}$$

$$R_{d_3}(\theta_2) = \frac{1}{2}\cdot 3 + \frac{1}{2}\cdot 2 = 2\frac{1}{2}$$

$$R_{d_4}(\theta_1) = \frac{1}{4}\cdot 4 + \frac{3}{4}\cdot 1 = 1\frac{3}{4}$$

$$R_{d_4}(\theta_2) = \frac{1}{2}\cdot 2 + \frac{1}{2}\cdot 3 = 2\frac{1}{2}$$

$$\therefore S_0 = \text{the set of risk points of all non-randomized rules}$$
$$= \left\{(1,3), (4,2), \left(3\frac{1}{4}, 2\frac{1}{2}\right), \left(1\frac{3}{4}, 2\frac{1}{2}\right)\right\}.$$

If $y_2 = my_1 + C$ using = lined points $m = -\frac{2}{9}$, $c = \frac{26}{9}$

Here to find a minimax rule means to find a rule with risk point $\left(\frac{26}{11}, \frac{26}{11}\right)$ (Fig. 7.10)

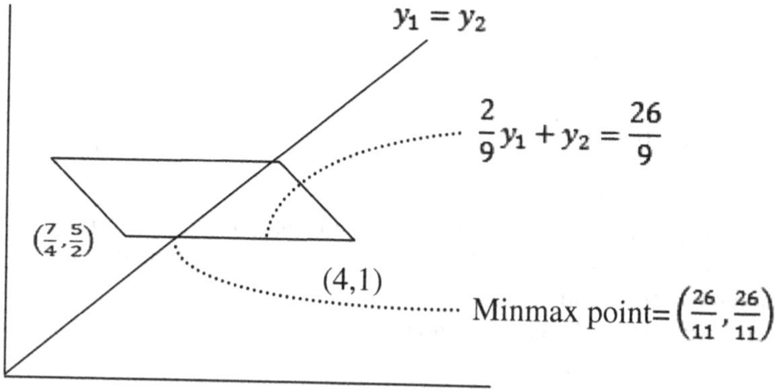

Fig. 7.10

Let $\delta \in \mathscr{D}$. For $X = x$

$$\begin{aligned} \delta &= a_1 \text{ with probability } \delta(x) \\ &= a_2 \text{ with probability } 1 - \delta(x) \end{aligned}$$

Let $\delta(0) = u, \delta(1) = v,\ \delta \cong (u, v), 0 \le u, v \le 1$

$$\delta(a_1/0) = u, \delta(a_1/1) = v$$

$$\delta(a_2/0) = 1 - u, \delta(a_2/1) = 1 - v.$$

$$\begin{aligned} R_\delta(\theta_1) &= \frac{1}{4}\{u \cdot 1 + (1-u) \cdot 4\} + \frac{3}{4}\{v \cdot 1 + (1-v)4\} \\ &= \frac{1}{4}(16 - 3u - 9v) \end{aligned}$$

$$\begin{aligned} R_\delta(\theta_2) &= \frac{1}{2}\{u \cdot 3 + (1-u) \cdot 2\} + \frac{1}{2}\{v \cdot 3 + (1-v)2\} \\ &= \frac{1}{2}(u + v + 4) \end{aligned}$$

$$R_\delta(\theta_1) = R_\delta(\theta_2) = \frac{26}{11}$$

$$\Rightarrow \frac{1}{4}(16 - 3u - 9v) = \frac{26}{11} \Rightarrow u + 3v = \frac{24}{11} \quad (7.12)$$

$$\text{and } \frac{1}{2}(u + v + 4) = \frac{26}{11} \Rightarrow u + v = \frac{8}{11} \quad (7.13)$$

(7.12), (7.13) gives the unique solution $u = 0$, $v = \frac{8}{11}$.
Thus, the unique minimax rule is given as

$$\delta(a_1/0) = 0,\ \delta(a_2/0) = 1,\ \delta(a_1/1) = \frac{8}{11},\ \delta(a_2/1) = \frac{3}{11}.$$

Note The unique minimax rule is purely randomized. Thus, unlike Bayes rules, a minimax rule may be purely randomized, i.e. although a minimax rule exists, no non-randomized rule is minimax.

Alternative (direct/or Algebraic approach)

Let us take the same Example 7.21 (Fig. 7.11)

Fig. 7.11

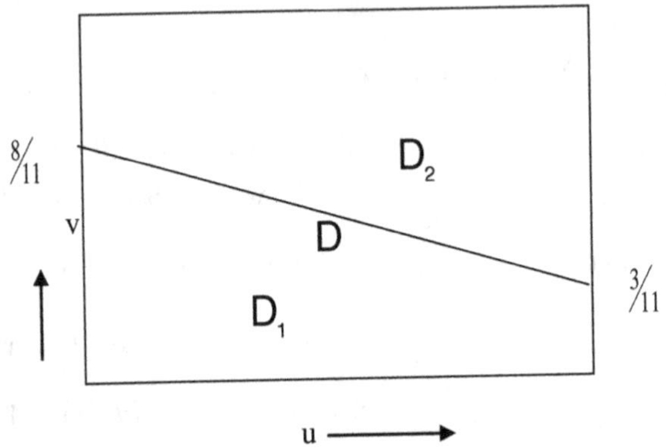

$$\underset{\theta\in\Omega}{\text{Sup}}\ R_\delta(\theta) = \max\{R_\delta(\theta_1), R_\delta(\theta_2)\} = \frac{1}{4}(16 - 3u - 9v)$$

if $\frac{1}{4}(16-3u-9v) \geq \frac{1}{2}(u+v+4)$, i.e. if $5u+11v \leq 8$ and $= \frac{1}{2}(u+v+4)$ if $\frac{1}{2}(u+v+4) \geq \frac{1}{4}(16-3u-9v)$, i.e. if $5u+11v \geq 8$

Let $\mathscr{D}_1 = \{\delta \equiv (u,v)/5u+11v \leq 8\}$

$$\mathscr{D}_2 = \{\delta \equiv (u,v)/5u+11v > 8\} \qquad \Rightarrow D_1 + D_2 = D$$

For $\delta \in \mathscr{D}_1$, $\underset{\theta\in\Omega}{\text{Sup}}\ R_\delta(\theta) = \frac{16-3u-9v}{4}$

Now $\underset{\delta\in D_1}{\text{Inf}}\ \underset{\theta\in\Theta}{\text{Sup}} R_\delta(\theta) = \underset{\substack{0\leq u,v\leq 1\\ 5u+11v\leq 8}}{\text{Inf}} \left(\frac{16-3u-9v}{4}\right)$

$$= \inf_{0\leq u\leq 1}\ \inf_{0\leq v\leq \frac{8-5u}{11}} \left(\frac{16-3u-9v}{4}\right) = \inf_{0\leq u\leq 1} \frac{1}{4}\left\{16 - 3u - \frac{9(8-5u)}{11}\right\}$$

$$= \inf_{0 \le u \le 1} \frac{1}{4}(12u + 104) = \frac{104}{44} = \frac{26}{11}$$

and inf attained for $u = 0$, $v = \frac{8-5.0}{11} = \frac{8}{11}$

Similarly, $\inf_{\delta \in \mathscr{D}_2} \operatorname{Sup}_{\theta \in \Theta} R_\delta(\theta) = \frac{26}{11}$, which is for $u = 0$, $v = \frac{8}{11}$

Finally, $\inf_{\delta \in \mathscr{D}} \operatorname{Sup}_{\theta \in \Theta} R_\delta(\theta)$

$$= \min\left\{ \inf_{\delta \in \mathscr{D}_1} \operatorname{Sup}_{\theta \in \Theta} R_\delta(\theta), \inf_{\delta \in \mathscr{D}_2} \operatorname{Sup}_{\theta \in \Omega} R_\delta(\theta) \right\} = \frac{26}{11}$$

and inf is attained if $u = 0$, $v = \frac{8}{11}$.

Thus, the unique minimax rule is given as $u = 0$, $v = \frac{8}{11}$

i.e. $\delta(a_1/0) = 0, \delta(a_2/0) = 1$, $\delta(a_1/1) = \frac{8}{11}, \delta(a_2/1) = \frac{3}{11}$

II. Use of Bayes rule

A rule δ_0 is said to be an equalizer rule if $R_{\delta_0}(\theta) = \text{Const}\ \forall \theta \in \Omega$.

Result 1 If an equalizer rule δ_0 is Bayes (w.r.t some prior τ), then δ_0 is minimax. If δ_0 is unique Bayes (w.r.t. τ), then δ_0 is unique minimax (and hence admissible).

Proof $R_{\delta_0}(\theta) = c\,\forall \theta \Rightarrow \operatorname{Sup}_{\theta \in \Theta} R_{\delta_0}(\theta) = c$ and $r(\tau, \delta_0) = c$

Minimaxiety: If possible let δ_0 be not minimax, so there exists a δ_1 such that

$$\begin{aligned} &\operatorname{Sup}_{\theta \in \Theta} R_{\delta_1}(\theta) < \operatorname{Sup}_{\theta \in \Theta} R_{\delta_0}(\theta) = c \\ &\Rightarrow R_{\delta_1}(\theta) \le \operatorname{Sup}_{\theta \in \Theta} R_{\delta_1}(\theta) = c \forall \theta \\ &\Rightarrow r(\tau, \delta_1) < c = r(\tau, \delta_0) \end{aligned}$$

But this contradicts that δ_0 is Bayes w.r.t. τ. Hence, δ_0 is minimax.

Unique minimaxiety

If possible let δ_0 be not unique minimax. So there exists another δ_1 which is also minimax, i.e. there exists another δ_1 such that

$$\begin{aligned} &\operatorname{Sup}_{\theta \in \Theta} R_{\delta_1}(\theta) = \operatorname{Sup}_{\theta \in \Theta} R_{\delta_1}(\theta) = c \\ &\Rightarrow R_{\delta_1}(\theta) \le \operatorname{Sup}_{\theta \in \Theta} R_{\delta_1}(\theta) = c \forall \theta \\ &\Rightarrow r(\tau, \delta_1) \le c = r(\tau, \delta_0) \end{aligned}$$

i.e. $r(\tau, \delta_1) = r(\tau, \delta_0)$ ($\because$ δ_0 is Bayes w.r.t. τ)

$\Rightarrow$ δ_1 is also Bayes w.r.t τ, but this contradicts that δ_0 is unique Bayes w.r.t. τ.

Hence δ_0 is unique minimax.

Example 7.22 Let $\begin{aligned} X &= 1 \text{ with probability} \theta \\ &= 0 \text{ with prob } 1-\theta. \qquad 0<\theta<1 \end{aligned}$

To estimate θ under squared error loss.
Let $d(x) = a$ non-randomized rule.
Let $d(1) = u$, $d(0) = v$, $0<u, v<1$.

$$d \equiv (u, v)$$

Equalizer rule $R_d(\theta) = \theta(u-\theta)^2 + (1-\theta)(v-\theta)^2$

$$= \theta^2(1+2v-2u) + \theta\left(u^2 - v^2 - 2v\right) + v^2$$

The rule is equalizer iff $1+2v-2u = 0$, or,

$$u = \frac{1+2v}{2} \tag{7.14}$$

and $u^2 - v^2 - 2v = 0$ or $\frac{(1+2v)^2}{4} - v^2 - 2v = 0$ (using 7.14)
Or $\frac{1}{4} - v = 0 \Rightarrow v = \frac{1}{4} \Rightarrow u = \frac{3}{4}$
Thus, the only equalizer non-randomized rule is

$$d(1) = \frac{3}{4},\ d(0) = \frac{1}{4}.$$

Bayes rule: Let $\tau =$ a prior distribution
$E(\theta) = m_1$ and $E\left(\theta^2\right) = m_2$

$$\therefore r(\tau, d) = ER_d(\theta) = m_2(1+2v-2u) + m_1\left(u^2 - v^2 - 2v\right) + v^2$$

Now $\frac{\partial r(\tau,d)}{\partial u} = 0 \Rightarrow -2m_2 + 2m_1 u = 0 \Rightarrow u = \frac{m_2}{m_1}$

$$\frac{\partial r(\tau, d)}{\partial v} = 0 \Rightarrow 2m_2 - 2m_1 v - 2m_1 + 2v = 0$$
$$\Rightarrow v = \frac{m_1 - m_2}{1 - m_1}$$

Thus, the unique Bayes rule w.r.t. τ is

$$d(1) = \frac{m_2}{m_1}, d(0) = \frac{m_1 - m_2}{1 - m_1} \text{ where } m_1 = E(\theta), m_2 = E\left(\theta^2\right)$$

Hence, the equalizer non-randomized rule is unique Bayes w.r.t. a τ such that $\frac{m_2}{m_1} = \frac{3}{4}$ and $\frac{m_1 - m_2}{1 - m_1} = \frac{1}{4}$.
$\Rightarrow m_1 = \frac{1}{2}$ and $m_2 = \frac{3}{8}$.

[For example, let $\tau = B\left(\frac{1}{2}, \frac{1}{2}\right)$ prior $\alpha = \beta$ $m_1 = \frac{\alpha}{\alpha+\beta} = \frac{1}{2}$ and $m_2 = \frac{\alpha(\alpha+1)}{(\alpha+\beta)(\alpha+\beta+1)} = \frac{3}{8}$ and the equalizer non-randomized rule is unique Bayes w.r.t. $B\left(\frac{1}{2}, \frac{1}{2}\right)$ prior].

Thus the non-randomized rule $d_0(1) = \frac{3}{4}, d_0(0) = \frac{1}{4}$ is equalizer as well as unique Bayes (w.r.t some prior) $\Rightarrow d_0(X)$ is minimax (unique).

Example 7.23

$$X \sim \text{Bin}(n, \theta), n \text{ known and } 0 < \theta < 1$$

To estimate θ under squared error loss.

$$\tau_{\alpha\beta} = B(\alpha, \beta) \text{ prior } \alpha, \beta > 0$$

The unique Bayes rule w.r.t. $\tau_{\alpha\beta}$ is

$$d_{\alpha\beta}(X) = \frac{X+\alpha}{n+\alpha+\beta}$$

$$R_{d_{\alpha\beta}}(\theta) = E_\theta\left\{\frac{X+\alpha}{n+\alpha+\beta} - \theta\right\}^2$$

$$= \frac{E_\theta\{(x-n\theta) - \theta(\alpha+\beta) + \alpha\}^2}{(n+\alpha+\beta)^2}$$

$$[\because E_\theta(x-n\theta) = 0] \Rightarrow \frac{E_\theta(x-n\theta)^2 + \theta^2(\alpha+\beta)^2 + \alpha^2 - 2\theta\alpha(\alpha+\beta)}{(n+\alpha+\beta)^2}$$

$$\left[\because E_\theta(x-n\theta)^2 = n\theta(1-\theta)\right] \Rightarrow \frac{\theta^2\left\{(\alpha+\beta)^2 - n\right\} + \theta\{n - 2\alpha(\alpha+\beta)\} + \alpha^2}{(n+\alpha+\beta)^2}$$

$d_{\alpha\beta}$ is equalizer iff

$$\left.\begin{array}{r}(\alpha+\beta)^2 = n \\ 2\alpha(\alpha+\beta) = n\end{array}\right\} \Leftrightarrow \begin{array}{l}\alpha = \frac{\sqrt{n}}{2} \\ \beta = \frac{\sqrt{n}}{2}\end{array}$$

Thus the rule

$$d_{\frac{\sqrt{n}}{2}, \frac{\sqrt{n}}{2}}(X) = \frac{X + \frac{\sqrt{n}}{2}}{n+\sqrt{n}}$$

is equalizer as well as unique Bayes (w.r.t $B\left(\frac{\sqrt{n}}{2}, \frac{\sqrt{n}}{2}\right)$ prior). Hence $\frac{X+\sqrt{n}/2}{n+\sqrt{n}}$ is the unique minimax estimator of θ.

Example 7.24 Let $X \sim \text{Bin}(n, \theta), n$ be known $0 < \theta < 1$

To estimate θ under loss function $L(\theta, a) = \frac{(\theta - a)^2}{\theta(1-\theta)}$

Let $d_0(X) = \frac{X}{n}$, $R_{d_0}(\theta) = \frac{E_\theta\left(\frac{X}{n} - \theta\right)^2}{\theta(1-\theta)} = \frac{1}{n} \quad \forall\theta$

i.e. d_0 is an equalizer rule.

Also, d_0 is unique Bayes w.r.t. $R(0,1)$ prior.

Hence $d_0(X) = \frac{X}{n}$ is the unique minimax estimator of θ.

Result 2 If an equalizer rule δ_0 is extended Bayes, then it is minimax.

Example 7.25 $X_1, X_2, \ldots, X_n$ i.i.d $\sim N(\theta, 1)$, $-\infty < \theta < \infty$

To estimate θ under squared error loss. Let $d_0 = \overline{X}$, $R_{d_0}(\theta) = \frac{1}{n} \, \forall\theta$, i.e. d_0 is equalizer. Also, d_0 is extended Bayes. Hence $\overline{X}$ is minimax.

Proof of Result 2

$$R_{\delta_0}(\theta) = c \ \forall\theta$$

So, $\sup_{\theta\in\Theta} R_{\delta_0}(\theta) = c \Rightarrow r(\tau, \delta_0) = c \ \forall\tau.$

Also, δ_0 is extended Bayes

$\Rightarrow$ given any $\in\, > 0$, there exists a prior $\tau_\in$ such that

$$\begin{aligned} c = r(\tau_\in, \delta_0) &\le \inf_{\delta\in D} r(\tau_\in, \delta) + \in \\ \text{or,} \ \inf_{\delta\in D} r(\tau_\in, \delta) &\ge c - \in \end{aligned} \tag{7.15}$$

if possible let δ_0 be not minimax.

So there exists a δ_1 such that

$$\sup_{\theta\in\Theta} R_{\delta_1}(\theta) < \sup_{\theta\in\Theta} R_{\delta_0}(\theta) = c \tag{7.16}$$

(7.16) implies there exists an $\in$ such that

$$\begin{aligned} &\sup_{\theta\in\Theta} R_{\delta_1}(\theta) < c - \in \\ &\Rightarrow R_{\delta_1}(\theta) < c - \in \ \forall\theta, \text{ since } R_\delta(\theta) \le \sup_{\theta\in\Theta} R_\delta(\theta) \\ &\Rightarrow r(\tau, \delta_1) < c - \in \ \text{ whatever be } \tau. \\ &\Rightarrow \inf_{\delta\in\mathscr{D}} r(\tau, \delta) < c - \in \ \text{ whatever be } \tau \end{aligned} \tag{7.17}$$

$$\left[\because \inf_{\delta\in\mathscr{D}} r(\tau, \delta) \le r(\tau, \delta_1)\right]$$

(7.17) contradicts (7.15). Hence δ_0 must be minimax. □

Result 3 Let δ_0 be such that

(i) $R_{\delta_0}(\theta) \leq c \, \forall\theta$ for some real constant c.
(ii) δ_0 is Bayes (unique Bayes) w.r.t. a prior τ_0 such that $r(\tau_0, \delta_0) = c$

Then δ_0 is minimax (unique minimax).

Corollary 1 *Let δ_0 be such that*
(i)′ $R_{\delta_0}(\theta) = c \, \forall\theta$ (This is in fact Result 1)
(ii)′ δ_0 is Bayes (unique Bayes) w.r.t. a prior τ_0.
Then δ_0 is minimax (unique minimax). (i)′, (ii)′ ⇒ (i), (ii)

Corollary 2 *Let $\hat{\delta}_0$ be such that*

$$(i)' \quad \begin{aligned} R_{\delta_0}(\theta) &= c \ \forall\theta \in \Theta_0(\subseteq\Theta) \\ &\leq c \quad \forall\theta \in \Theta - \Theta_0 \end{aligned}$$

(ii)′ δ_0 is Bayes (unique Bayes) w.r.t. a τ_0 such that $\Pr\{\theta \in \Theta_0\} = 1$
Then δ_0 is minimax (unique minimax)
(i)′, (ii)′, ⇒ (i), (ii)

Note For $\Theta_0 = \Theta$, Corollary 2 ⇒ Corollary 1

Proof of Result 3 For any δ and any τ,

$$\operatorname*{Sup}_{\theta\in\Omega} R_\delta(\theta) \geq r(\tau, \delta) \tag{7.18}$$

$$\left[\text{As } R_\delta(\theta) \leq \operatorname*{Sup}_{\theta\in\Theta} R_\delta(\theta) \forall\theta \Rightarrow r(\tau, \delta) \leq \operatorname*{Sup}_{\theta\in\Theta} R_\delta(\theta)\right]$$

For $\delta = \delta_0$ and $\tau = \tau_0$, (7.18)

$$\Rightarrow r(\tau_0, \delta_0) \leq \operatorname*{Sup}_{\theta\in\Theta} R_{\delta_0}(\theta) \quad \text{by (ii)} \tag{7.19}$$

$$\text{Also (i)} \Rightarrow \operatorname*{Sup}_{\theta\in\Theta} R_{\delta_0}(\theta) \leq c \tag{7.20}$$

(7.19), (7.20)

$$\Rightarrow \operatorname*{Sup}_{\theta\in\Theta} R_{\delta_0}(\theta) = c \tag{7.21}$$

So, minimaxiety of δ_0:

$$
\begin{aligned}
\text{For any, } \delta,\ \sup_{\theta\in\Theta} R_\delta(\theta) &\geq r(\tau_0,\delta) && \text{by (7.18)}\\
&\geq r(\tau_0,\delta_0) && \text{(Since, } \delta_0 \text{ is Bayes w.r.t. } \tau_0)\\
&= c(\text{by(ii)})\\
&= \sup_{\theta\in\Theta} R_{\delta_0}(\theta) && \text{by (7.21)}
\end{aligned}
$$

$\Rightarrow \delta_0$ is minimax.
Unique minimaxiety of δ_0: For any $\delta(\neq \delta_0)$

$$
\begin{aligned}
\sup_{\theta\in\Omega} R_\delta(\theta) &\geq r(\tau_0,\delta)\ (\text{by(7.18)})\\
&> r(\tau_0,\delta_0)\ (\text{Since } \delta_0 \text{ is unique Bayes w.r.t.} \tau_0)\\
&= c\ (\text{by (ii)})\\
&= \sup_{\theta\in\Omega} R_{\delta_0}(\theta)\ \text{by (7.21)}
\end{aligned}
$$

Thus $\sup\limits_{\theta\in\Omega} R_\delta(\theta) > \sup\limits_{\theta\in\Omega} R_{\delta_0}(\theta)$
$\forall\delta(\neq \delta_0) \Rightarrow \delta_0$ is unique minimax. □

Example 7.26 Let $X \sim \text{Bin}(n,\theta_1)$ n be known.
$Y \sim \text{Bin}(n,\theta_2)\ 0<\theta_1,\theta_2<1; \theta_1,\theta_2$ are unknown.

To estimate $\theta_1-\theta_2$ under squared error loss, we can expect a rule of the form $aX+bY+c$ to be minimum. However, no rule of this form is an equalizer rule. So Result 1 (or Corollary 1) cannot be applied. But Corollary 2 can be applied as follows:

Step 1: To find an equalizer Bayes rule in some $\Theta_0(\subseteq\Theta)$. Let $\Theta_0 = \{\theta_1,\theta_2/0<\theta_1,\theta_2<1,\theta_1+\theta_2=1\}$. Restricting to Θ_0, let us write $\theta_1=\theta$, $\theta_2 = 1-\theta$.

Thus, we have,

$$
\left.\begin{aligned}
&X \sim \text{Bin}(n,\theta)\\
&Y \sim \text{Bin}(n,1-\theta)\\
&\text{or } n-Y \sim \text{Bin}(n,\theta)
\end{aligned}\right]\ \text{independent.}
$$

Without any loss of generality we may restrict ourselves to rules based on $Z = X+(n-Y) \sim \text{Bin}(2n,\theta)$ (Sufficient statistic)

If $X\sim\text{Bin}(n,\theta)$, an equalizer and unique Bayes (w.r.t. $\text{Bin}\left(\frac{\sqrt{n}}{2},\frac{\sqrt{n}}{2}\right)$ prior) estimator of θ under squared error loss is $\frac{X+\frac{\sqrt{n}}{2}}{n+\sqrt{n}}$.

If $Z\sim\text{Bin}(2n,\theta)$, an equalizer and unique Bayes (w.r.t. $\text{Bin}\left(\frac{\sqrt{2n}}{2},\frac{\sqrt{2n}}{2}\right)$ prior) estimator of θ under squared error loss is $\frac{Z+\frac{\sqrt{2n}}{2}}{2n+\sqrt{2n}}$.

To estimate now $\theta_1 - \theta_2 = 2\theta - 1$, consider the following:

Lemma *Under squared error loss, if δ_0 is an equalizer Bayes (unique) estimator of $g(\theta)$, then $\delta_0^* = a\delta_0 + b$ is an equalizer Bayes (unique) estimator of $g^*(\theta) = ag(\theta) + b$.*

Proof For any estimator δ of $g(\theta)$ we can define an induced estimator, viz. $\delta^* = a\delta_0 + b$ of $g^*(\theta) = ag(\theta) + b$ and vice versa.

Under squared error loss, $R_\delta(\theta) = a^2 R_{\delta^*}(\theta)$

$$r(\tau, \delta) = a^2 r(\tau, \delta^*)$$

Hence, δ_0 is equalizer $\Rightarrow \delta^* = a\delta_0 + b$ is equalizer. □

δ_0 is Bayes (unique) w.r.t. $\tau \Rightarrow \delta_0^* = a\delta_0 + b$ is Bayes (unique).

By the Lemma, an equalizer Bayes (unique) estimator of $2\theta - 1$ is

$$\frac{2\left(z + \frac{\sqrt{2n}}{2}\right)}{2n + \sqrt{2n}} = \frac{2(X - Y)}{2n + \sqrt{2n}}$$

Thus, if we restrict to Θ_0, an equalizer Bayes (unique) estimator of $\theta_1 - \theta_2$ is $\frac{2(X-Y)}{2n+\sqrt{2n}} = d_0(\text{say})$

Step 2: $R_{d_0}(\theta_1, \theta_2) \le c \ \forall (\theta_1, \theta_2) \in \Theta$ where $c = R_{d_0}(\theta_1, \theta_2)$ for $(\theta_1, \theta_2) \in \Theta_0$.

Proof For $(\theta_1, \theta_2) \in \Theta$

$$\begin{aligned}
R_{d_0}(\theta_1, \theta_2) &= E_{\theta_1, \theta_2}\left\{\frac{2(X - Y)}{2n + \sqrt{2n}} - (\theta_1 - \theta_2)\right\}^2 \\
&= E_\theta\left\{2(X - n\theta_1) - 2(Y - n\theta_2) - \sqrt{2n}(\theta_1 - \theta_2)\right\}^2 \Big/ \left(2n + \sqrt{2n}\right)^2 \\
&= \frac{4E_\theta(X - n\theta_1)^2 + 4E_\theta(Y - n\theta_2)^2 + 2n(\theta_1 - \theta_2)^2}{\left(2n + \sqrt{2n}\right)^2} \\
&= \frac{2\theta_1(1 - \theta_1) + 2\theta_2(1 - \theta_2) + (\theta_1 - \theta_2)^2}{\left(1 + \sqrt{2n}\right)^2} = \frac{\text{Numerator}}{\text{Dinominator}}.
\end{aligned}$$

$$\begin{aligned}
&\text{Now Numerator} = 2\theta_1 + 2\theta_2 - \theta_1^2 - \theta_2^2 - 2\theta_1\theta_2 \\
&= 1 - \{1 - \theta_1 - \theta_2\}^2 \le 1 \\
&{}'='\ \text{holds iff } \theta_1 + \theta_2 = 1
\end{aligned}$$

Hence,
$$\begin{aligned}
R_{d_0}(\theta_1, \theta_2) &= \frac{1}{\left(1 + \sqrt{2n}\right)^2} = c \quad \forall (\theta_1, \theta_2) \in \Theta_0 \\
&< c \ \forall (\theta_1, \theta_2) \in \Theta - \Theta_0
\end{aligned}$$
□

By Corollary 2, Step 1 + Step 2 gives us $d_0 = \frac{2(X-Y)}{2n+\sqrt{2n}}$ is the unique minimax estimator of $\theta_1 - \theta_2$.

Result 4 Let δ_0 be such that

(i) $R_{\delta_0}(\theta) \leq c \ \forall \theta \in \Theta$, c = a real constant
(ii) There exists a sequence of Bayes rules $\{\delta_n\}$ w.r.t. sequence of priors $\{\tau_n\}$ such that $r\{\tau_n, \delta_n\} \to c$. Then δ_0 is a minimax.

Proof For any δ and any τ,

$$\operatorname*{Sup}_{\theta \in \Theta} R_\delta(\theta) \geq r(\tau, \delta) \tag{7.22}$$

(as was in the Proof of Result 3) □
(7.22) ⇒ For any δ,

$$\operatorname*{Sup}_{\theta \in \Theta} R_\delta(\theta) \geq r(\tau_n, \delta) \geq r(\tau_n, \delta_n) \to c \text{ by (ii)}$$

$$\text{(Since, } \delta_n \text{ is Bayes w.r.t. } \tau_n \text{ prior)} \tag{7.23}$$

For $\delta = \delta_0$
(7.23) ⇒ $\operatorname*{Sup}_{\theta \in \Theta} R_{\delta_0}(\theta) \geq c$ and also condition (i) ⇒ $\operatorname*{Sup}_{\theta \in \Theta} R_{\delta_0}(\theta) \leq c$

$$\Rightarrow \operatorname*{Sup}_{\theta \in \Theta} R_{\delta_0}(\theta) = c \tag{7.24}$$

Then (7.23), (7.24) ⇒ for any δ,

$$\operatorname*{Sup}_{\theta \in \Theta} R_\delta(\theta) \geq c = \operatorname*{Sup}_{\theta \in \Theta} R_{\delta_0}(\theta)$$

i.e. δ_0 is minimax.

Example 7.27 Let $X_1, X_2, .., X_n$ i.i.d $\sim N(\theta, 1), -\infty < \theta < \infty$
To estimate θ under squared error loss,
Let $d_0 = \overline{X}$, $R_{d_0}(\theta) = \frac{1}{n} \ \forall \theta$

(i) is satisfied with $c = \frac{1}{n}$.

Let $\tau_\sigma : N(0, \sigma^2)$ prior
d_σ = Bayes estimator of θ w.r.t. $\tau_\sigma = \frac{n\sigma^2}{1 + n\sigma^2} \overline{X}$
$r(\tau_\sigma, d_\sigma) = \frac{\sigma^2}{1 + n\sigma^2} \to \frac{1}{n} = c$ as $\sigma^2 \to \infty$
Thus (ii) is satisfied.
Hence $d_0 = \overline{X}$ is minimax.

Example 7.28 Let $X \sim$ Poisson (θ), $0 < \theta < \alpha$.

To estimate θ with $L(\theta, a) = \frac{(\theta - a)^2}{\theta}$.

(Apply Result 4 to prove that $d_0 = X$ is minimax)

Hint $R_{d_0}(\theta) = \frac{E_\theta(X-\theta)^2}{\theta} = 1 \Rightarrow$ (i) is satisfied with $c = 1$. Take $\tau_{\alpha\beta}(\theta) \infty e^{-\alpha\theta} \cdot \theta^{\beta-1}; 0 < \theta < \infty$. $d_{\alpha\beta}(X) =$ Bayes estimator of θ w.r.t. $\tau_{\alpha\beta} = \frac{x+\beta-1}{1+\alpha} r(\tau_{\alpha\beta}, d_{\alpha\beta}) \to 1 = c$ as $\alpha \to 0$, $\beta \to 1$. Hence $d_0 = X$ is minimax.

Other Methods: Use of Cramer-Rao inquality.

Result 1 If an equalizer rule δ_0 is admissible, then δ_0 is minimax.

Proof $R_{d_0}(\theta) = c \,\forall\theta \Rightarrow \operatorname*{Sup}_{\theta\in\Theta} R_{d_0}(\theta) = c$.

If possible let δ_0 be not minimax. Then there exists a δ_1 such that $\operatorname*{Sup}_{\theta\in\Theta} R_{\delta_1}(\theta) < \operatorname*{Sup}_{\theta\in\Theta} R_{\delta_0}(\theta) = c$

$$\Rightarrow R_{\delta_1}(\theta) < C = R_{\delta_0}(\theta) \;\forall\theta \tag{7.25}$$

(7.25) $\Rightarrow \delta_1 > \delta_0$, which contradicts that δ_0 is admissible. Hence, δ_0 is minimax. To estimate a real-valued parameter θ under squared error loss. $\Theta =$ an open interval of R_1. Without any loss of generality we can restrict ourselves to non-randomized rules only (since the loss function is convex). □

Let $d(X) =$ a non-randomized rule.

$$b_d(\theta) = E_\theta(d(X)) - \theta = \text{Bias of } d(X)$$

$$\begin{aligned}\text{By C--R inequality } R_d(\theta) &= \text{MSE}_\theta(d(X)) \\ &= b_d^2(\theta) + V_\theta(d(X)) \\ &\geq b_d^2(\theta) + \left\{1 + b_d'(\theta)\right\}^2 / \text{I}(\theta) \quad \forall\theta \\ &= C_d(\theta) \qquad \text{(say)}\end{aligned}$$

$$\text{I}(\theta) = \text{ Fisher's information function.}$$

Result 2 Let d_0 be a non-randomized rule such that

(i) MSE of d_0 attains C–R lower bound, i.e.

$$R_{d_0}(\theta) = C_{d_0}(\theta) \quad \forall\theta$$

(ii) For any non-randomized rule d_1,

$$C_{d_1}(\theta) \leq C_{d_0}(\theta) \quad \forall\theta$$
$$\Rightarrow b_{d_1}(\theta) = b_{d_0}(\theta) \quad \forall\theta$$

Then d_0 is admissible.
If further, d_0 is equalizer, then d_0 is minimax.

Proof Result I $\Rightarrow$ proves that it is minimax □

Proof of admissibility If possible let d_0 be inadmissible.
Then there exists a d_1 such that

$$R_{d_1}(\theta) \leq R_{d_0}(\theta) \quad \forall\theta \text{ with strict inequality for at least one } \theta \tag{7.26}$$

(7.26) $\Rightarrow$

$$\underbrace{C_{d_1}(\theta) \leq R_{d_1}(\theta)} \leq \underbrace{R_{d_0}(\theta) = C_{d_0}(\theta)} \quad \forall\theta \tag{7.27}$$

by C–R inequality and by (i)
(7.27) $\Rightarrow$

$$b_{d_1}(\theta) = b_{d_0}(\theta) \quad \forall\theta \quad \text{by (ii)}$$
$$\Rightarrow C_{d_1}(\theta) = C_{d_0}(\theta) \quad \forall\theta \tag{7.28}$$

(7.27) and (7.28) $\Rightarrow$

$$C_{d_0}(\theta) \leq R_{d_1}(\theta) \leq R_{d_0}(\theta) = C_{d_0}(\theta) \quad \forall\theta \tag{7.29}$$

We must have equality in (7.29) everywhere, implying that $R_{d_1}(\theta) = R_{d_0}(\theta) \forall\theta$. Thus, strict inequality in (7.26) cannot hold for any θ, i.e. there cannot be any d_1 such that $d_1 > d_0$.

Hence d_0 is admissible. □

Example 7.29 Let $x_1, x_2 \ldots x_n$ i.i.d $\sim N(\theta, 1), -\infty < \theta < \infty$. To estimate θ under squared error loss.

$\bar{X}$ is sufficient $\Rightarrow$ it is enough to restrict to n.r. rules based on $\bar{X}$ only.
Let $d_0 = d_0(\bar{X}) = \bar{X}$.
$R_{d_0}(\theta) = \frac{1}{n} \forall\theta$, i.e. d_0 is equalizer.
Also, $b_{d_0}(\theta) = 0 \forall\theta$, i.e. d_0 is unbiased.

$$R_{d_0}(\theta) = C_{d_0}(\theta) = \frac{1}{n} \forall\theta$$

i.e. condition (i) of Result 2 is satisfied [Here $I(\theta) = n$].
Let $d = d(\bar{X})$ be any n.r rule based on $\bar{X}$.

Lemma $C_d(\theta) \le C_{d_0}(\theta)\ \forall\ \theta$.
$\Rightarrow b_d(\theta) = 0\,\forall\,\theta$, *i.e. d is also unbiased.*
Lemma $\Rightarrow$ *Condition (ii) of Result 2 is also satisfied.*
Hence, (i) d_0 *is admissible.*
(ii) d_0 *is minimax.*
Also, (iii) d_0 *is unique minimax.*
[Proof of (iii): Let $d_1 = d_1(x)$ *be another minimax rule.*
Then

$$\sup_{\theta\in\Theta} R_{d_1}(\theta) = \sup_{\theta\in\Theta} R_{d_0}(\theta) = \frac{1}{n} = C_{d_0}(\theta)$$
$$\Rightarrow \underbrace{C_{d_1}(\theta) \le R_{d_1}(\theta)} \le \sup_{\theta\in\Theta} R_{d_1}(\theta) = C_{d_0}(\theta)\forall\theta$$

By C–R inequality
$\Rightarrow C_{d_1}(\theta) \le C_{d_0}(\theta)\ \forall\ \theta \Rightarrow b_{d_1}(\theta) = 0\,\forall\,\theta$ *(By Lemma).*
$\therefore$ d_1 *is an unbiased estimator of* θ. *But since* $\bar{X}$ *is complete* d_0 *is the unique unbiased estimator of* θ, *i.e.,* $d_1 = d_0$, *Hence* $d_0 = \bar{X}$ *is the unique minimax estimator of* θ*]*

Proof of Lemma Writing $b_d(\theta) = b(\theta)$
Let $C_d(\theta) \le C_{d_0}(\theta) = \frac{1}{n}\,\forall\,\theta$

$$\text{i.e., } b^2(\theta) + \{1 + b'(\theta)\}^2 \big/ n \le {}^1\!/_n\,\forall\,\theta \tag{7.30}$$

$$(7.30) \Rightarrow b'(\theta) \le 0\,\forall\,\theta \text{ i.e., } b(\theta) \text{ is non-increasing} \tag{7.31}$$

$$\left[\text{as } (7.30) \Rightarrow \frac{1}{n} + \frac{2b'(\theta)}{n} \le b^2(\theta) + \{1 + b'(\theta)\}^2 \big/ n \le {}^1\!/_n\right.$$
$$\left.\Rightarrow \frac{2b'(\theta)}{n} \le 0 \Rightarrow b'(\theta) \le 0\right]$$

$$\text{Also } (7.30) \Rightarrow b^2(\theta) + 2b'(\theta) \le 0 \tag{7.32}$$

$$\left[\text{As } (7.30) \Rightarrow nb^2(\theta) + b'^2(\theta) + 2b'(\theta) \le 0\right.$$
$$\left.\Rightarrow b^2(\theta) + 2b'(\theta) \le nb^2(\theta) + b'^2(\theta) + 2b'(\theta) \le 0\right]$$

Now $(7.32) \Rightarrow -\frac{b'(\theta)}{b'^2(\theta)} \ge \frac{1}{2}\ \forall\ \theta$ such that $b(\theta) \ne 0$

$$\text{Or } \frac{d}{d\theta} b^{-1}(\theta) \geq \frac{1}{2} \quad \forall\ \theta \text{ such that } b(\theta) \neq 0 \tag{7.33}$$

$$(7.31), (7.33) \Rightarrow b(\theta) \to 0 \text{ as } \theta \to \pm\infty \tag{7.34}$$

Finally (7.31), (7.34) $\Rightarrow b(\theta) = 0\ \forall\ \theta$, which proves the Lemma. □

7.6 Minimax Rule: Some Theoretical Aspects

A statistical decision problem ≡ A game between statistician and nature.

$$\Theta = \text{ the set of possible actions for nature.}$$

$$Œ = \text{ the set of possible actions for statistician.}$$

$L(\theta, a) =$ Loss (to the statistician) if the statistician chooses an action 'a' and nature chooses an action 'θ'.

A randomized action for the statistician = a probability distribution over Œ.

The statistician observes the value of a r.v. X. If $X = x$ is observed, the statistician chooses a randomized action $\delta(x)$.

$$\delta(x) = \text{ a randomized rule for statistician.}$$

$\tau =$ a prior distribution. $=$ a probability distribution over Θ.

$=$ a randomized action for the nature.

If the statistician chooses a randomized rule δ and the nature chooses a randomized action τ, then the statistician's expected loss is $\gamma(\tau, \delta) =$ Bayes risk of δ w.r.t. τ.

Result 1 For any $\delta \in \mathscr{D}$,

$\underset{\theta \in \Theta}{\text{Sup}}\ R_\delta(\theta) = \underset{\tau \in \Theta^*}{\text{Sup}}\ \gamma(\tau, \delta)$ where Θ^* = the set of all possible τ's.

Proof

$$\begin{aligned} R_\delta(\theta) &\leq \underset{\theta \in \Theta}{\text{Sup}}\, R_\delta(\theta)\ \forall\ \theta \\ \Rightarrow \gamma(\tau, \delta) &\leq \underset{\theta \in \Theta}{\text{Sup}}\, R_\delta(\theta)\ \forall\ \tau \\ \Rightarrow \underset{\tau \in \Theta^*}{\text{Sup}}\ \gamma(\tau, \delta) &\leq \underset{\theta \in \Theta}{\text{Sup}}\, R_\delta(\theta) \end{aligned} \tag{7.35}$$

Consider a prior τ_0 which chooses a particular value θ with probability 1.

Then $r(\tau_0, \delta) = R_\delta(\theta)$
Hence, $\sup\limits_{\tau \in \Theta^*} r(\tau, \delta) \geq r(\tau_0, \delta) = R_\delta(\theta) \; \forall \; \theta$
Thus $R_\delta(\theta) \leq \sup\limits_{\tau \in \Theta^*} r(\tau, \delta) \; \forall \; \theta$

$$\Rightarrow \sup_{\theta \in \Theta} R_\delta(\theta) \leq \sup_{\tau \in \Theta^*} r(\tau, \delta) \tag{7.36}$$

(7.35), (7.36) $\Rightarrow \sup\limits_{\theta \in \Theta} R_\delta(\theta) = \sup\limits_{\tau \in \Theta^*} r(\tau, \delta)$, hence the proof.

A rule δ_0 is minimax if it minimizes

$$\sup_{\theta \in \Omega} R_\delta(\theta) \text{w.r.t } \delta \in \mathscr{D}$$

$$\text{Or, } \sup_{\tau \in \Theta^*} \gamma(\tau, \delta) \text{ w.r.t } \delta \in \mathscr{D} \text{ [by Result 1]}$$

i.e. if $\sup\limits_{\tau \in \Theta^*} r(\tau, \delta) = \inf\limits_{\delta \in \mathscr{D}} \sup\limits_{\tau \in \Theta^*} r(\tau, \delta) = \bar{v}$ (say)

$$\bar{v} = \text{ Upper value of the game.}$$

Thus, if a statistician chooses a minimax rule δ_0, his expected loss is at most $\bar{v}$ whatever be the action chosen by nature.

Similarly, a prior τ_0 is said to be a maximum rule for the nature or a least favourable prior for the statistician if τ_0 maximizes $\inf\limits_{\delta} r(\tau, \delta)$w.r.t τ, i.e. if

$$\inf_{\delta} r(\tau_0, \delta) = \sup_{\tau} \inf_{\delta} r(\tau, \delta) = \underline{v} \text{ (Say)}$$

$$\underline{v} = \text{ Lower value of the game.}$$

If nature chooses a least favourable τ_0, then expected loss (of the statistician) is at least $\underline{v}$ whatever be the rule the statistician chooses. □

Result 2 $\underline{v} \leq \bar{v}$

Proof

$$r(\tau, \delta) \leq \sup_{\tau} r(\tau, \delta) \; \forall \; \tau, \delta$$
$$\Rightarrow \inf_{\delta} r(\tau, \delta) \leq \inf_{\delta} \sup_{\tau} r(\tau, \delta) = \bar{v} \; \forall \; \tau$$
$$\Rightarrow \sup_{\tau} \inf_{\delta} r(\tau, \delta) \leq \bar{v}$$
$$\Rightarrow \underline{v} \leq \bar{v}$$

The statistical game is said to have a value v if $\underline{v} = \bar{v} = v$, □

Result 3 if the statistical game has a value and a least favourable prior τ_0 and a minimax rule δ_0 exists, then δ_0 is Bayes w.r.t. τ_0.

Proof $\underline{v} = \inf_\delta r(\tau_0, \delta) \le r(\tau_0, \delta_0) \le \operatorname{Sup}_\tau r(\tau, \delta_0) = \bar{v}$

If $\underline{v} = \bar{v}$, then '=' must hold every where implying $\inf_\delta r(\tau_0, \delta) = r(\tau_0, \delta_0) \Rightarrow \delta_0$ is Bayes w.r.t. τ_0. □

Minimax theorem Let Θ be finite and the risk set S be bounded below. Then the statistical game will have a value and a least favourable prior τ_0 exists.

If further, S is closed from below an admissible minimax rule δ_0 exists and δ_0 Bayes w.r.t. τ_0.

Thus if Θ is finite and S is bounded below as well as closed from below, then

(i) A minimax rule exists
(ii) An admissible minimax rule exists and
(iii) A minimax rule is Bayes (w.r.t least favourable prior τ_0).

Result 4 Suppose there exists a rule δ_0 such that

(i) $R_{\delta_0}(\theta) \le c \; \forall \; \theta$
(ii) δ_0 is Bayes w.r.t. some τ_0 and $r(\tau_0, \delta_0) = c$,

then

(a) δ_0 is minimax
(b) τ_0 is least favourable prior.

Proof

(a) Proved earlier
(b) To show $\inf_\delta r(\tau_0, \delta) \ge \inf_\delta r(\tau, \delta) \; \forall \; \tau \qquad (b)$

Now (i) $\Rightarrow r(\tau, \delta_0) \le c \; \forall \; \tau$

$\Rightarrow \inf_\delta r(\tau, \delta) \le r(\tau, \delta_0) \le c = r(\tau_0, \delta_0) = \inf_\delta r(\tau_0, \delta) \; \forall \; \tau \qquad$ by (ii)

This proves (b). □

7.7 Invariance

Many statistical decision problems are invariant w.r.t. some transformations of X. In such case it seems reasonable to restrict to decision rules, which are also invariant w.r.t. similar transformations. Such a decision rule is called an invariant decision rule and in many problems a best rule exists within the class of invariant rules.

Example 7.30 $X \sim N(\theta, 1), -\infty < \theta < \infty$

We are to estimate θ under the squared error loss.

Suppose one considers a transformation of X, viz., $X' = X + c$, c = a given constant and considers the problem of estimating $\theta' = \theta + c$ on the basis of $X' \sim N(\theta', 1)$ under the squared error loss.

For an action 'a' for the first problem, there is an action $a' = a + c$ for the second problem and vice versa with $L(\theta, a) = L(\theta', a')$. Thus the two problems may be considered to be equivalent in the sense that $(\Theta, \mathcal{Æ}, L) \equiv (\Theta', \mathcal{Æ}', L')$.

Now let $d = d(X) =$ a reasonable estimator of θ on the basis of X. Then $d(X') = d(X + c)$ should be a reasonable estimator of θ' on the basis of X'. Also, if $d(x) =$ a reasonable estimate of θ on the basis of $X = x$ then $d(x) + c$ should be a reasonable estimate for θ'. The two estimates are identical if

$$d(x + c) = d(x) + c \tag{7.37}$$

An estimator $d(X)$ is said to be a location invariant or an equivariant if (7.37) holds $\forall x \forall c$.

$d(X)$ is an equivariant estimator iff $d(X) = X + K = d_K(X)$ (say) for some constant K.

[If $d(X) = X + K$, then (7.37) is satisfied $\forall x \forall c$. Let (7.37) be satisfied $\forall x \forall c$. For $c = -x$, $(i) \Rightarrow d_0 = d(x) - x$; or $d(x) = x + K$, $K = d(0)$ $R_{d_k}(\theta) = E(X + K - \theta)^2 = 1 + K^2$ which is minimum when $K = 0$. Thus $R_{d_0}(\theta) \le R_{d_k}(\theta) \forall \theta \forall K$.

$\Rightarrow d_0(X) = X$ is the best within the class of equivariant estimators.]

Invariant statistical decision problems

$(\Theta, \mathcal{Æ}, L)$ X = a r.v. and x = observed value of $X \in \mathcal{X}$ (=sample space)

P_θ = A probability distribution over $\mathcal{X}$ depending on θ.

$P = \{P_\theta / \theta \in \Theta\}$ = family of probability distribution.

A statistical decision problem $\equiv (\Theta, a, L)$ and P,

Groups of transformation of X(or $\mathcal{X}$)

$Y = g(X)$ = a transformation of X

$g(x) =$ a single valued function of x.

$g : \mathcal{X} \rightarrow \mathcal{X}^*$, g = a transformation on $\mathcal{X}$

We assume that g is measurable so that $g(x)$ is an r.v. g is said to be an onto transformation if the range of $g(x)$ is $\mathcal{X}$, i.e. $\mathcal{X}^*$ is $\mathcal{X}$.

g is said to be 1:1 if $g(x_1) = g(x_2) \Rightarrow x_1 = x_2$.

Example 7.31 $\mathcal{X} = R_1$; $g(x) = x + c, c = a$ real constant. This g is 1:1 and onto.

The identity transformation e is defined as $e(x) = x$. Let g_1, g_2 be two transformations on $\mathcal{X}$. Then the composition of g_2, g_1, denoted by $g_2 g_1$ is defined as $g_2 g_1(x) = g_2[g_1(x)]$.

Example 7.32 $\mathcal{X} = R_1$

$g_1(x) = x + c_1$ and $g_2(x) = c_2$, c_1, c_2 are real constants. $g_1 g_2(x) = x + c_1 + c_2$

Clearly, $g_1g_2g_3 = g_1(g_2g_3) = (g_1g_2)g_3$
Also $ge = eg = g$

If g is a transformation on $\mathcal{X}$, then the inverse transformation of g, denoted by g^{-1}, is the transformation g such that

$gg^{-1} = g^{-1}g = e.$

In the example, $g_1^{-1}(x) = x - c_1$.

Note g^{-1} exists iff g is 1:1 and onto.

Let G = a class of transformation on $\mathcal{X}$

Definition G is called a group of transformations if G is closed under the compositions and inverses, i.e. if

i. $g_1, g_2 \in G \Rightarrow g_2g_1 \in G$
ii. $g \in G \Rightarrow g^{-1} \in G$.

Note Let G be a group of transformations, then every $g \in G$ is 1:1 and onto (since g^{-1} exists).

Also, the identity transformation e always $\in G$ [if $g \in G$, then $g^{-1} \in G$, $e = g^{-1}g \in G$].

Example 7.33 $\mathcal{X} = R_1$

$g_c(x) = x + c, c = a$ real constant.

Let $G = \{g_c / -\infty < c < \infty\}$

$$g_{c_1}, g_{c_2} \in G \Rightarrow g_{c_1}g_{c_2} \in G[As g_{c_1}g_{c_2}(x) = x + c_1 + c_2; c_1 + c_2 = c]$$

$$g_c \in G \Rightarrow g_c^{-1} \in G[As g_c^{-1}(x) = x + (-c)]$$

Hence, G is a group of transformation which is Additive or Location group.

Example 7.34 $\mathcal{X} = R_1$, $g_c(x) = cx$ where c = a positive real constant

$$g_{c_1}g_{c_2}(x) = c_1c_2x$$

$$g_c^{-1}(x) = \frac{1}{c}x$$

Let $G = \{g_e / 0 < c < \infty\}$

$$g_{c_1}, g_{c_2} \in G \Rightarrow g_{c_1}g_{c_2} \in G$$

$$g_c \in G \Rightarrow g_c^{-1} \in G$$

Thus G is a group of transformations.
These are multiplicative or group under scale transformation.

Example 7.35 $\mathscr{X} = R_1$, $g_{a,b} = a + bx$

$$G = \left\{ g_{a,b} / -\infty < a < \infty, 0 < b < \infty \right\}$$

G is a group transformation.
It is a group under both location and scale transformation.

Example 7.36 $\mathscr{X} = \{0, 1, 2 \ldots n\}$
Let $g(x) = n - x$

$$G = \{e, g\}$$

$$eg = g \in G; g^{-1}(x) = x = e(x) \in G$$

Also $e^{-1} \in G$ [Trivially]
Hence, G is a group of transformation.

Example 7.37 $\mathscr{X} = (x_1, x_2, x_3, \ldots\ldots x_n)$
$\mathscr{X}_0$ = The set of possible values of x_i

$$\mathscr{X} = \mathscr{X}_0 x \mathscr{X}_0 x \ldots\ldots\ldots x \mathscr{X}_0$$

Let $i = (i_1, i_2, i_3, \ldots\ldots i_n)$ be a permutation of $1, 2 \ldots n$
Let $g_i(x) = (x_{i_1}, x_{i_2} \ldots\ldots x_{i_n})$

$$G = \{g_i / i \in \text{ the set of all possible permutation of } (1, 2 \ldots n)\}$$

G is a group of transformations. It is a permutation group.
The invariance of a statistical decision problem is considered to be w.r.t a given group transformations G on $\mathscr{X}$.

Invariance of P Let G = a given group of transformations on $\mathscr{X}$.

Definition $P = \{P_\theta / \theta \in \Theta\}$ is said to be invariant w.r.t G if for any $g \in G$ and any $\theta \in \Theta$ (i.e., any $P_\theta \in P$) there exists a unique $\theta' \in \Theta$ (i.e. a unique $P_{\theta'} \in P$) such that probability distribution of $y = g(x)$ is $P_{\theta'}$ when the probability distribution of X is P_θ.

This unique θ' determined by g and θ is denoted by $\bar{g}(\theta)$.

Example 7.38 $X \sim N(\theta, 1), -\infty < \theta < \infty$

$$P = \{N(\theta, 1) / -\infty < \theta < \infty\}$$

Let $G = \{g_c / -\infty < c < \infty\}$ where $g_c(x) = x + c$
If $X \sim N(\theta, 1)$ then $Y = g_c(x) \sim N(\theta + c = \theta', 1)$

θ' is uniquely determined by c and θ.
Thus P is invariant under G with
$\bar{g}_c(\theta) = \theta + c$.

Example 7.39 $X \sim \exp(\theta), 0<\theta<\infty$
P.d.f of X under θ is $\frac{1}{\theta}e^{-\frac{x}{\theta}}, x > 0$

$$P = \{\exp(\theta)/0<\theta<\infty\}$$

Let $G = \{g_c/0<c<\infty\}$ where $g_c(x) = cx$
If $X \sim \exp(\theta)$, then $g_c(x) \sim \exp(c\theta)$, i.e. $c\theta = \theta'$. θ' is uniquely determined by c and θ. Thus P is invariant under G with $\bar{g}_c(\theta) = c\theta$.

Example 7.40 Let $X \sim \text{Bin}(n, \theta)$, n known, $0<\theta<1$

$$P = \{\text{Bin}(n, \theta)/0<\theta<1\}$$

Let G = a group of transformations on $\mathscr{X} = \{e, g\}$ where $g(x) = n - x$
If $X \sim \text{Bin}(n, \theta)$ then $e(x) \sim \text{Bin}(n, \theta = \theta')$ and $g(x) \sim \text{Bin}(n, 1 - \theta = \theta')$
θ' is uniquely determined by θ and member of G. Thus P is invariant under G with $\bar{e}(\theta) = \theta, \bar{g}(\theta) = 1 - \theta$.

Invariance of loss function

Let G = a group of transformations on $\mathscr{X}$
Let P be invariant w.r.t G with induced group of transformations on Θ as $\bar{G} = \{\bar{g}/g \in G\}$.

Definition The loss function L is said to be invariant w.r.t G if for each $g \in G$ and each $a \in Œ$, there exists a unique $a' \in Œ$ such that

$$L(\theta, a) = L(\bar{g}(\theta), a') \; \forall \theta \in \Theta.$$

This unique a' determined by g and 'a' is denoted by $\bar{g}(a)$.

Example 7.41 $X \sim N(\theta, 1), -\infty<\theta<\infty$

$$G = \{g_c/-\infty<c<\infty\}; g_c = x + c$$

P is invariant w.r.t
G with $\bar{G} = \{\bar{g}_c/-\infty<c<\infty\}, \bar{g}_c(\theta) = c + \theta$.
To estimate θ under $L(\theta, a) = (\theta - a)^2$
For any $g_c \in G, a \in Œ$, there is an $a' = a + c \in Œ$
such that $L(\theta, a) = L(\bar{g}_c(\theta), a') \; \forall \theta \in \Omega$.
a' is uniquely determined by a and c. Hence the loss function is invariant w.r.t G.

Example 7.42 $X \sim \exp(\theta), 0 < \theta < \infty$

$$G = \{g_c/0 < c < \infty\}, g_c(x) = cx$$

P is invariant w.r.t. G with
$\bar{G} = \{\bar{g}_c/0 < c < \infty\}$, $\bar{g}_c(\theta) = c\theta$.
To estimate θ with $L(\theta, a) = \left(1 - \frac{a}{\theta}\right)^2$
For $a' = ca$, $L(\theta, a) = L(\bar{g}_c(\theta), a')\ \forall \theta \in \Omega$.
This a' is uniquely determined by a and c. Hence the loss function is invariant w. r.t. G.

Example 7.43 $X \sim \text{Bin}(n, \theta)$, $0 < \theta < 1$

$$G = \{e, g\}, e(x) = x, g(x) = n - x$$

P is invariant w.r.t. G with
$\bar{G} = \{\bar{e}, \bar{g}\}$, $\bar{e}(\theta) = \theta$, $\bar{g}(\theta) = 1 - \theta$.
To estimate θ under squared error loss.
Then $L(\theta, a) = L(\bar{e}(\theta), a')$ where $a' = a$
and $L(\theta, a) = L(\bar{g}(\theta), a')$ where $a' = 1 - a$. a' is uniquely determined by a member of G. Thus L is invariant w.r.t. G.
Invariance of a statistical decision problem:
A statistical decision problem $\equiv (\Theta, Œ, L)$ and P
G = A group of transformation of $\mathcal{X}$.

Definition A Statistical decision problem is said to be invariant under G if
(i) P is invariant under G
and (ii) L is invariant under G.
Thus as already shown

i. $X \sim N(\theta, 1)$ to estimate θ under squared error loss

$$G = \{g_e/ - \infty < c < \infty\}, g_e(x) = x + c$$

the problem is invariant under G.

ii.
$$X \sim \exp(\theta), 0 < \theta < \infty$$
To estimate θ under $L(\theta, a) = \left(1 - \frac{a}{\theta}\right)^2, g_e(x) = cx$ the problem is invariant under G.

iii. $X \sim \text{Bin}(n, \theta)$, n is known, $0 < \theta < 1$
To estimate θ under squared error loss with $G = \{e, g\}$
$e(x) = x$, $g(x) = n - x$, the problem is invariant under G.

Example 7.44 $X \sim N(\mu, \sigma^2), -\infty < \mu < \infty, \sigma^2 > 0$
To test $H_0 : \mu \leq 0$ against $H_1 : \mu > 0$, i.e. $\theta \in \Theta_0$ against $\theta \in \Theta_1$

$$\Theta_0 = \{\theta = (\mu, \sigma^2)/\mu \leq 0\}$$

$$\Theta_1 = \{\theta = (\mu, \sigma^2)/\mu > 0\}, \Theta = \Theta_0 + \Theta_1$$

Let $G = \{g_e/0 < c < \infty\}, g_c(x) = cx$
= A group of transformation on $\mathcal{X}$

$$X \sim N(\mu, \sigma^2)$$

$$\Rightarrow g_c(x) \sim N(c\,\mu, c^2\sigma^2) \in P$$

P is invariant under G with $\bar{g}_c(\theta) \sim (c\,\mu, c^2\sigma^2)\ \theta \in \Theta_i \Leftrightarrow$

Note $\bar{g}_e(\theta) \in \Theta_i, i = 0, 1, 2, \ldots \ldots$(i)
i.e. both P_0 and P_1 are invariant under G
where $P_i = \{P_\theta/\theta \in \Theta_i\}, i = 0, 1.$
Also, $L(\theta, a) = L(\bar{g}_c(\theta), a_i'), i = 0, 1 \forall \theta \in \Theta$ by (i)
$\Rightarrow$ Loss is invariant under G

Note To test $H_0 : \theta \in \Theta_0$ against $H_1 : \theta \in \Theta_1, \Theta_0, \Theta_1$, disjoint, $\Theta_0 + \Theta_1 = \Theta$

$$a = \{a_0, a_1\}, a_i = \text{accept}\, H_i.$$

	a_0	a_1
$\theta \in \Theta_0$	0	L_0
$\theta \in \Theta_1$	L_1	0

Let the loss function be 0–L_i
Let G = a group of transformation on $\mathcal{X}$

$$P = \{P_\theta/\theta \in \Theta\}; P_i = \{P_\theta/\theta \in \Theta_i\}$$

Let both P_0 and P_1 be invariant under G, then P is invariant under G.
Also, $\theta \in \Theta_i \Leftrightarrow \bar{g}(\theta) \in \Theta_i, i = 0, 1$
Hence, $L(\theta, a_i) = L(\bar{g}(\theta), a_i), i = 0, 1 \forall \theta \in \Theta$
L is invariant under G
A test of hypothesis problem (with 0–L_i loss) is said to be invariant under G if both P_0 and P_1 are invariant under G.

Invariant decision rule

Let G = a group of transformation on $\mathcal{X}$. The problem is invariant under G with corresponding group of induced transformations on Θ and a.

Let $g \in G$

Original problem (in term of X)	Transformed problem (in terms of g(X)
$\theta \in \Theta, a \in Œ$	$\theta' = \bar{g}(\theta) \in \Theta, a' = \bar{g}(a) \in Œ$
$L(\theta, a)$	$L(\theta, a) = L(\theta', a')$
$P = \{P_\theta / \theta \in \Theta\}$	$P = \{P_{\theta'} / \theta' \in \Theta\}$

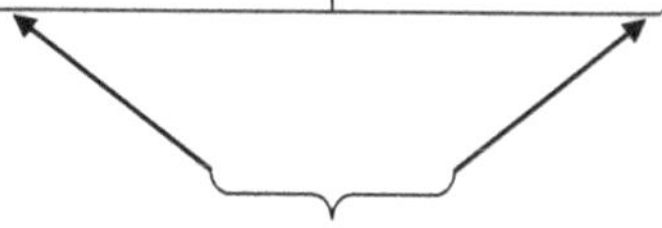

Equivalent Problem.

Let $d(X) = a$ be reasonable n.r. rule for the original problem. $d(g(x))$ should be a reasonable rule for the transformed problem. Also if for $X = x$, $d(x) \in Œ$ is a reasonable action for the original problem, then for $g(X) = g(x), \tilde{g}(d(X))$ should be a reasonable action in the transformed problem.

These two agree if $d(g(x)) = \tilde{g}(d(x))\ldots\ldots(ii)$

A non-randomized rule is said to be an invariant non-randomized rule if (ii) holds $\forall x \in \mathcal{X} \forall g \in G$.

We thus get a class of n.r. decision rules as

D_{I} = the class of invariant n.r. rules.

Appendix

A.1 Exact Tests Related to Binomial Distribution

A.1.1 We have an infinite population for which π = unknown proportion of individuals having certain character, say A. We are to test $H_0 : \pi = \pi_0$.

For doing this we draw a sample of size n. Suppose x = no. of individuals in the sample have character A. The sufficient statistic x is used for testing $H_0 : \pi = \pi_0$. Suppose x_0 is the observed value of x. Then $x \sim \text{bin}(n, \pi)$.

(a) $H_1 : \pi > \pi_0; \omega_0 : P[x \geq x_0/H_0] \leq \alpha$ i.e., $\sum_{x \geq x_0} \binom{n}{x} \pi_0^x (1 - \pi_0)^{n-x} \leq \alpha$

(b) $H_2 : \pi < \pi_0; \omega_0 : P[x \leq x_0/H_0] \leq \alpha$ i.e., $\sum_{x \leq x_0} \binom{n}{x} \pi_0^x (1 - \pi_0)^{n-x} \leq \alpha$

(c) $H_3 : \pi \neq \pi_0$; where $\pi_0 = \frac{1}{2}$ may be of our interest.

$$\omega_0 : P\left[\left|x - \frac{n}{2}\right| \geq d_0/H_0\right] \leq \alpha$$

$$\text{i.e., } P\left[x \geq \frac{n}{2} + d_0/H_0\right] + P\left[x \leq \frac{n}{2} - d_0/H_0\right] \leq \alpha$$

$$\text{i.e., } \sum_{x \geq \frac{n}{2} + d_0} \binom{n}{x} \left(\frac{1}{2}\right)^n + \sum_{x \leq \frac{n}{2} - d_0} \binom{n}{x} \left(\frac{1}{2}\right)^n \leq \alpha \text{ where } d_0 = \left|x_0 - \frac{n}{2}\right|$$

Note

(1) For other values of π_0 the exact test cannot be obtained as binomial distribution is symmetric only when $\pi = \frac{1}{2}$.
(2) For some selected n and π the binomial probability sums considered above are given in Table 37 of Biometrika (Vol. 1)

P.K. Sahu et al., *Estimation and Inferential Statistics*,
DOI 10.1007/978-81-322-2514-0

A.1.2 Suppose we have two infinite populations with π_1 and π_2 as the unknown proportion of individuals having character A. We are to test $H_0 : \pi_1 = \pi_2$.

To do this we draw two samples from two populations having sizes n_1 and n_2. Suppose x_1 and x_2 as the random variables denoting the no. of individuals in the 1st and 2nd samples with character A.

To test $H_0 : \pi_1 = \pi_2$ we make use of the statistics x_1 and x_2 such that $x_1 + x_2 = x$ (constant), say.

Under $H_0 : \pi_1 = \pi_2 = \pi$ (say),

$$\begin{aligned} f(x_1) &= \text{p.m.f. of } x_1 = \binom{n_1}{x_1}\pi^{x_1}(1-\pi)^{n_1-x_1} \\ f(x_2) &= \text{p.m.f. of } x_2 = \binom{n_2}{x_2}\pi^{x_2}(1-\pi)^{n_2-x_2} \\ f(x) &= \text{p.m.f. of } x = \binom{n_1+n_2}{x}\pi^{x}(1-\pi)^{n_1+n_2-x}. \end{aligned}$$

The conditional distribution of x_1 given x has p.m.f.

$$f(x_1/x) = \frac{\binom{n_1}{x_1}\binom{n_2}{x_2}}{\binom{n_1+n_2}{x}}, \text{ which is hypergeometric and independent of } \pi.$$

Suppose the observed values of x_1 and x are x_{10} and x_0 respectively.

(a) $H_1 : \pi_1 > \pi_2,\ \omega_0 : P[x_1 \geq x_{10}/x = x_0] \leq \alpha$

$$\text{i.e., } \sum_{x_1 \geq x_{10}} \frac{\binom{n_1}{x_1}\binom{n_2}{x_0 - x_1}}{\binom{n_1+n_2}{x_0}} \leq \alpha$$

(b) $H_2 : \pi_1 < \pi_2,\ \omega_0 : P[x_1 \leq x_{10}/x = x_0] \leq \alpha$

$$\text{i.e., } \sum_{x_1 \leq x_{10}} \frac{\binom{n_1}{x_1}\binom{n_2}{x_0 - x_1}}{\binom{n_1+n_2}{x_0}} \leq \alpha$$

(c) $H_3 : \pi_1 \neq \pi_2$, exact test is not available.

Note The above probabilities can be obtained from the tables of hypergeometric distributions (Standard University Press).

A.2 Exact Tests Related to Poisson Distribution

A.2.1 Suppose we have a Poisson population with unknown parameter λ. We draw a random sample $(x_1, x_2, \ldots, x_n)$ of size n from this population. Here, we are to test $H_0 : \lambda = \lambda_0$.

To develop a test we make use of the sufficient statistic $y = \sum_{i=1}^{n} x_i$, which is itself distributed as Poisson with parameter $n\lambda$. The p.m.f. of y under H_0 is therefore $f(y) = e^{-n\lambda_0}\frac{(n\lambda_0)^y}{y!}, y = 0, 1, 2\ldots$

Suppose y_0 is the observed value of y.

(a) $H_1 : \lambda > \lambda_0, \ \omega_0 : P[y \geq y_0/\lambda = \lambda_0] \leq \alpha$

$$\text{i.e.,} \sum_{y \geq y_0} e^{-n\lambda_0}\frac{(n\lambda_0)^y}{y!} \leq \alpha.$$

(b) $H_2 : \lambda < \lambda_0, \ \omega_0 : P[y \leq y_0/\lambda = \lambda_0] \leq \alpha$

$$\text{i.e.,} \sum_{y \leq y_0} e^{-n\lambda_0}\frac{(n\lambda_0)^y}{y!} \leq \alpha.$$

(c) $H_3 : \lambda \neq \lambda_0$: exact test is not available.

Note These probabilities may be obtained from Table 7 of Biometrika (Vol. 1)

A.2.2 Suppose we have two populations $P(\lambda_1)$ and $P(\lambda_2)$. We draw a random sample $(x_{11}, x_{12}, \ldots, x_{1n_1})$ of size n_1 from $P(\lambda_1)$ and another random sample $(x_{21}, x_{22}, \ldots, x_{2n_2})$ of size n_2 from $P(\lambda_2)$. We are to test $H_0 : \lambda_1 = \lambda_2 = \lambda$ (say). Here we note that $y_1 = \sum_{i=1}^{n_1} x_{1i} \sim P(n_1\lambda_1)$ and $y_2 = \sum_{i=1}^{n_2} x_{2i} \sim P(n_2\lambda_2)$.

To develop a test we shall make use of the sufficient statisticsy$_1$ and y_2 but shall concentrate only on those for which $y = y_1 + y_2$ = constant. Under H_0 the p.m.f. of y_1, y_2 and y are

$$f(y_1) = e^{-n_1\lambda}\frac{(n_1\lambda)^{y_1}}{y_1!}; f(y_2) = e^{-n_2\lambda}\frac{(n_2\lambda)^{y_2}}{y_2!} \text{ and } f(y) = e^{-(n_1+n_2)\lambda}\frac{\{(n_1+n_2)\lambda\}^y}{y!}$$

The conditional distribution of y_1 given y has the p.m.f. as

$$f(y_1/y) = \frac{e^{-n_2\lambda}\frac{(n_2\lambda)^{y-y_1}}{(y-y_1)!}\cdot e^{-n_1\lambda}\frac{(n_1\lambda)^{y_1}}{y_1!}}{e^{-(n_1+n_2)\lambda}\frac{\{(n_1+n_2)\lambda\}^y}{y!}}$$

$$= \frac{y!}{y_1!y_2!}\frac{n_1^{y_1}n_2^{y_2}}{(n_1+n_2)^y}$$

$$= \binom{y}{y_1}\left(\frac{n_1}{n_1+n_2}\right)^{y_1}\left(1-\frac{n_1}{n_1+n_2}\right)^{y_2} \sim \text{bin}\left(y, \frac{n_1}{n_1+n_2}\right) \text{ free of } \lambda.$$

So this may be regarded as sufficient statistic. Suppose the observed values of y_1 and y are y_{10} and y_0 respectively. We consider the conditional p.m.f. $f(y_1/y_0)$ for testing H_0.

(a) $H_1 : \lambda_1 > \lambda_2; \omega_0 : P[y_1 \geq y_{10}/y = y_0] \leq \alpha$

$$\text{i.e.,} \sum_{y_1 \geq y_{10}} \binom{y_0}{y_1}\left(\frac{n_1}{n_1+n_2}\right)^{y_1}\left(\frac{n_2}{n_1+n_2}\right)^{y_0-y_1} \leq \alpha$$

(b) $H_2 : \lambda_1 < \lambda_2; \quad \omega_0 : P[y_1 \leq y_{10}/y = y_0] \leq \alpha$

$$\text{i.e.,} \sum_{y_1 \leq y_{10}} \binom{y_0}{y_1}\left(\frac{n_1}{n_1+n_2}\right)^{y_1}\left(\frac{n_2}{n_1+n_2}\right)^{y_0-y_1} \leq \alpha.$$

(c) $H_3 : \lambda \neq \lambda_0$: exact test is not available.

A.3 A Test for Independence of Two Attributes

In many investigations one is faced with the problem of judging whether two qualitative characters, say A and B, may be said to be independent. Let us denote the forms of A by $A_i\{i = 1(1)k\}$ and the forms of B by $B_j\{j = 1(1)l\}$, and the probability associated with the cell A_iB_j in the two-way classification of the population by p_{ij}. The probability associated with A_i is then $p_{i0} = \sum_j p_{ij}$ and that associated with B_j is $p_{0j} = \sum_i p_{ij}$. We show the concerned distribution in the following table:

A	B						Total
	B_1	B_2	....	B_j	....	B_l	
A_1	p_{11}	p_{12}	....	p_{ij}	....	p_{1l}	p_{10}
A_2	p_{21}	p_{22}	....	p_{2j}	....	p_{2l}	p_{20}
.	.	.		.		.	.
.	.	.		.		.	.
A_i	p_{i1}	p_{i2}	....	p_{ij}	....	p_{il}	p_{i0}
.	.	.		.		.	.
.	.	.		.		.	.
A_k	p_{k1}	p_{k2}	....	p_{kj}	....	p_{kl}	p_{k0}
Total	p_{01}	p_{02}	....	p_{0j}	....	p_{0l}	1

where $p_{ij} = P\left[A = A_i, B = B_j\right] \cdot \forall(i,j)$

$$p_{i0} = P(A = A_i) \text{ and } p_{0j} = P\left(B = B_j\right)$$

We are to test H_0 : A and B are independent $\Leftrightarrow H_0 : p_{ij} = p_{i0} \times p_{0j}\ \forall(i,j)$

To do this we draw a random sample of size n. Let n_{ij} = observed frequency for the cell A_iB_j. The marginal frequency of A_i is $n_{i0} = \sum_j n_{ij}$ and that of B_j is $n_{0j} = \sum_i n_{ij}$. Note that the joint p.m.f. of n_{ij} is multinomial, i.e.

$$f\left(n_{ij}, \begin{matrix} i = 1(1)k \\ j = 1(1)l \end{matrix} \middle/ p_{ij}; \begin{matrix} i = 1(1)k \\ j = 1(1)l \end{matrix}\right) = \frac{n!}{\prod_i \prod_j (n_{ij})!} \prod_i \prod_j (p_{ij})^{n_{ij}}.$$

Under $H_0 : p_{ij} = p_{io} \times p_{oj} \forall(i,j)$

$$f\left(n_{ij}, \begin{matrix} i = 1(1)k \\ j = 1(1)l \end{matrix}\right) = \frac{n!}{\prod_i \prod_j (n_{ij})!} \prod_i (p_{io})^{n_{io}} \prod_j (p_{oj})^{n_{oj}}$$

$$f(n_{i0}) = \frac{n!}{\prod_i (n_{i0})!} \prod_i (p_{i0})^{n_{i0}} \forall i = 1(1)k$$

$$f(n_{0j}) = \frac{n!}{\prod_j (n_{0j})!} \prod_j (p_{0j})^{n_{0j}} \forall j = 1(1)l$$

The conditional distribution of n_{ij} keeping marginals fixed is, under H_0, $\frac{f(n_{ij})}{f(n_{i0}) f(n_{0j})} = \frac{\prod_i (n_{i0})! \prod_j (n_{0j})!}{n! \prod_i \prod_j (n_{ij})!}$

This may be used for testing H_0. Keeping marginal frequencies fixed we change the cell-frequencies and calculate the corresponding probabilities. If the sum of the probabilities $\leq \alpha$, then we reject H_0.

A.4 Problems Related to Univariate Normal Distribution

Suppose we have a normal population with mean μ and standard deviation σ. We draw a random sample $(x_1, x_2, \ldots, x_n)$ of size n from this population. Here $\bar{x} = \frac{1}{n}\sum_1^n x_i$, $s^2 = \frac{1}{n}\sum_i (x_i - \bar{x})^2$ and $s'^2 = \frac{1}{n-1}\sum_i (x_i - \bar{x})^2$.

A.4.1 To test $H_0 : \mu = \mu_0$.

Case I σ known: we note that $\frac{\sqrt{n}(\bar{x}-\mu)}{\sigma} \sim N(0,1)$

Under H_0, $\tau = \frac{\sqrt{n}(\bar{x}-\mu_0)}{\sigma} \sim N(0,1)$.

$$H_1 : \mu > \mu_0; \omega_0 : \tau > \tau_\alpha$$
$$H_2 : \mu < \mu_0; \omega_0 : \tau < -\tau_\alpha$$
$$H_3 : \mu \neq \mu_0; \omega_0 : |\tau| > \tau_{\alpha/2}$$

$100(1-\alpha)\%$ confidence interval for μ (when H_0 is rejected) is $\left(\bar{x} \mp \frac{\sigma}{\sqrt{n}}\tau_{\alpha/2}\right)$

Case II σ unknown: Here we estimate σ by s' and $\frac{\sqrt{n}(\bar{x}-\mu)}{s'} \sim t_{n-1}$.

Under H_0 $t = \frac{\sqrt{n}(\bar{x}-\mu_0)}{s'} \sim t_{n-1}$.

$$H_1 : \mu > \mu_0; \omega_0 : t > t_{\alpha,n-1}$$
$$H_2 : \mu < \mu_0; \omega_0 : t < -t_{\alpha,n-1}$$
$$H_3 : \mu \neq \mu_0; \omega_0 : |t| > t_{\alpha/2,n-1}$$

$100(1-\alpha)\%$ confidence interval for μ is $\left(\bar{x} \mp \frac{s'}{\sqrt{n}} t_{\alpha/2}, n-1\right)$

A.4.2 To test $H_0 : \sigma = \sigma_0$.

Case I μ known: we know $\frac{\sum(x_i-\mu)^2}{\sigma^2} \sim \chi_n^2$, under H_0, $\chi^2 = \frac{\sum(x_i-\mu)^2}{\sigma_0^2} \sim \chi_n^2$.

$$H_1 : \sigma > \sigma_0; \ \omega_0 : \chi^2 > \chi^2_{\alpha,n}$$
$$H_2 : \sigma < \sigma_0; \ \omega_0 : \chi^2 < \chi^2_{1-\alpha,n}$$
$$H_3 : \sigma \neq \sigma_0; \ \omega_0 : \chi^2 > \chi^2_{\alpha/2,n}$$

or,

$$\chi^2 < \chi^2_{1-\alpha/2,n}$$

$$P\left[\chi^2_{1-\alpha/2,n} < \frac{\sum (x_i - \mu)^2}{\sigma^2} < \chi^2_{\alpha/2,n}\right] = 1 - \alpha$$

$$\text{i.e., } P\left[\frac{\sum (x_i - \mu)^2}{\chi^2_{\alpha/2,n}} < \sigma^2 < \frac{\sum (x_i - \mu)^2}{\chi^2_{1-\alpha/2,n}}\right] = 1 - \alpha$$

$\therefore 100(1-\alpha)\%$ confidence interval for σ^2 when μ is known is $\left[\frac{\sum (x_i-\mu)^2}{\chi^2_{\alpha/2,n}}, \frac{\sum (x_i-\mu)^2}{\chi^2_{1-\alpha/2,n}}\right]$.

Case II μ unknown: we know $\frac{\sum (x_i - \bar{x})^2}{\sigma^2} \sim \chi^2_{n-1}$ under H_0, $\chi^2 = \frac{\sum (x_i-\bar{x})^2}{\sigma_0^2} \sim \chi^2_{n-1}$

$$H_1 : \sigma > \sigma_0;\ \omega_0 : \chi^2 > \chi^2_{\alpha,n-1}$$
$$H_2 : \sigma < \sigma_0;\ \omega_0 : \chi^2 < \chi^2_{1-\alpha,n-1}$$
$$H_3 : \sigma \neq \sigma_0;\ \omega_0 : \chi^2 > \chi^2_{\alpha/2,n-1}.$$

or,

$$\chi^2 > \chi^2_{1-\alpha/2,n-1}$$

$$P\left[\chi^2_{1-\alpha/2,n-1} < \frac{\sum (x_i - \bar{x})^2}{\sigma^2} < \chi^2_{\alpha/2,n-1}\right] = 1 - \alpha$$

$$\text{i.e., } P\left[\frac{\sum (x_i - \bar{x})^2}{\chi^2_{\alpha/2,n-1}} < \sigma^2 < \frac{\sum (x_i - \bar{x})^2}{\chi^2_{1-\alpha/2,n-1}}\right] = 1 - \alpha$$

$\therefore 100(1-\alpha)\%$ confidence interval for σ^2 when μ is unknown is $\left[\frac{\sum (x_i-\bar{x})^2}{\chi^2_{\alpha/2,n-1}}, \frac{\sum (x_i-\bar{x})^2}{\chi^2_{1-\alpha/2,n-1}}\right]$.

A.5 Problems Relating Two Univariate Normal Distributions

Suppose we have two independent populations $N(\mu, \sigma_1^2)$ and $N(\mu_2, \sigma_2^2)$. We draw a random sample $(x_{11}, x_{12}, \ldots, x_{1n_1})$ of size n_1 from the first population and another random sample $(x_{21}, x_{22}, \ldots, x_{2n_2})$ of size n_2 from the second population.

Now, we have for the 1st and the 2nd samples

$$\bar{x}_1 = \frac{1}{n_1} \sum_{i=1}^{n_1} x_{1i} \qquad \text{and} \qquad \bar{x}_2 = \frac{1}{n_2} \sum_{i=1}^{n_2} x_{2i}$$

$$s_1'^2 = \frac{1}{n_1 - 1} \sum_{i=1}^{n_1} (x_{1i} - \bar{x}_1)^2 \qquad s_2'^2 = \frac{1}{n_2 - 1} \sum_{i=1}^{n_2} (x_{2i} - \bar{x}_2)^2$$

respectively.

(I) $H_0 : 1_1\mu_1 + 1_2\mu_2 = 1_3$.

Case I σ_1, σ_2 known:

We find that $\dfrac{1_1\bar{x}_1 + 1_2\bar{x}_2 - (1_1\mu_1 + 1_2\mu_2)}{\sqrt{\dfrac{1_1^2\sigma_1^2}{n_1} + \dfrac{1_2^2\sigma_2^2}{n_2}}} \sim N(0, 1)$

Under H_0, $\tau = \dfrac{1_1\bar{x}_1 + 1_2\bar{x}_2 - 1_3}{\sqrt{\dfrac{1_1^2\sigma_1^2}{n_1} + \dfrac{1_2^2\sigma_2^2}{n_2}}} \sim N(0, 1)$

$$\therefore H_1 : 1_1\mu_1 + 1_2\mu_2 > 1_3; \omega_0 : \tau > \tau_\alpha$$
$$H_2 : 1_1\mu_1 + 1_2\mu_2 < 1_3; \omega_0 : \tau < -\tau_\alpha$$
$$H_3 : 1_1\mu_1 + 1_2\mu_2 \neq 1_3; \omega_0 : |\tau| > \tau_{\alpha/2}$$

Also, $(1 - \alpha)100\%$ confidence interval for $(1_1\mu_1 + 1_2\mu_2)$ is

$$\left[1_1\bar{x}_1 + 1_2\bar{x}_2 \mp \sqrt{\frac{1_1^2\sigma_1^2}{n_1} + \frac{1_2^2\sigma_2^2}{n_2}} \cdot \tau_{\alpha/2} \right]$$

Case II σ_1, σ_2 unknown:

Fisher's t-test: We assume $\sigma_1 = \sigma_2 = \sigma$, say.

σ^2 is estimated by $\dfrac{(n_1-1)s_1'^2 + (n_2-1)s_2'^2}{(n_1+n_2-2)} = s'^2$ say

Also, $\dfrac{1_1\bar{x}_1 + 1_2\bar{x}_2 - (1_1\mu_1 + 1_2\mu_2)}{s'\sqrt{\dfrac{1_1^2}{n_1} + \dfrac{1_2^2}{n_2}}} \sim t_{n_1 + n_2 - 2}$

Under H_0, $t = \dfrac{1_1\bar{x}_1 + 1_2\bar{x}_2 - 1_3}{s'\sqrt{\dfrac{1_1^2}{n_1} + \dfrac{1_2^2}{n_2}}} \sim t_{n_1 + n_2 - 2}$

This t is known as Fisher's t when $1_1 = 1$, $1_2 = -1$.

$$H_1 : 1_1\mu_1 + 1_2\mu_2 > 1_3; \quad \omega_0 : t > t_{\alpha,n_1+n_2-2}$$
$$H_2 : 1_1\mu_1 + 1_2\mu_2 < 1_3; \quad \omega_0 : t < -t_{\alpha,n_1+n_2-2}$$
$$H_3 : 1_1\mu_1 + 1_2\mu_2 \neq 1_3; \quad \omega_0 : |t| > t_{\alpha/2,n_1+n_2-2}$$

Also 100(1 − α)% confidence interval for $1_1\mu_1 + 1_2\mu_2$ is

$$\left(1_1\bar{x}_1 + 1_2\bar{x}_2 \mp s'\sqrt{\frac{1_1^2}{n_1} + \frac{1_2^2}{n_2}}t_{\alpha/2,n_1+n_2-2}\right).$$

Note–I The above procedure may also be applicable when σ_1 and σ_2 are not equal provided $\left|1 - \frac{\sigma_1^2}{\sigma_2^2}\right| < 0.4$—theoretical investigation in this area verifies this.

Note–II when homoscedasticity assumption $\sigma_1 = \sigma_2$ is not tenable then we require the alternative procedure and the corresponding problem is known as the Fisher-Behren problem.

Note–III For $1_1 = 1$ and $1_2 = -1$ we get the test procedure for the difference between the two means. Also for testing the ratio of the means, i.e. for testing $H_0 : \frac{\mu_1}{\mu_2} = k$, say, we start with $(\bar{x}_1 - k\bar{x}_2)$.

(II) $H_0 : \frac{\sigma_1}{\sigma_2} = \xi_0$:

Case I μ_1, μ_2 known: $\frac{\frac{1}{n_1}\sum(x_{1i}-\mu_1)^2}{\frac{1}{n_1}\sum(x_{2i}-\mu_2)^2} \cdot \frac{1}{\left(\frac{\sigma_1^2}{\sigma_2^2}\right)} \sim F_{n_1,n_2}$

$\therefore$ Under H_0, $F = \frac{\sum(x_{1i}-\mu_1)^2/n_1}{\sum(x_{2i}-\mu_2)^2/n_2} \cdot \frac{1}{\xi_0^2} \sim F_{n_1,n_2}$

$$H_1 : \frac{\sigma_1}{\sigma_2} > \xi_0; \quad \omega_0 : F > F_{\alpha,n_1,n_2}$$
$$H_2 : \frac{\sigma_1}{\sigma_2} < \xi_0; \quad \omega_0 : F < F_{1-\alpha,n_1,n_2}$$
$$H_3 : \frac{\sigma_1}{\sigma_2} \neq \xi_0; \quad \omega_0 : F > F_{\alpha/2,n_1,n_2} \quad \text{or,} \quad F < F_{1-\alpha/2,n_1,n_2}.$$

Also, $P\left[F_{1-\alpha/2,n_1,n_2} < \frac{\sum(x_{1i}-\mu_1)^2/n_1}{\sum(x_{2i}-\mu_2)^2/n_2} \cdot \frac{\sigma_2^2}{\sigma_1^2} < F_{\alpha/2,n_1,n_2}\right] = 1 - \alpha$

Or, $P\left[\sqrt{\frac{n_2\sum(x_{1i}-\mu_1)^2}{n_1\sum(x_{2i}-\mu_2)^2 F_{\alpha/2,n_1,n_2}}} < \frac{\sigma_1}{\sigma_2} < \sqrt{\frac{n_2\sum(x_{1i}-\mu_1)^2}{n_1\sum(x_{2i}-\mu_2)^2 F_{1-\alpha/2,n_1,n_2}}}\right] = 1 - \alpha$

This provides the $100(1-\alpha)\%$ confidence interval for $\frac{\sigma_1}{\sigma_2}$ when μ_1, μ_2 are known.

Case II μ_1, μ_2 unknown:

We have $\frac{\frac{1}{n_1-1}\sum(x_{1i}-\bar{x}_1)^2}{\frac{1}{n_2-1}\sum(x_{2i}-\bar{x}_2)^2} \cdot \frac{1}{\left(\frac{\sigma_1^2}{\sigma_2^2}\right)} \sim F_{n_1-1,n_2-1}$

$$\text{i.e.,}\ \frac{s_1'^2}{s_2'^2} \cdot \frac{\sigma_2^2}{\sigma_1^2} \sim F_{n_1-1,n_2-1}$$

under H_0, $F = \frac{s_1'^2}{s_2'^2} \cdot \frac{1}{\xi_o^2} \sim F_{n_1-1,n_2-1}$

$$\therefore H_1 : \frac{\sigma_1}{\sigma_2} > \xi_0, \omega_0 : F > F_{\alpha,n_1-1,n_2-1}$$

$$H_2 : \frac{\sigma_1}{\sigma_2} < \xi_0, \omega_0 : F < F_{1-\alpha,n_1-1,n_2-1}$$

$$H_3 : \frac{\sigma_1}{\sigma_2} \neq \xi_0, \omega_0 : F > F_{\alpha/2,n_1-1,n_2-1} \quad \text{or} \quad F < F_{1-\alpha/2;n_1-1,n_2-1}.$$

$$\text{Also, } P\left[F_{1-\alpha/2,n_1-1,n_2-1} < \frac{s_1'^2}{s_2'^2} \cdot \frac{1}{\left(\frac{\sigma_1}{\sigma_2}\right)^2} < F_{\alpha/2,n_1-1,n_2-1}\right] = 1 - \alpha$$

$$\text{Or, } P\left[\sqrt{\frac{s_1'^2}{s_2'^2 F_{\alpha/2,n_1-1,n_2-1}}} < \frac{\sigma_1}{\sigma_2} < \sqrt{\frac{s_1'^2}{s_2'^2 F_{1-\alpha/2,n_1-1,n_2-1}}}\right] = 1 - \alpha$$

i.e., $100(1-\alpha)\%$ confidence interval for $\frac{\sigma_1}{\sigma_2}$, when μ_1, μ_2 are unknown, is

$$\left[\frac{s_1'/s_2'}{\sqrt{F_{\alpha/2,n_1-1,n_2-1}}}, \frac{s_1'/s_2'}{\sqrt{F_{1-\alpha/2,n_1-1,n_2-1}}}\right].$$

A.6 Problems Relating to Bivariate Normal Distributions

Suppose in a given population the variables x and y are distributed in the bivariate normal form $N_2(\mu_x,\mu_y;\sigma_x,\sigma_y;\rho)$. Let $(x_1,y_1),(x_2,y_2),\ldots,(x_n,y_n)$ be the values of x and y observed in a sample of size n drawn from this population. We shall suppose that the n pairs of sample observations are random and independent. We shall also assume that all the parameters are unknown.

We have for the sample observations

$$\bar{x} = \frac{1}{n}\sum_i x_i,\ \bar{y} = \frac{1}{n}\sum_i y_i,\ s_x'^2 = \frac{1}{n-1}\sum_i (x_i - \bar{x})^2,$$

$$s_y'^2 = \frac{1}{n-1}\sum_i (y_i - \bar{y})^2, \text{ and } r_{xy} = \frac{\frac{1}{n-1}\sum_i (x_i - \bar{x})^2 (y_i - \bar{y})^2}{s_x' s_y'}$$

(1) To test $H_0 : \rho = 0$:

We know when $\rho = 0,\ t = \frac{r\sqrt{n-2}}{\sqrt{1-r^2}} \sim t_{n-2}$

$$\begin{aligned} &H_1 : \rho > 0, \quad \omega_0 : t > t_{\alpha,n-2} \\ &H_2 : \rho < 0, \quad \omega_0 : t > -t_{\alpha,n-2} \\ &H_3 : \rho \neq 0, \quad \omega_0 : |t| > t_{\alpha/2,n-2} \end{aligned}$$

Note For testing $\rho = \rho_0(\neq 0)$, exact test is difficult to get as for $\rho \neq 0$ the distribution of r is complicated in nature. But for moderately large n one can use the large sample test which will be considered later.

(2) $H_0 : \mu_x - \mu_y = \xi_0$

Define $z = x - y \Rightarrow \mu_z = \mu_x - \mu_y$ i.e., we are to test $H_0 : \mu_z = \xi_0$. Also note that $\frac{\sqrt{n}(\bar{z}-\mu_z)}{s'_z} \sim t_{n-1}$ where $s'^2_z = \frac{1}{n-1}\sum_i (z_i - \bar{z})^2 = s'^2_x + s'^2_y - 2s'_{xy}$ $s'_{xy} = \frac{1}{n-1}\sum_i (x_i - \bar{x})^2 (y_i - \bar{y})^2$. Under $H_0,\ t = \frac{\sqrt{n}(\bar{z}-\xi_0)}{s'_z} \sim t_{n-1}$.

For $H_1 : \mu_x - \mu_y > \xi_0, \omega_0 : t > t_{\alpha,n-1}$

$$\begin{aligned} &H_2 : \mu_x - \mu_y < \xi_0, \quad \omega_0 : t < -t_{\alpha,n-1} \\ &H_3 : \mu_x - \mu_y \neq \xi_0, \quad \omega_0 : |t| > t_{\alpha/2,n-1} \end{aligned}$$

Also, $100(1-\alpha)\%$ confidence interval for $\mu_z = \mu_x - \mu_y$ is $\left(\bar{z} \mp \frac{s'_z}{\sqrt{n}} t_{\alpha/2,n-1}\right)$

(3) $H_0 : \frac{\mu_x}{\mu_y} = \eta_0$: we write $\eta = \frac{\mu_x}{\mu_y}$.

To test $H_0 : \eta = \eta_0$, we take $z = x - \eta y \Rightarrow \mu_z = \mu_x - \eta\mu_y = 0$.

$\bar{z} = \bar{x} - \eta\bar{y}$ = a function of η.

$s'^2_z = s'^2_z + \eta^2 s'^2_y - 2\eta s'_{xy}$ = a function of η.

Now, $\frac{\sqrt{n}(\bar{z}-\mu_z)}{s'_z} \sim t_{n-1}$. i.e., $\frac{\sqrt{n}\bar{z}}{s'_z} \sim t_{n-1} (\because \mu_z = 0)$

Under $H_0,\ t = \frac{\sqrt{n}\bar{z}_0}{s'_{z_0}} \sim t_{n-1}$ where $\bar{z}_0 = \bar{x} - \eta_0\bar{y}$

$$s'^2_{z_0} = s'^2_x + \eta_0 s'^2_y - 2\eta_0 s'_{xy}$$

So for $H_1 : \frac{\mu_x}{\mu_y} > \eta_0;\quad \omega_0 : t > t_{\alpha,n-1}$

$$\begin{aligned} &H_2 : \frac{\mu_x}{\mu_y} < \eta_0; \ \omega_0 : t < -t_{\alpha,n-1} \\ &H_3 : \frac{\mu_x}{\mu_y} \neq \eta_0; \ \omega_0 : |t| > t_{\alpha/2,n-1}. \end{aligned}$$

Again $P\left[-t_{\alpha/2,n-1} < \frac{\sqrt{n}\bar{z}}{s_z'} < t_{\alpha/2,n-1}\right] = 1-\alpha$

i.e., $P\left[\left|\frac{\sqrt{n}\bar{z}}{s_z'}\right| < t_{\alpha/2,n-1}\right] = 1-\alpha$ or $P[\psi(\eta) < 0] = 1-\alpha$.

Solving the equation $\psi(\eta) = \frac{n\bar{z}^2}{s_z'^2} - \left(t_{\alpha/2,n-1}\right)^2 = 0$ which is a quadratic equation in η, one can get two roots η_1 and $\eta_2(>\eta_1)$. Now if $\psi(\eta)$ is a convex function and η_1 and η_2 are real, then $P[\eta_1 < \eta < \eta_2] = 1-\alpha$. If $\psi(\eta)$ is a concave function, then $P[\eta < \eta_1, \eta > \eta_2] = 1-\alpha$. But if η_1 and η_2 be imaginary then from the given sample $100(1-\alpha)\%$Confidence interval does not exist.

(4) Test for the ratio $\xi = \frac{\sigma_x}{\sigma_y}$:

We write $u = x + \xi y, \quad v = x - \xi y$

$$\therefore \mathrm{Cov}(u,v) = \sigma_x^2 - \xi^2\sigma_y^2 \Rightarrow \rho_{uv} = 0$$

Then, $\frac{r_{uv}\sqrt{n-2}}{\sqrt{1-r_{uv}^2}} \sim t_{n-2}$

where $r_{uv} = \frac{\frac{1}{n}\sum(u_i-\bar{u})(v_i-\bar{v})}{s_u s_v}$ = a function of ξ. We are to test $H_0 : \frac{\sigma_x}{\sigma_y} = \xi_0$, i.e. $H_0 : \xi = \xi_0$.

$\therefore$ under H_0, $t = \frac{r_{uv}^0\sqrt{n-2}}{\sqrt{1-r_{uv}^{02}}} \sim t_{n-2}$

where r_{uv}^0 = value of r_{uv} under $\xi = \xi_0$.

For $H_1 : \xi > \xi_0; \omega_0 : t > t_{\alpha,n-2}$

$$H_2 : \xi < \xi_0; \omega_0 : t < -t_{\alpha,n-2}$$
$$H_3 : \xi \neq \xi_0; \omega_0 : |t| > t_{\alpha/2,n-2}.$$

Also, $P\left[-t_{\alpha/2,n-2} < \frac{r_{uv}\sqrt{n-2}}{\sqrt{1-r_{uv}^2}} < t_{\alpha/2,n-2}\right] = 1-\alpha$

Solving the equation $\psi(\xi) = \frac{r_{uv}^2(n-2)}{1-r_{uv}^2} - t_{\alpha/2,n-2}^2 = 0$, (which is a quadratic in ξ) one can get two roots ξ_1 and $\xi_2(>\xi_1)$. If these roots are real and $\psi(\xi)$ is a convex function, then $P(\xi_1 < \xi < \xi_2) = 1-\alpha$. Again if $\psi(\xi)$ is concave, $P(\xi < \xi_1, \xi > \xi_2) = 1-\alpha$. But if ξ_1 and ξ_2 are not real, then $100(1-\alpha)\%$ Confidence interval does not exist so far as the given sample is concerned.

(5) σ_x, σ_y, ρ are known:

$H_0 : \mu_x = \mu_x^0,\ \mu_y = \mu_y^0$ against $H_1 : H_0$ is not true. We know that

$$Q(x,y) = \frac{1}{1-\rho^2}\left[\left(\frac{x-\mu_x}{\sigma_x}\right)^2 - 2\rho\left(\frac{x-\mu_x}{\sigma_x}\right)\left(\frac{y-\mu_y}{\sigma_y}\right) + \left(\frac{y-\mu_y}{\sigma_y}\right)^2\right] \sim \chi_2^2$$

$$(\bar{x},\bar{y}) \sim N_2\left(\mu_x, \mu_y, \frac{\sigma_x^2}{n}, \frac{\sigma_y^2}{n}, \rho\right)$$

$$\therefore Q(\bar{x},\bar{y}) = \frac{n}{1-\rho^2}\left[\left(\frac{\bar{x}-\mu_x}{\sigma_x}\right)^2 - 2\rho\left(\frac{\bar{x}-\mu_x}{\sigma_x}\right)\left(\frac{\bar{y}-\mu_y}{\sigma_y}\right) + \left(\frac{\bar{y}-\mu_y}{\sigma_y}\right)^2\right] \sim \chi_2^2$$

Under H_0,

$$\chi^2 = \frac{n}{1-\rho^2}\left[\left(\frac{\bar{x}-\mu_x^0}{\sigma_x}\right)^2 - 2\rho\left(\frac{\bar{x}-\mu_x^0}{\sigma_x}\right)\left(\frac{\bar{y}-\mu_y^0}{\sigma_y}\right) + \left(\frac{\bar{y}-\mu_y^0}{\sigma_y}\right)^2\right] \sim \chi_2^2$$

Hence, the critical region is $\omega_0 : \chi^2 > \chi^2_{\alpha,2}$.

A.7 Problems Relating to k-Univariate Normal Distributions

Suppose there are k-populations $N(\mu_1, \sigma_1^2), N(\mu_2, \sigma_2^2), \ldots N(\mu_k, \sigma_k^2)$. We draw a random sample of size n_i from the ith population with n_i (≥ 2 for at least one i).

Define

$x_{ij} = j$th observation of ith sample, $i = 1,2,\ldots,k$; $j = 1,2,\ldots, n_i$

$\bar{x}_i = i$th sample mean $= \frac{1}{n_i}\sum_{j=1}^{n_i} x_{ij}$

$s_i'^2 = i$th sample variance $= \frac{1}{n_i - 1}\sum_{j=1}^{n_i}\left(x_{ij} - \bar{x}_i\right)^2$

(I) We are to test $H_0 : \mu_1 = \mu_2 = \cdots = \mu_k (= \mu)$, say against H_1. There is at least one inequality in H_0.

Assumption $\sigma_1 = \sigma_2 = \cdots = \sigma_k (= \sigma)$ say.

Note that $\bar{x}_i \sim N\left(\mu_i, \frac{\sigma^2}{n_i}\right)$

$\therefore \frac{\sqrt{n_i}(\bar{x}_i - \mu_i)}{\sigma} \sim N(0, 1)\ \forall i$ and are independent.

Also, $\frac{(n_i - 1)s_i'^2}{\sigma^2} \sim \chi^2_{n_i - 1}$ ($\bar{x}_i$ and s_i' are independent.)

Under H_0

$$\left.\begin{aligned} &\sum_{i=1}^{k} \frac{n_i(\bar{x}_i - \mu)^2}{\sigma^2} \sim \chi_k^2 \\ \text{and } &\sum_{i=1}^{k} \frac{(n_i - 1)s_i'^2}{\sigma^2} \sim \chi^2_{n-k} \end{aligned}\right\} \text{ these two } \chi^2 \text{ are independent.}$$

But the unknown μ is estimated by

$$\hat{\mu} = \frac{1}{n}\sum n_i \bar{x}_i = \bar{x}(\text{say}); n = \sum_i n_i$$

$\therefore$ Under H_0, $\sum_{i=1}^{k} n_i(\bar{x}_i - \bar{x})^2 \sim \sigma^2\chi^2_{k-1}$ and $\sum_{i=1}^{k}(n_i - 1)s_i'^2 \sim \sigma^2\chi^2_{n-k}$.

$\therefore$ Under H_0, $F = \dfrac{\sum n_i(\bar{x}_i - \bar{x})^2 / k-1}{\sum_i (n_i - 1)s_i'^2 / n-k} \sim F_{k-1,n-k}$.

$\omega_0 : F > F_{\alpha;k-1,n-k}$. If H_0 is rejected, then we may be interested to test H_0: $\mu_i = \mu_j$ against $H_1 : \mu_i \neq \mu_j \forall (i,j)$.

$$(\bar{x}_i - \bar{x}_j) \sim N\left(\mu_i - \mu_j, \sigma^2\left(\frac{1}{n_i} + \frac{1}{n_j}\right)\right)$$
$$\Rightarrow \frac{\bar{x}_i - \bar{x}_j - (\mu_i - \mu_j)}{\sigma\sqrt{\frac{1}{n_i} + \frac{1}{n_j}}} \sim N(0, 1)$$

Unknown σ^2 is estimated by $\hat{\sigma}^2 = \frac{\sum (n_i-1)s_i'^2}{n-k} = s'^2$, say $\therefore \frac{(\bar{x}_i-\bar{x}_j)-(\mu_i-\mu_j)}{s'\sqrt{\frac{1}{n_i}+\frac{1}{n_j}}} \sim t_{n-k}$.

$\therefore$ under H_0, $t = \frac{(\bar{x}_i-\bar{x}_j)}{s'\sqrt{\frac{1}{n_i}+\frac{1}{n_j}}} \sim t_{n-k}$.

$\therefore \omega_0 : |t| > t_{\alpha/2,n-k}$. Also, $100(1-\alpha)\%$ confidence interval for $(\mu_i - \mu_j)$ is $\left\{(\bar{x}_i-\bar{x}_j) \mp s'\sqrt{\frac{1}{n_i} + \frac{1}{n_j}} t_{\alpha/2,n-k}\right\}$.

(II)Bartlett's test To test $H_0 : \sigma_1 = \sigma_2 = \cdots = \sigma_k (= \sigma)$, say against H_1: There is at least one inequality in H_0.

Define $\gamma_i = n_i - 1$ and $\gamma = \sum_{i=1}^{k} \gamma_i = n - k$. Bartlett's test statistic M is such that

$$M = \gamma \log_e \left\{\sum_{i=1}^{k} \frac{\gamma_i s_i'^2}{\gamma}\right\} - \sum_{i=1}^{k} \gamma_i \log_e s_i'^2$$

Under H_0 $M \sim \chi^2_{k-1}$ (approximately) provided none of γ_i is small. For small samples $M' = \frac{M}{\left\{1+\frac{c_1}{3(k-1)}\right\}} \sim \chi^2_{k-1}$ under H_0 where $c_1 = \sum_{i=1}^{k} \frac{1}{\gamma_i} - \frac{1}{\gamma}$ and $\omega_0 : M' > \chi^2_{\alpha,k-1}$.

A.8 Test for Regression

Suppose the sample values of x and y are arranged in arrays of y according to the fixed values of x as given below:

x_1	x_2	$\ldots$	x_i	$\ldots$	x_k
y_1	y_{21}	$\ldots$	y_{i1}	$\ldots$	y_{k1}
y_{12}	y_{22}	$\ldots$	y_{i2}		y_{k2}
.	.	$\ldots$			
.	.				
.	.				
y_{1n_1}	y_{2n_1}		y_{in_i}	$\ldots$	y_{kn_k}

Define $\bar{y}_{i0} = \frac{1}{n_i}\sum_{j=1}^{n_i} y_{ij}, \quad \bar{y}_{00} = \frac{1}{n}\sum_i n_i\bar{y}_{i0} = \bar{y}$

$$\bar{x} = \frac{1}{n}\sum_i n_i x_i, \quad n = \sum_i n_i$$

$$e_{yx}^2 = \frac{\sum_i n_i(\bar{y}_{i0} - \bar{y}_{00})^2}{\sum_i \sum_j (\bar{y}_{ij} - \bar{y}_{00})^2}$$

$$e_{yx} = +\sqrt{e_{yx}^2} = \text{ sample correlation ratio.}$$

$$r = \frac{\frac{1}{n}\sum_i \sum_j (y_{ij} - \bar{y}_{00})(x_i - \bar{x})}{\sqrt{\left\{\frac{1}{n}\sum_i \sum_j (y_{ij} - \bar{y}_{00})^2\right\}\left\{\frac{1}{n}\sum_i n_i(x_i - \bar{x})^2\right\}}}$$

We assume $y_{ij}/x_i \sim N_1(\mu_i, \sigma^2)$, i.e. $E(y_{ij}/x_i) = \mu_{i.}$.

(I) Test for regression: H_0 There does not exist any regression of y on x.

$$\Leftrightarrow H_0 : \mu_1 = \mu_2 = \cdots = \mu_k.$$

Define $\eta_{yx}^2 = \frac{V(E(y/x))}{V(y)}$; $\quad \eta_{yx} = +\sqrt{\eta_{yx}^2}$ = population correlation ratio.

$\therefore$ To test H_0 is equivalent to test $H_0 : \eta_{yx}^2 = 0$ against $H_1 : \eta_{yx}^2 > 0$

We note that

$$\sum_i\sum_j (y_{ij} - \bar{y}_{00})^2 = \sum_i\sum_j (y_{ij} - \bar{y}_{i0})^2 + \sum_i n_i(\bar{y}_{i0} - \bar{y}_{00})^2$$

Under H_0

$$SS_B = e_{yx}^2 \sum_i\sum_j (y_{ij} - \bar{y}_{00})^2 = \sum_i n_i(\bar{y}_{i0} - \bar{y}_{00})^2 \sim \sigma^2 \cdot \chi_{k-1}^2$$

$$SS_w = \left(1 - e_{yx}^2\right)\sum_i\sum_j (y_{ij} - \bar{y}_{00})^2 = \sum_i\sum_j (y_{ij} - \bar{y}_{i0})^2 \sim \sigma^2 . \chi_{n-k}^2$$

$\therefore$ Under H_0 :$F = \frac{e_{yx}^2/(k-1)}{(1-e_{yx}^2)/n-k} \sim F_{k-1,n-k}.\left[F = \frac{SS_B/(k-1)}{SS_W/n-k}\right]$

$$\therefore \omega_0 : F > F_{\alpha;k-1,n-k}.$$

(II) If H_0 is rejected then we may be interested in testing whether the regression is linear, i.e. we are to test

$$H_0 : \mu_i = \alpha + \beta x_i \quad \forall i$$
$$H_1 : \mu_i \neq \alpha + \beta x_i$$

We note that, $e_{yx}^2\sum_i\sum_j(y_{ij}-\bar{y}_{00})^2=\sum_i n_i(\bar{y}_{i0}-\bar{y}_{00})^2$

Also, $r^2\sum_i\sum_j(y_{ij}-\bar{y}_{00})^2=\frac{\left\{\sum_i\sum_j(y_{ij}-\bar{y}_{00})(x_i-\bar{x})\right\}^2}{\sum_i n_i(x_i-\bar{x})^2}=\hat{\beta}^2\sum n_i(x_i-\bar{x})^2$

where $\hat{\beta}=\frac{\sum_i\sum_j(y_{ij}-\bar{y}_{00})(x_i-\bar{x})}{\sum_i n_i(x_i-\bar{x})^2}$

$\therefore\left(e_{yx}^2-r^2\right)\sum_i\sum_j(y_{ij}-\bar{y}_{00})^2=\sum_i n_i(\bar{y}_{i0}-\bar{y}_{00})^2-\hat{\beta}^2\sum_i n_i(x_i-\bar{x})^2\sim\sigma^2.\chi_{k-2}^2$ under H_0.

Also, $e_{yx}^2\sum_i\sum_j(y_{ij}-\bar{y}_{00})^2$ and $\left(e_{yx}^2-r^2\right)\sum_i\sum_j(y_{ij}-\bar{y}_{00})^2$ are independent.

$\therefore$ under H_0, $F=\frac{\left(e_{yx}^2-r^2\right)/(k-2)}{\left(1-e_{yx}^2\right)/n-k}\sim F_{k-2,n-k}$

$$\therefore\omega_0:F>F_{\alpha;k-2,n-k}$$

A.9 Tests Relating to Simple Linear Regression Equation

Regression of y on x is established and it is linear, i.e. $E(y/x)=\alpha+\beta x$, say

$$\therefore E(y/x=x_i)=\alpha+\beta x_i, i=1(1)n.$$
$$y/x\sim N(\alpha+\beta x,\sigma^2)$$

Least square (LS) regression line is given by $Y=a+bx$, where a, b are the LS estimates of α and β, i.e. $a=\bar{y}-b\bar{x}$ and $b=\frac{\sum(y_i-\bar{y})(x_i-\bar{x})}{\sum(x_i-\bar{x})^2}=\frac{S_{xy}}{S_{xx}}$.

$\therefore\bar{y}\sim N\left(\alpha+\beta\bar{x},\frac{\sigma^2}{n}\right)$ and $b\sim N\left(\beta,\frac{\sigma^2}{S_{xx}}\right)$. Also they are independent.

$\therefore$ 'a' is normal with $E(a)=E(\bar{y})-\bar{x}E(b)=\alpha$.

$$V(a)=V(\bar{y})+\bar{x}^2V(b)=\frac{\sigma^2}{n}+\bar{x}^2\frac{\sigma^2}{S_{xx}}=\frac{\sigma^2}{nS_{xx}}\left(S_{xx}+n\bar{x}^2\right)=\frac{\sigma^2}{ns_{xx}}\left(\sum x_i^2\right)$$

i.e., $a\sim N\left(\alpha,\sigma^2\left(\frac{1}{n}+\frac{\bar{x}^2}{S_{xx}}\right)\right)$

$H_{01}:\alpha=\alpha_0$: under H_{01}, $t=\frac{a-\alpha_0}{\hat{\sigma}\sqrt{\frac{1}{n}+\frac{\bar{x}^2}{S_{xx}}}}\sim t_{n-2}$

where $\hat{\sigma}^2=\sum(y_i-a-bx_i)^2/(n-2)$

$$\therefore H_{11} : \alpha > \alpha_0, \omega_0 : t > t_{\alpha,n-2}$$
$$H_{21} : \alpha < \alpha_0, \omega_0 : t < -t_{\alpha,n-2}$$
$$H_{31} : \alpha \neq \alpha_0, \omega_0 : |t| > t_{\alpha/2,n-2}.$$

Also, $100(1-\alpha)\%$ confidence interval for α is $\left(a \mp \hat{\sigma}\sqrt{\frac{1}{n} + \frac{\bar{x}^2}{S_{xx}}} t_{\alpha/2}, n-2\right)$.
$H_{02} : \beta = \beta_0$: under H_{02}, $t = \frac{(b-\beta_0)\sqrt{S_{xx}}}{\hat{\sigma}} \sim t_{n-2}$

$$\therefore H_{12} : \beta > \beta_0, \quad \omega_0 : t > t_{\alpha,n-2}$$
$$H_{22} : \beta < \beta_0, \quad \omega_0 : t < -t_{\alpha,n-2}$$
$$H_{32} : \beta \neq \beta_0, \quad \omega_0 : |t| > t_{\alpha/2,n-2}.$$

Also, $100(1-\alpha)\%$ confidence interval for β is

$$\left(b \mp \frac{\hat{\sigma}}{\sqrt{S_{xx}}} \cdot t_{\alpha/2,n-2}\right)$$

$$H_{03} : \alpha = \alpha_0, \beta = \beta_0 : \ \text{Cov}(a,b) = \text{Cov}\ (\bar{y} - b\bar{x}, b)$$

$$= -\bar{x}V(b) = -\bar{x}\frac{\sigma^2}{S_{xx}}.$$

$$\therefore \begin{pmatrix} a \\ b \end{pmatrix} \sim N_2\left\{\begin{pmatrix} \alpha \\ \beta \end{pmatrix}, \begin{pmatrix} \frac{\sigma^2 \sum x_i^2}{nS_{xx}} & -\frac{\sigma^2 \bar{x}}{S_{xx}} \\ -\frac{\sigma^2 \bar{x}}{S_{xx}} & \frac{\sigma^2}{S_{xx}} \end{pmatrix}\right\}$$

i.e., $\begin{pmatrix} a \\ b \end{pmatrix} \sim N_2\left\{\begin{pmatrix} \alpha \\ \beta \end{pmatrix}, \frac{\sigma^2}{nS_{xx}}\begin{pmatrix} \sum x_i^2 & -\bar{x}\cdot n \\ -\bar{x}\cdot n & n \end{pmatrix}\right\}$

$$\left[\text{Let } \frac{\sigma^2}{nS_{xx}}\begin{pmatrix} \sum x_i^2 & -\bar{x}\cdot n \\ -\bar{x}\cdot n & n \end{pmatrix} = \sum\right]$$

$$\therefore \begin{pmatrix} a-\alpha \\ b-\beta \end{pmatrix}' \sum^{-1} \begin{pmatrix} a-\alpha \\ b-\beta \end{pmatrix} \sim \chi_2^2.$$

Now, $\sum^{-1} = \frac{\text{adj}\sum}{|\sum|} = \frac{\frac{\sigma^2}{nS_{xx}}\begin{pmatrix} n & n\bar{x} \\ n\bar{x} & \sum x_i^2 \end{pmatrix}}{\left(\frac{\sigma^2}{nS_{xx}}\right)^2\left(n\sum x_i^2 - n^2\bar{x}^2\right)}$

$$= \frac{nS_{xx}}{\sigma^2 nS_{xx}} \begin{pmatrix} n & n\bar{x} \\ n\bar{x} & \sum x_i^2 \end{pmatrix} = \frac{1}{\sigma^2} \begin{pmatrix} n & n\bar{x} \\ n\bar{x} & \sum x_i^2 \end{pmatrix}$$

$$\therefore \begin{pmatrix} a-\alpha \\ b-\beta \end{pmatrix}' \sum^{-1} \begin{pmatrix} a-\alpha \\ b-\beta \end{pmatrix} = \frac{1}{\sigma^2} \begin{pmatrix} a-\alpha \\ b-\beta \end{pmatrix}' \begin{pmatrix} n & n\bar{x} \\ n\bar{x} & \sum x_i^2 \end{pmatrix} \begin{pmatrix} a-\alpha \\ b-\beta \end{pmatrix}$$

$$\Rightarrow \left[n(a-\alpha)^2 + 2n\bar{x}(a-\alpha)(b-\beta) + (b-\beta)^2 \sum x_i^2 \right] \sim \sigma^2 \chi_2^2$$

Again, $\sum_1^n (y_i - a - bx_i)^2 \sim \sigma^2 \cdot \chi_{n-2}^2$
$\therefore$ under H_{03},

$$F = \frac{\left\{ n(a-\alpha_0)^2 + 2n\bar{x}(a-\alpha_0)(b-\beta_0) + (b-\beta_0)^2 \sum x_i^2 \right\} / 2}{\sum (y_i - a - bx_i)^2 / (n-2)} \sim F_{2,n-2}$$

$\therefore w_0 : F > F_{\alpha;2,n-2}$.

A.10 Tests Relating to Multiple and Partial Correlation Coefficient

Suppose $\underset{\sim}{x}^{px1} \sim N_p\left(\underset{\sim}{\mu}, \sum^{pxp}\right)$

$\rho_{1.23\ldots p}$ = population multiple correlation coefficient of X_1 on $X_2, X_3, \ldots, X_p$

$r_{1.23\ldots p}$ = sample multiple correlation coefficient of X_1 on $X_2, X_3, \ldots, X_p$ based on a sample of size n $(\geq p+1)$

$$= \left(1 - \frac{|R|}{R_{11}}\right)^{1/2} \text{ where } R = \begin{pmatrix} 1 & r_{12} & r_{13} & \ldots & r_{1p} \\ & 1 & r_{23} & \ldots & r_{1p} \\ & & & \ldots & \ldots \\ & & & \ldots & \ldots \\ & & & & 1 \end{pmatrix} \text{ and } R_{11} = \text{cofactor of } r_{11}$$

in R.

If $\rho_{1.23\ldots p} = 0$ then $F = \frac{r_{1.23\ldots p}^2/(p-1)}{(1-r_{1.23\ldots p}^2)/(n-p)} \sim F_{p-1,n-p}$.

To test
$H_0 : \rho_{1.23\ldots p} = 0$ against $H_1 : \rho_{1.23\ldots p} > 0$

$$\therefore w_0 : F > F_{\alpha;p-1,n-p}.$$

$\rho_{12.34\ldots p}$ = population partial correlation coefficient of X_1 and X_2 eliminating the effect of $X_3, \ldots, X_p$.

$r_{12.34\ldots p}$ = sample partial correlation coefficient of X_1 and X_2 eliminating the effect of $X_3, \ldots, X_p$

$= -\frac{R_{12}}{\sqrt{R_{11}R_{22}}}$. If $\rho_{12.34\ldots p}$ then

$$t = \frac{r_{12.34\ldots p}\sqrt{n-p}}{\sqrt{1-r^2_{12.34\ldots p}}} \sim t_{n-p}$$

Thus for testing $H_0 : \rho_{12.34\ldots p} = 0$ against

$$H_1 : \rho_{12.34\ldots p} > 0; \quad \omega_0 : t > t_{\alpha,n-p}$$
$$H_2 : \rho_{12.34\ldots p} < 0; \quad \omega_0 : t < -t_{\alpha,n-p}$$
$$H_3 : \rho_{12.34\ldots p} \neq 0; \quad \omega_0 : |t| > t_{\alpha/2,n-p}.$$

A.11 Problems Related to Multiple Regression

We consider a set of variables $(y; x_1, x_2, \ldots, x_p)$, where y is stochastic and $(x_1, x_2, \ldots, x_p)$ are nonstochastic. Let the multiple regression of y on $x_1, x_2, \ldots, x_p$ be

$$E(y/x_1, x_2, \ldots, x_p) = \beta_0 + \beta_1 x_1 + \beta_2 x_2 .. + \beta_p x_p \tag{A.1}$$

where $\beta_0, \beta_1, \beta_2, \beta_p$ are constants. In fact,

β_i = partial regression coefficient of y on x_i eliminating the effects of $x_j,\ j \neq i = 1, 2, \ldots p$.

Define $\sigma_{iy} = \text{Cov}(x_i, y), \sigma_{ij} = \text{Cov}(x_i, x_j),\ \sigma_{yy} = v(y),\ \rho_{iy} =$ correlation of $(x_i, y),\ \rho_{ij} =$ correlation of $(x_i, x_j), i = 1, 2, ..p$ and $j = 1(1)p$

We write $\underset{\sim(1)}{\sigma}^{px1} = (\sigma_{1y}, \sigma_{2y}, \ldots, \sigma_{py},)'$

$$\sum^{pxp} = \begin{pmatrix} \sigma_{11} & \sigma_{12} & \ldots & \sigma_{1p} \\ \sigma_{21} & \sigma_{22} & \ldots & \sigma_{2p} \\ \ldots & \ldots & \ldots & \ldots \\ \sigma_{p1} & \sigma_{p2} & \ldots & \sigma_{pp} \end{pmatrix} = \text{variance-covariance matrix of } x_1, x_2, .., x_p$$

We write

$$\sum_0^{\overline{p+1}x\overline{p+1}} = \begin{pmatrix} \sigma_{yy} & \sigma_{y1} & \sigma_{y2}\ldots & \sigma_{yp} \\ \sigma_{1y} & \sigma_{11} & \sigma_{12}\ldots & \sigma_{1p} \\ \sigma_{2y} & \sigma_{21} & \sigma_{22}\ldots & \sigma_{2p} \\ \ldots & \ldots & \ldots & \ldots \\ \sigma_{py} & \sigma_{p1} & \sigma_{p2}\ldots & \sigma_{pp} \end{pmatrix}$$

$$= \begin{pmatrix} \sigma_{yy} & \underset{\sim(1)}{\sigma}' \\ \underset{\sim(1)}{\sigma} & \sum^{pxp} \end{pmatrix} = \text{variance–covariance matrix of } y, x_1, x_2, \ldots, x_p.$$

Similarly, we write

$$\rho_0^{\overline{p+1}x\overline{p+1}} = \begin{pmatrix} \rho_{yy} & \rho_{y1} & \rho_{y2\cdots} & \rho_{yp} \\ \rho_{1y} & \rho_{11} & \rho_{12\cdots} & \rho_{1p} \\ \rho_{2y} & \rho_{21} & \rho_{22\cdots} & \rho_{2p} \\ \cdots & \cdots & \cdots & \cdots \\ \rho_{py} & \rho_{p1} & \rho_{p2\cdots} & \rho_{pp} \end{pmatrix} = \text{correlation matrix of } y,$$

$x_1, x_2, \ldots, x_p$.

Now, $|\sum_0| =$ (product of the diagonal element of $\sum_0)|\rho_0|$

$$= (\sigma_{yy}\sigma_{11}\sigma_{22}\ldots\sigma_{pp})|\rho_0|$$

$\therefore |\rho_0| = \frac{|\sum_0|}{(\sigma_{yy}\sigma_{11}\sigma_{22}\ldots\sigma_{pp})}$. Also, $|\sum| = (\sigma_{11}\sigma_{22}\ldots\sigma_{pp})x$ Cofactor of ρ_{yy} in ρ_0.

$\therefore$ Cofactor of ρ_{yy} in $\rho_0 = \frac{|\sum|}{\sigma_{11}\sigma_{22}\ldots\sigma_{pp}}$

$$\therefore \rho^2_{y.12\ldots p} = 1 - \frac{|\rho_0|}{\text{Cofactor of } \rho_{yy} \text{ in } \rho_0}$$

$$= 1 - \frac{|\sum_0|/(\sigma_{yy}\sigma_{11}\sigma_{22}\ldots\sigma_{pp})}{|\sum|/(\sigma_{11}\sigma_{22}\ldots\sigma_{pp})} = 1 - \frac{|\sum_0|}{\sigma_{yy}|\sum|}$$

$$= 1 - \frac{\sigma_{yy} - \underset{\sim(1)}{\sigma'}\sum^{-1}\underset{\sim(1)}{\sigma}}{\sigma_{yy}} = \frac{\sigma'_{(1)}\sum^{-1}\sigma_{(1)}}{\sigma_{yy}} = \frac{\sigma'_{(1)}\underset{\sim}{\beta}}{\sigma_{yy}} \text{ as } \underset{\sim}{\beta} = \sum^{-1}\underset{\sim(1)}{\sigma}.$$

$$\therefore \rho^2_{y.12\ldots p} = \frac{\underset{\sim(1)}{\sigma'}\underset{\sim}{\beta}}{\sigma_{yy}} = \frac{\underset{\sim}{\beta}'\sum\underset{\sim}{\beta}}{\sigma_{yy}}, \qquad \left[\underset{\sim}{\beta} = \sum^{-1}\underset{\sim(1)}{\sigma} \Rightarrow \sum\underset{\sim}{\beta} = \underset{\sim(1)}{\sigma} \Rightarrow \underset{\sim(1)}{\sigma'}\underset{\sim}{\beta} = \underset{\sim}{\beta}'\sum\underset{\sim}{\beta}\right]$$

Suppose we are given the set of observations

$$(y_\alpha, x_{1\alpha}, x_{2\alpha}, \ldots, x_{p\alpha}), \ \alpha = 1(1)n, \qquad n > p+1.$$

Define $\bar{x}_i = \frac{1}{n}\sum_{\alpha=1}^n x_{i\alpha}$, $S_{ij} = \sum_{\alpha=1}^n (x_{i\alpha} - \bar{x}_i)(x_{j\alpha} - \bar{x}_j)$

$$S_{iy} = \sum_{\alpha=1}^n (x_{i\alpha} - \bar{x}_i)(y_\alpha - \bar{y}_j). \quad \forall i,j = 1(1)p$$

$$S^{pxp} = \begin{pmatrix} S_{11} & S_{12} & \cdots & S_{1p} \\ S_{21} & S_{22} & \cdots & S_{2p} \\ \cdots & \cdots & \cdots & \cdots \\ S_{p1} & S_{p2} & \cdots & S_{pp} \end{pmatrix} \text{ which is positive definite.}$$

Estimated regression equation of y on $x_1, x_2, \ldots, x_p$ is $y = \hat{\beta}_0 + \hat{\beta}_1 x_1 + \hat{\beta}_2 x_2 + \cdots + \hat{\beta}_p x_p$

where $\hat{\beta}_0, \hat{\beta}_1, \hat{\beta}_2, \ldots, \hat{\beta}_p$ are the solutions of the following normal equations:

$$\left.\begin{array}{llllll} S_{1y} & = \hat{\beta}_1 S_{11} & \hat{\beta}_2 S_{12} & + \cdots + & \hat{\beta}_p S_{1p} \\ S_{2y} & = \hat{\beta}_1 S_{21} & \hat{\beta}_2 S_{22} & + \cdots + & \hat{\beta}_p S_{2p} \\ \cdots & \cdots & \cdots & & \\ S_{py} & = \hat{\beta}_1 S_{p1} & \hat{\beta}_2 S_{p2} & + \cdots + & \hat{\beta}_p S_{pp} \end{array}\right\} \tag{A.2}$$

and $\hat{\beta}_0 = \bar{y} - \hat{\beta}_1\bar{x}_1 - \hat{\beta}_2\bar{x}_2 - \cdots - \hat{\beta}_p\bar{x}_p$

We write $\underset{\sim}{y}^{nx1} = (y_1, y_2, \ldots, y_n)'$

$$K^{nxp} = \begin{pmatrix} x_{11} - \bar{x}_1 & x_{21} - \bar{x}_2 & \ldots & x_{p1} - \bar{x}_p \\ x_{12} - \bar{x}_1 & x_{22} - \bar{x}_2 & \ldots & x_{p2} - \bar{x}_p \\ \cdots & \cdots & \cdots & \cdots \\ x_{1n} - \bar{x}_1 & x_{2n} - \bar{x}_2 & \ldots & x_{pn} - \bar{x}_p \end{pmatrix}$$

$$\underset{\sim}{\hat{\beta}}^{px1} = \left(\hat{\beta}_1, \hat{\beta}_2, .., \hat{\beta}_p\right)'$$

Note that $S_{iy} = \sum_{\alpha=1}^{n} (x_{i\alpha} - \bar{x}_i) y_\alpha$, (A.2) reduces to

$$S\underset{\sim}{\hat{\beta}} = K'\underset{\sim}{y} \Rightarrow \underset{\sim}{\hat{\beta}} = S^{-1}K'\underset{\sim}{y}$$

$\Rightarrow \hat{\beta}_1, \hat{\beta}_2, \ldots, \hat{\beta}_p$ are linear functions of $y_1, y_2, \ldots, y_n$ which are normal.

$$\therefore \underset{\sim}{\hat{\beta}} \sim N_p\left(E\left(\hat{\beta}\right), D\left(\underset{\sim}{\hat{\beta}}\right)\right)$$

Now, $\underset{\sim}{\hat{\beta}} = S^{-1}K'\underset{\sim}{y} = S^{-1}K'\left(\underset{\sim}{y} - \bar{y}\underset{\sim}{\in}\right)$

where $\underset{\sim}{\in} = (1, 1, \ldots, 1)'$ and $K'\underset{\sim}{\in} = \underset{\sim}{0}$

$$\therefore E\left(\underset{\sim}{\hat{\beta}}\right) = S^{-1}K'E\left(\underset{\sim}{y} - \bar{y}\underset{\sim}{\in}\right)$$

$$E(y_\alpha) = \beta_0 + \beta_1 x_{1\alpha} + \cdots + \beta_p x_{p\alpha}$$

$$E(\bar{y}) = \beta_0 + \beta_1\bar{x}_1 + \cdots + \beta_p\bar{x}_p$$

$$E(y_\alpha - \bar{y}) = \beta_1(x_{1\alpha} - \bar{x}_1) + \cdots + \beta_p(x_{p\alpha} - \bar{x}_p)$$

$$E\left(\underset{\sim}{y} - \bar{y}\underset{\sim}{\in}\right) = E\begin{pmatrix} y_1 & - & \bar{y} \\ y_2 & - & \bar{y} \\ & \vdots & \\ y_n & - & \bar{y} \end{pmatrix} = K\underset{\sim}{\beta}$$

$$\therefore E\left(\hat{\underset{\sim}{\beta}}\right) = S^{-1}K'K\underset{\sim}{\hat{\beta}} = S^{-1}S\underset{\sim}{\beta} = \underset{\sim}{\beta} \quad [\because K'K = S]$$

$$D\left(\hat{\beta}\right) = S^{-1}K'\sigma^2 I_n KS^{-1} = \sigma^2 S^{-1}K'KS^{-1} = \sigma^2 S^{-1}SS^{-1} = \sigma^2 S^{-1}$$

$$\therefore \underset{\sim}{\hat{\beta}} = S^{-1}K'\underset{\sim}{y} \sim N_p\left(\underset{\sim}{\beta}, \sigma^2 S^{-1}\right)$$

We write $S^{-1} = ((S^{ij})) \qquad \therefore V(\hat{\beta}_i) = \sigma^2 S^{ii}$
and

$$\mathrm{Cov}\left(\hat{\beta}_i, \hat{\beta}_j\right) = \sigma^2 S^{ij} \qquad \forall i,j = 1(1)p$$

$$\therefore \hat{\beta}_i \sim N_1(\beta_i, \sigma^2 S^{ii}) \quad i = 1(1)p$$

Again, $\hat{\beta}_0 = \bar{y} - \hat{\beta}_1\bar{x}_1 - \hat{\beta}_2\bar{x}_2 - \hat{\beta}_p\bar{x}_p$

$$\therefore E\left(\hat{\beta}_0\right) = E(\bar{y}) - \sum_{i=1}^{p} E\left(\hat{\beta}_i\right)\bar{x}_i = \left(\beta_0 + \sum_{i=1}^{p} \beta_i\bar{x}_i\right) - \sum_{i=1}^{p} \beta_i\bar{x}_i = \beta_0$$

$$V\left(\hat{\beta}_0\right) = V\left(\bar{y} - \sum \hat{\beta}_i\bar{x}_i\right)$$

$$= V\left(\bar{y} - \underset{\sim}{\bar{x}}'\underset{\sim}{\hat{\beta}}\right); \quad \underset{\sim}{\bar{x}}' = (\bar{x}_1, \bar{x}_2, \ldots, \bar{x}_p)$$

$= \frac{\sigma^2}{n} + \underset{\sim}{\bar{x}}'D\left(\underset{\sim}{\hat{\beta}}\right)\underset{\sim}{\bar{x}}$ (as $\bar{y}$ and $\underset{\sim}{\hat{\beta}}$ are independent)

$$= \frac{\sigma^2}{n} + \underset{\sim}{\bar{x}}'\sigma^2 S^{-1}\underset{\sim}{\bar{x}} = \sigma^2\left[\frac{1}{n} + \underset{\sim}{\bar{x}}'S^{-1}\underset{\sim}{\bar{x}}\right].$$

Thus $\hat{\beta}_0$ is also a linear combination of normal variables.

$$\therefore \hat{\beta}_0 \sim N_1\left(\beta_0, \sigma^2\left[\frac{1}{n} + \underset{\sim}{\bar{x}}'S^{-1}\underset{\sim}{\bar{x}}\right]\right)$$

Again $Y = \hat{\beta}_0 + \sum_{1}^{p} \hat{\beta}_i x_i, \quad \therefore Y \sim N_1(E(Y), V(Y))$

where $E(Y) = E\left(\hat{\beta}_0\right) + \sum E\left(\hat{\beta}_i\right)x_i = \beta_0 + \sum \beta_i x_i = \xi_x$, (say)

$$V(Y) = V\left(\hat{\beta}_0 + \sum_{i=1}^{p} \hat{\beta}_i x_i\right) = V\left[\bar{y} - \sum_i \hat{\beta}_i \bar{x}_i + \sum_i \hat{\beta}_i x_i\right]$$

$$= V\left[\bar{y} + \sum_i \hat{\beta}_i (x_i - \bar{x}_i)\right] = V(\bar{y}) + V\left(\sum_i \hat{\beta}_i (x_i - \bar{x}_i)\right)$$

$$= \frac{\sigma^2}{n} + \sum_1^p \sum_1^p (x_i - \bar{x}_i)(x_j - \bar{x}_j) \mathrm{Cov}\left(\hat{\beta}_i, \hat{\beta}_j\right)$$

$$= \frac{\sigma^2}{n} + \sum_1^p \sum_1^p (x_i - \bar{x}_i)(x_j - \bar{x}_j) \sigma^2 S^{ij} = \sigma^2 \left[\frac{1}{n} + \left(\underset{\sim}{x} - \bar{x}\right)' S^{-1} (\underset{\sim}{x} - \bar{x})\right]$$

$$\therefore Y \sim N_1\left(\beta_0 + \sum \beta_i x_i = \xi_x, \sigma^2 \left[\frac{1}{n} + \left(\underset{\sim}{x} - \bar{x}\right)' S^{-1} (\underset{\sim}{x} - \bar{x})\right]\right)$$

To get different test procedures σ^2 is estimated as

$$\hat{\sigma}^2 = \frac{1}{n-p-1} \sum_{\alpha=1}^{p} \left(y_\alpha - \hat{\beta}_0 - \hat{\beta}_1 x_{1\alpha} + \ldots + \hat{\beta}_p x_{p\alpha}\right)^2$$

$$= \frac{1}{n-p-1} \sum_{\alpha=1}^{n} \left\{(y_\alpha - \bar{y}) - \sum_i \hat{\beta}_i (x_{i\alpha} - \bar{x}_i)\right\}^2$$

$$= \frac{1}{n-p-1} \left[S_{yy} - \sum_{\alpha=1}^{n} \sum_i \sum_j \hat{\beta}_i \hat{\beta}_j (x_{i\alpha} - \bar{x}_i)(x_{i\alpha} - \bar{x}j)\right]$$

$$= \frac{1}{n-p-1} \left[S_{yy} - \sum_i \sum_j \hat{\beta}_i \hat{\beta}_j S_{ij}\right] = \frac{1}{n-p-1} \left[S_{yy} - \underset{\sim}{\hat{\beta}}' S \underset{\sim}{\hat{\beta}}\right]$$

(Note that $\rho^2_{y.12\ldots p} = \frac{\underset{\sim}{\beta}' \sum \underset{\sim}{\beta}}{\sigma_{yy}}$)

(1) $H_{01} : \beta_1 = \beta_2 = \cdots = \beta_p = 0$

$\Rightarrow x_1, x_2, \ldots, x_p$ are not worthwhile in predicting y.

$$\because \rho^2_{y.12\ldots p} = \frac{\underset{\sim}{\hat{\beta}}' \sum \underset{\sim}{\hat{\beta}}}{\sigma_{yy}} \quad \therefore \beta_1 = \beta_2 = \cdots = \beta_p = 0 \Rightarrow \rho^2_{y.12\ldots p} = 0$$

So the problem is to test $H_{01} : \rho^2_{y.12\ldots p} = 0$ against $H_1 : \rho^2_{y.12\ldots p} > 0$

Now $S_{yy}\left(1 - r^2_{y.12\ldots p}\right) = S_{yy} - \underset{\sim}{\hat{\beta}}' \sum \underset{\sim}{\hat{\beta}}$

$$= \sum_{\alpha=1}^{n} \left(y_\alpha - \hat{\beta}_0 - \hat{\beta}_1 x_{1\alpha} - \cdots - \hat{\beta}_p x_{p\alpha}\right) \sim \sigma^2 \chi^2_{n-p-1}$$

Also, $S_{yy}r^2_{y.12\ldots p} = \hat{\underset{\sim}{\beta}}' S \hat{\underset{\sim}{\beta}} = S_{yy} - \left(S_{yy} - \hat{\underset{\sim}{\beta}}' S \hat{\underset{\sim}{\beta}}\right)$

$$\therefore S_{yy} = \left(S_{yy} - \hat{\underset{\sim}{\beta}}' S \hat{\underset{\sim}{\beta}}\right) + S_{yy}r^2_{y.12\ldots p}$$

$$S_{yy} \sim \sigma^2\chi^2_{n-1} \qquad \therefore S_{yy}r^2_{y.12\ldots p} \sim \sigma^2\chi^2_p$$

$$\therefore F_1 = \frac{r^2_{y.12\ldots p}\Big/p}{\left(1 - r^2_{y.12\ldots p}\right)\Big/(n-1-p)} \sim F_{p,n-p-1}$$

$$\therefore \omega_0 : F_1 > F_{\alpha;p,n-p-1}$$

(2) $H_0 : \beta_0 = \beta$ against $H_1 : \beta_0 \neq \beta$

Under H_0, $t = \dfrac{\hat{\beta}_0 - \beta}{\hat{\sigma}\sqrt{\dfrac{1}{n} + \underset{\sim}{\bar{x}}' S^{-1} \underset{\sim}{\bar{x}}}} \sim t_{n-p-1}$

where $\hat{\sigma}^2 = \frac{1}{n-p-1}\left[S_{yy} - \hat{\underset{\sim}{\beta}}' S \hat{\underset{\sim}{\beta}}\right] = S'^2_{y.12\ldots p}$, say

$$\text{and } \hat{\beta}_0 = \bar{y} - \sum \hat{\beta}_i \bar{x}_i = \bar{y} - \underset{\sim}{\bar{x}}' \hat{\underset{\sim}{\beta}}$$

$$\omega_0 : |t| > t_{\alpha/2,n-p-1}$$

(3) $H_0 : \beta_i = \beta_i^0$ against $H_1 : \beta_i \neq \beta_i^0 \ \forall i = 1(1)p$

$$\hat{\beta}_i \sim N_1\left(\beta_i, \sigma^2 S^{ii}\right)$$

Under H_0, $t = \frac{\hat{\beta}_i - \beta_i^0}{\hat{\sigma}\sqrt{S^{ii}}} \sim t_{n-p-1}$.

$$\omega_0 : |t| > t_{\alpha/2,n-p-1}$$

$100(1-\alpha)\%$ confidence interval for β_i is

$$\left(\hat{\beta}_i \mp \hat{\sigma}\sqrt{S^{ii}}\, t_{\alpha/2,n-p-1}\right)$$

(4) $H_0 : \beta_i - \beta_j = \delta_0$ against $H_1 : \beta_i - \beta_j \neq \delta_0$. $\forall i \neq j = 1(1)p$

$$\hat{\beta}_i - \hat{\beta}_j \sim N_1\left(\beta_i - \beta_j, \sigma^2\left(S^{ii} + S^{jj} - 2S^{ij}\right)\right)$$

$\therefore$ under H_0, $t = \frac{\left(\hat{\beta}_i - \hat{\beta}_j\right) - \delta_0}{\hat{\sigma}\sqrt{S^{ii} + S^{jj} - 2S^{ij}}} \sim t_{n-p-1}$

$$\therefore \omega_0 : |t| > t_{\alpha/2,n-p-1}$$

$100(1-\alpha)\%$ confidence interval for $(\beta_i - \beta_j)$ is

$$\left(\left(\hat{\beta}_i - \hat{\beta}_j\right) \mp \hat{\sigma}\sqrt{S^{ii} + S^{jj} - 2S^{ij}}\, t_{\alpha/2,n-p-1}\right)$$

(5) $H_0 : E(Y) = \xi_x = \xi^0$

Under H_0, $t = \dfrac{Y-\xi^0}{\hat{\sigma}\sqrt{\frac{1}{n} + \left(\underset{\sim}{x} - \underset{\sim}{\bar{x}}\right)' S^{-1}\left(\underset{\sim}{x} - \underset{\sim}{\bar{x}}\right)}} \sim t_{n-p-1}$

$$\omega_0 : |t| > t_{\alpha/2,n-p-1}.$$

$100(1-\alpha)\%$ confidence interval for ξ_x is

$$\left(Y \mp \hat{\sigma}\sqrt{\frac{1}{n} + \left(\underset{\sim}{x} - \underset{\sim}{\bar{x}}\right)' S^{-1}\left(\underset{\sim}{x} - \underset{\sim}{\bar{x}}\right)}\, t_{\alpha/2,n-p-1}\right)$$

where $Y = \hat{\beta}_0 + \sum_{i=1}^{p} \hat{\beta}_i x_i$

A.12 Distribution of the Exponent of the Multivariate Normal Distribution

Let $\underset{\sim}{x}^{px1} \sim N_p\left(\underset{\sim}{\mu}^{px1}, \sum^{pxp}\right)$, $\quad \sum$ is positive definite.

The p.d.f. of $\underset{\sim}{x}$ is

$$f\left(\underset{\sim}{x}\right) = \frac{1}{(2\pi)^{p/2}\sqrt{|\sum|}} e^{-\frac{1}{2}\left(\underset{\sim}{x} - \underset{\sim}{\mu}\right)' \sum^{-1}\left(\underset{\sim}{x} - \underset{\sim}{\mu}\right)}, \quad \begin{matrix} -\infty < x_i < \infty \\ -\infty < \mu_i < \infty \end{matrix} \text{ and } 0 < \sigma_i < \infty$$

$$Q(\underset{\sim}{x}) = (\underset{\sim}{x} - \underset{\sim}{\mu})' \sum^{-1} (\underset{\sim}{x} - \underset{\sim}{\mu})$$

Since $\sum$ is positive definite, there exists a nonsingular matrix V^{pxp} such that $\sum^{-1} = VV'$.

$\therefore Q(\underset{\sim}{x}) = (\underset{\sim}{x} - \underset{\sim}{\mu})' VV' (\underset{\sim}{x} - \underset{\sim}{\mu}) = \underset{\sim}{y}'\underset{\sim}{y}$ where $\underset{\sim}{y} = V'(\underset{\sim}{x} - \underset{\sim}{\mu})$

$$= \sum_{i=1}^{p} y_i^2.$$

$$|J| = \left|\frac{\partial(x_1, x_2, \ldots, x_p)}{\partial(y_1, y_2, \ldots, y_n)}\right| = \frac{1}{|V|} = \frac{1}{\sqrt{|\sum^{-1}|}} = \sqrt{|\sum|}$$

$$\therefore \text{ p.d.f. of } \underset{\sim}{y} \text{ is } f(\underset{\sim}{y}) = \frac{1}{(2\pi)^{p/2}\sqrt{|\sum|}} e^{-\frac{1}{2}\underset{\sim}{y}'\underset{\sim}{y}} \cdot \sqrt{|\sum|}$$

$$= \frac{1}{(2\pi)^{p/2}} e^{-\frac{1}{2}\sum_1^P y_1^2}.$$

Now $y_1, y_2, \ldots, y_p$ are i.i.d $N(0, 1)$

$$\therefore \sum_1^p y_i^2 \sim \chi_p^2, \text{ i.e., } Q(\underset{\sim}{x}) \sim \chi_p^2$$

If we now want to find the distribution of $Q^*(\underset{\sim}{x}) = \underset{\sim}{x}'\sum^{-1} x$, since $\sum$ is positive definite, there exists a non-singular matrix V^{pxp} such that $\sum^{-1} = VV'$.

$\therefore Q^*(\underset{\sim}{x}) = \underset{\sim}{x}'VV'x = \underset{\sim}{z}'\underset{\sim}{z}$ where $\underset{\sim}{Z} = V'\underset{\sim}{x}$.

Here also $|J| = \sqrt{|\sum|}$.

$$\therefore (\underset{\sim}{x} - \underset{\sim}{\mu})'\sum^{-1}(\underset{\sim}{x} - \underset{\sim}{\mu}) = (\underset{\sim}{x} - \underset{\sim}{\mu})'VV'(\underset{\sim}{x} - \underset{\sim}{\mu})$$

$$= \left(V'\underset{\sim}{x} - V'\underset{\sim}{\mu}\right)' I_p \left(V'\underset{\sim}{x} - V'\underset{\sim}{\mu}\right)$$

$$= \left(\underset{\sim}{z} - V'\underset{\sim}{\mu}\right)' I_p \left(\underset{\sim}{z} - V'\underset{\sim}{\mu}\right)$$

$$\therefore f(z) = \frac{1}{(2\pi)^{p/2}} e^{-\frac{1}{2}\left(\underset{\sim}{z} - V'\underset{\sim}{\mu}\right)' I_p \left(\underset{\sim}{z} - V'\underset{\sim}{\mu}\right)}$$

$\therefore z_1, z_2, \ldots, z_p$ are normal with common variance unity but with means given by $E\left(\underset{\sim}{z}\right) = V'\underset{\sim}{\mu}$.

$\therefore \sum_1^p z_i^2 \sim$ non-central χ_p^2 with non-centrality parameter $\left(V'\underset{\sim}{\mu}\right)'\left(V'\underset{\sim}{\mu}\right) = \underset{\sim}{\mu}'VV'\underset{\sim}{\mu} = \underset{\sim}{\mu}'\sum^{-1}\mu$.

A.13 Large Sample Distribution of Pearsonian Chi-Square

Events	A_1	A_2	....	A_i	......	A_k	Total
Probability	P_1	P_2	....	P_i	......	P_k	1
Frequency	n_1	n_2	....	n_i	......	n_k	n

$$\therefore f(n_1, n_2, \ldots, n_k) = \frac{n!}{\prod_i n_i!} \prod_{i=1}^{k} p_i^{n_i}$$

$$n_i \sim \text{Bin}(n, p_i)$$

Pearsonian chi-square statistic is $\chi^2 = \sum_{i=1}^{k} \frac{(n_i - np_i)^2}{np_i}$
Using Stirling's approximation to factorials

$$f(n_1, n_2, \ldots, n_k) \simeq \frac{\sqrt{2\pi} e^{-n} n^{n+\frac{1}{2}}}{\prod_1^k \sqrt{2\pi} e^{-n_i} n_i^{n_i+\frac{1}{2}}} \prod_1^k p_i^{n_i}$$

$$= \frac{n^{n+\frac{1}{2}} \prod_1^k p_i^{n_i}}{(2\pi)^{\frac{k-1}{2}} \prod_1^k n_i^{n_i+\frac{1}{2}}}$$

$$= \frac{\sqrt{n}}{(2\pi)^{\frac{k-1}{2}} \prod \sqrt{np_i}} \prod_1^k \left(\frac{np_i}{n_i}\right)^{n_i+\frac{1}{2}}$$

$$\therefore \log_e f(n_1, n_2, \ldots, n_k) \simeq C + \sum_{i=1}^{k} \left(n_i + \frac{1}{2}\right) \log_c \left(\frac{np_i}{n_i}\right) \tag{A.3}$$

where $C = \log_e \left[\frac{\sqrt{n}}{(2\pi)^{\frac{k-1}{2}} \prod_1^k \sqrt{np_i}}\right]$

We write $\delta_i = \frac{n_i - np_i}{\sqrt{np_i q_i}}, q_i = 1 - p_i$

$$\Rightarrow n_i = np_i + \delta_i\sqrt{np_iq_i} \Rightarrow \frac{n_i}{np_i} = 1 + \delta_i\sqrt{\frac{q_i}{np_i}}$$

$$\therefore \frac{np_i}{n_i} = \left(1 + \delta_i\sqrt{\frac{q_i}{np_i}}\right)^{-1}$$

$$\therefore \log_e f(n_1, n_2, \ldots, n_k) = C - \sum_1^k \left(np_i + \frac{1}{2} + \delta_i\sqrt{np_iq_i}\right)\log_e\left(1 + \delta_i\sqrt{\frac{q_i}{np_i}}\right)$$

$$= C - \sum_1^k \left(np_i + \frac{1}{2} + \delta_i\sqrt{np_iq_i}\right)\left(\delta_i\sqrt{\frac{q_i}{np_i}} - \frac{\delta_i^2 q_i}{2np_i} + \frac{\delta_i^3 q_i^{3/2}}{3(np_i)^{3/2}} - \cdots\right),$$

Provided $\left|\delta_i\sqrt{\frac{q_i}{np_i}}\right| < 1$

$$= C - \sum_1^k \left(\delta_i\sqrt{np_iq_i} + \frac{1}{2}\delta_i\sqrt{\frac{q_i}{np_i}} - \frac{1}{2}\delta_i^2 q_i - \frac{1}{4}\delta_i^2\frac{q_i}{np_i} + \delta_i^2 q_i + \frac{\delta_i^3}{\sqrt{n}}(\cdots) + \cdots\right)$$

$$= C - \sum_1^k \left(\delta_i\sqrt{np_iq_i} + \frac{1}{2}\delta_i\sqrt{\frac{q_i}{np_i}} + \frac{1}{2}\delta_i^2 q_i - \frac{1}{4}\delta_i^2\frac{q_i}{np_i} + \frac{\delta_i^3}{\sqrt{n}}(\cdots)\right)\cdots \quad \text{(A.4)}$$

Note that $\sum \delta_i\sqrt{np_iq_i} = \sum_1^k (n_i - np_i) = n - n = 0$,
we assume that $\delta_i^3 = 0(\sqrt{n})$ i.e., $\frac{\delta_i^3}{\sqrt{n}} \to 0, \frac{\delta_i}{\sqrt{n}} \to 0 \Rightarrow \frac{\delta_i^2}{n} \to 0$

$\therefore$ All the terms in the R.H.S of (A.4) tends to zero except $\frac{1}{2}\delta_i^2 q_i$, thus (A.4) implies

$$\log_e f \simeq C - \frac{1}{2}\sum_1^k \delta_i^2 q_i \Rightarrow f \simeq e^C \cdot e^{-\frac{1}{2}\sum_1^k \delta_i^2 q_i}$$

$$\Rightarrow f \simeq \frac{\sqrt{n}}{(2\pi)^{\frac{k-1}{2}}\prod_1^k \sqrt{np_i}} e^{-\frac{1}{2}\sum_{i=1}^k \frac{(n_i - np_i)^2}{np_i}}$$

$$= \frac{1}{(2\pi)^{\frac{k-1}{2}}\sqrt{p_k}} e^{-\frac{1}{2}\sum_{i=1}^k \frac{(n_i - np_i)^2}{np_i}} \cdot \frac{1}{\prod_1^{k-1}\sqrt{np_i}} \quad \text{(A.5)}$$

We note that $\sum_1^k (n_i - np_i) = 0$
i.e., $n_k - np_k = -\sum_1^{k-1}(n_i - np_i)$

$$\therefore \sum_{i=1}^k \frac{(n_i - np_i)^2}{np_i} = \sum_{i=1}^{k-1} \frac{(n_i - np_i)^2}{np_i} + \frac{(n_k - np_k)^2}{np_k}$$

$$= \sum_{1}^{k-1} \frac{(n_i - np_i)^2}{np_i} + \frac{\left\{\sum_1^{k-1}(n_i - np_i)\right\}^2}{np_k} \tag{A.6}$$

We use the transformation $(n_1, n_2, \ldots, n_{k-1}) \rightarrow (x_1, x_2, \ldots, x_{k-1})$ where $x_i = \frac{n_i - np_i}{\sqrt{np_i}}, \quad i = 1(l)\overline{k-1}$.

$$|J| = \left|\frac{\partial(n_1, n_2, \ldots, n_{k-1})}{\partial(x_1, x_2, \ldots, x_{k-1})}\right| = \left|\text{Diag}\left(\sqrt{np_1} \ldots \sqrt{np_{k-1}}\right)\right|$$
$$= \prod^{k-1} \sqrt{np_i}$$

$$(A.6) \Rightarrow \sum_1^k \frac{(n_i - np_i)^2}{np_i} = \sum_1^{k-1} x_i^2 + \frac{\left(\sum_1^{k-1}\sqrt{np_i}x_i\right)^2}{np_k}$$
$$= \sum_1^{k-1} x_i^2 + \frac{1}{p_k}\left[\sum_1^{k-1} p_i x_i^2 + \sum_{i \neq j = 1}^{k-1}\sum \sqrt{p_i p_j} x_i x_j\right]$$
$$= \sum_1^{k-1}\left(1 + \frac{p_i}{p_k}\right)x_i^2 + \sum_{i \neq j = 1}^{k-1}\sum \frac{\sqrt{p_i p_j}}{p_k} x_i x_j$$
$$= \underset{\sim}{x}' A \underset{\sim}{x}$$

where

$$A^{\overline{k-1}x\overline{k-1}} = \begin{pmatrix} 1 + \frac{p_1}{p_k} & \frac{\sqrt{p_1 p_2}}{p_k} & \frac{\sqrt{p_1 p_3}}{p_k} \ldots & \frac{\sqrt{p_1 p_{k-1}}}{p_k} \\ & 1 + \frac{p_2}{p_k} & \frac{\sqrt{p_2 p_3}}{p_k} \ldots & \frac{\sqrt{p_2 p_{k-1}}}{p_k} \\ & & \ldots & \ldots \\ & & & 1 + \frac{p_{k-1}}{p_k} \end{pmatrix}$$

$$= \begin{pmatrix} 1 + a_1^2 & a_1 a_2 & a_1 a_3 \ldots & a_1 a_{k-1} \\ a_1 a_2 & 1 + a_2^2 & a_2 a_3 \ldots & a_2 a_{k-1} \\ & & \ldots & \ldots \\ a_1 a_{k-1} & a_2 a_{k-1} & a_3 a_{k-1} & 1 + a_{k-1}^2 \end{pmatrix} \text{ where } a_i = \sqrt{\frac{p_i}{p_k}}\ \forall i = 1(1)\overline{k-1}$$

Now

$$|A| = (a_1 a_2 .. a_{k-1}) \begin{vmatrix} a_1 + \frac{1}{a_1} & a_2 & a_3 \ldots & a_{k-1} \\ a_1 & a_2 + \frac{1}{a_2} & a_3 \ldots & a_{k-1} \\ \ldots. & \ldots & \ldots & \ldots \\ a_1 & a_2 & a_3 & a_{k-1} + \frac{1}{a_{k-1}} \end{vmatrix};\ \left(\frac{\text{Rows}}{a_i}\right)$$

$$= (a_1 a_2 \cdots a_{k-1})^2 \begin{vmatrix} 1+\frac{1}{a_1^2} & 1 & 1\ldots & 1 \\ 1 & 1+\frac{1}{a_2^2} & 1\ldots & 1 \\ 1 & 1 & 1+\frac{1}{a_3^2} & 1 \\ \ldots & \ldots & \ldots & \ldots \\ 1 & 1 & 1 & 1+\frac{1}{a_{k-1}^2} \end{vmatrix}$$

$$= \begin{vmatrix} a_1^2+1 & a_1^2 & \ldots & a_1^2 \\ a_2^2 & a_2^2+1 & \ldots & a_2^2 \\ \ldots & \ldots & \ldots & \\ a_{k-1}^2 & a_{k-1}^2 & \ldots & a_{k-1}^2+1 \end{vmatrix} \quad (i\text{th row } X\ a_i^2)$$

$$= \begin{vmatrix} 1+\sum_1^{k-1} a_i^2 & 1+\sum_1^{k-1} a_i^2 & \ldots & 1+\sum_1^{k-1} a_i^2 \\ a_2^2 & 1+a_2^2 & \ldots & a_2^2 \\ \ldots & \ldots & \ldots & \\ a_{k-1}^2 & a_{k-1}^2 & \ldots & 1+a_{k-1}^2 \end{vmatrix}$$ (1st row $R_1 = \sum R_i =$ sum of all rows)

$$= \left(1+\sum_1^{k-1} a_i^2\right) = \begin{vmatrix} 1 & 1 & \ldots & 1 \\ a_2^2 & a_2^2+1 & \ldots & a_2^2 \\ \ldots & \ldots & \ldots & \\ a_{k-1}^2 & a_{k-1}^2 & \ldots & 1+a_{k-1}^2 \end{vmatrix};$$

$$= \left(1+\sum_1^{k-1} a_i^2\right) = \begin{vmatrix} 1 & 1 & \ldots & 1 \\ 0 & 1 & \ldots & 0 \\ \ldots. & \ldots. & \ldots & \ldots \\ 0 & 0 & \ldots & 1 \end{vmatrix};$$

$$= 1 + \sum^{k-1} a_i^2 = 1 + \sum_1^{k-1} \frac{p_i}{p_k} = \frac{\sum_1^k p_i}{p_k} = \frac{1}{p_k}$$

$$\therefore \text{(A.5)} \Rightarrow f(x_1, x_1, \ldots, x_{k-1}) = \frac{1}{(2\pi)^{\frac{k-1}{2}}\sqrt{p_k}} e^{-\frac{1}{2}\underset{\sim}{x}'A\underset{\sim}{x}} \frac{1}{\prod_1^{k-1}\sqrt{np_i}} |J|$$

$$= \frac{\sqrt{|A|}}{(2\pi)^{\frac{k-1}{2}}} e^{-\frac{1}{2}\underset{\sim}{x}'A\underset{\sim}{x}}$$

$$= \frac{1}{(2\pi)^{\frac{k-1}{2}}\left|\sum\right|^{1/2}} e^{-\frac{1}{2}\underset{\sim}{x}'\sum^{-1}\underset{\sim}{x}} \text{ where } A^{-1} = \sum.$$

Since $\sum^{-1}$ is positive definite therefore there exists a non-singular V such that $\sum^{-1} = VV'$.

$\therefore \underset{\sim}{x}' \sum^{-1} \underset{\sim}{x} = \underset{\sim}{x}' vv' \underset{\sim}{x} = \underset{\sim}{y}' \underset{\sim}{y}$ where $\underset{\sim}{y} = v' \underset{\sim}{x}$.

Using transformation $(x_1, x_2, \ldots, x_{k-1}) \to (y_1, y_2, \ldots, y_{k-1})$

$$|J| = \frac{1}{|V|} = \left|\sum\right|^{1/2}$$

$$\therefore f(y_1, y_2, \ldots, y_{k-1}) = \frac{1}{(2\pi)^{\frac{k-1}{2}}} e^{-\frac{1}{2}\underset{\sim}{y}'\underset{\sim}{y}} \quad \Rightarrow y_1, y_2, \ldots, y_{k-1} \text{ are i.i.d. } N(0,\ 1)$$

$$\therefore \underset{\sim}{y}' \underset{\sim}{y} \sim \chi^2_{k-1}$$

$$\Rightarrow \underset{\sim}{x}' \sum^{-1} \underset{\sim}{x} \sim \chi^2_{k-1} \Rightarrow \sum_{i=1}^{k} \frac{(n_i - np_i)^2}{np_i} \sim \chi^2_{k-1}$$

Note This approximate distribution is valid if $\left|\delta_i \sqrt{\frac{q_i}{np_i}}\right| < 1$

i.e., $\delta_i^2 q_i < np_i \Rightarrow$ if $\delta_i^2 < \frac{np_i}{q_i}$, i.e. if $\text{Max}\delta_i^2 < \frac{np_i}{q_i}$

Again $\delta_i = \frac{n_i - np_i}{\sqrt{np_i q_i}}$, using normal approximation the effective range of δ_i is $(-3,\ 3)$ $\therefore \delta_i^2 \leq 9$

i.e.,

$$\text{Max}\delta_i^2 = 9$$

So the approximate distribution will be valid if $9 < \frac{np_i}{q_i}$, i.e. if $np_i > 9(1 - p_i)$, i.e. if $np_i > 9$. So the approximation is valid if the expected frequency for each event is at least 10.

Again, if we consider the effective range of δ_i as $(-2,\ 2)$, then the approximation is valid if the expected frequency for each event is at least 5.

It has been found by enquiry that if the expected frequencies are greater than 5 then the approximation is good enough.

If the expected frequencies of some classes be not at least 5 then some of the adjacent classes are pooled such that the expected frequencies of all classes after coalition are at least 5. If k^* be the no. of classes after coalition, then $\sum_{i=1}^{k^*} \frac{(n_i^* - np_i^*)^2}{np_i^*} \sim \chi^2_{k^*-1}$,

where n_i^* = observed frequency after coalition,

np_i^* =expected frequency after coalition.

Uses of Pearsonian-χ^2:

(1) Test for goodness of fit:

Classes	Probability	Frequency
A_1	p_1	n_1
A_2	p_2	n_2
.	.	.
.	.	.
.	.	.
A_i	p_i	n_i
:	:	:
A_k	p_k	n_k
Total	1	n

We are to test $H_0 : p_i = p_i^0 \cdot \forall i$

Under H_0, expected frequencies are np_i^0. We assume $np_i^0 \geq 5 \forall i$.

$\therefore$ Under H_0, $\sum_{i=1}^{k} \frac{\left(n_i - np_i^0\right)^2}{np_i^0} \sim \chi^2_{k-1}$

i.e. $\sum_{i=1}^{k} \frac{n_i^2}{np_i^0} - n \sim \chi^2_{k-1}$.

i.e. $\chi^2 = \sum_{i=1}^{k} \frac{O^2}{E} - n \sim \chi^2_{k-1}$

where O = observed frequency (n_i)

E = Expected frequency (np_i^0)

$$\therefore \omega_0 : \chi^2 > \chi^2_{\alpha, k-1}$$

Note Suppose the cell probabilities $p_1, p_2, \ldots, p_k$ depend on unknown parameters $\underset{\sim}{\theta}^{s \times 1} = (\theta_1, \theta_2, \ldots, \theta_s)'$ and suppose $\hat{\underset{\sim}{\theta}}$ be an efficient estimator of $\underset{\sim}{\theta}$. Then $\sum_{i=1}^{k} \frac{\left\{n_i - np_i(\hat{\underset{\sim}{\theta}})\right\}^2}{np_i\left(\hat{\underset{\sim}{\theta}}\right)} \sim \chi^2_{(k-1-s)}$.

(2) Test for homogeneityof similarly classified populations

Classes	Population					
	P_1	P_2	....	P_j	....	P_l
A_1	p_{11}	p_{12}	....	p_{1j}	....	p_{1l}
A_2	p_{21}	p_{22}	....	p_{2j}	....	p_{2l}
.	.	.	....	.	....	.
.	.	.	....	.	....	.
A_i	p_{i1}	p_{i2}		p_{ij}		p_{ij}
.	.	.		.		.
.	.	.		.		.
.				.		
A_k	p_{k1}	p_{k2}		p_{kj}		p_{kl}
Total	1	1	....	1	....	1

where p_{ij} = the probability that an individual selected from jth population will belong to ith class.

We are to test $H_0 : p_{i1} = p_{i2} = \cdots = p_{il}\ (= p_i \text{say})\ \forall i = 1(1)k$. To do this we draw a sample of size n and classify as shown below:

Classes	Population						Total
	P_1	P_2	....	P_j	....	P_l	
A_1	n_{11}	n_{12}		n_{1j}		n_{1l}	n_{10}
A_2	n_{21}	n_{22}		n_{2j}		n_{21}	n_{20}
.	.	.	.	.	.	.	.
.	.	.	.	.	.	.	.
A_i	n_{i1}	n_{i2}		n_{ij}		n_{il}	n_{i0}
.	.	.	.	.	.	.	.
.	.	.	.	.	.	.	.
A_k	n_{kl}	n_{k2}	....	n_{kj}	....	n_{kl}	n_{k0}
Total	n_{01}	n_{01}	....	n_{0j}	....	n_{0l}	n

For the jth population the Pearsonian chi-square statistic is

$$\sum_{i=1}^{k} \frac{\left\{n_{ij} - n_{0j}p_{ij}\right\}^2}{n_{0j}p_{ij}} \sim \chi^2_{(k-1)} \cdot \forall j = 1(1)1$$

$$\therefore \sum_{j=1}^{l} \sum_{i=1}^{k} \frac{\left\{n_{ij} - n_{0j}p_{ij}\right\}^2}{n_{0j}p_{ij}} \sim \chi^2_{1(k-1)}$$

$\therefore$ Under H_0, $\chi^2 = \sum_{j=1}^{l} \sum_{i=1}^{k} \frac{\left\{n_{ij} - n_{0j}p_i\right\}^2}{n_{0j}p_i} \sim \chi^2_{1(k-1)}$

p_i's are unknown and they are estimated by $\hat{p}_i = \frac{n_{i0}}{n} \forall i = 1(1)k$.

$\therefore$ under H_0, $\chi^2 = \sum_{j=1}^{1} \sum_{i=1}^{k} \frac{\left\{n_{ij} - \frac{n_{0j}n_{i0}}{n}\right\}}{n_{0j}\frac{n_{i0}}{n}} \sim \chi^2_{1(k-1)-(k-1)} = \chi^2_{(k-1)(l-1)}$

as the d.f. will be reduced by $(k-1)$ since we are to estimate any $(k-1)$ of $p_1, p_2, \ldots, p_k$ as $\sum_1^k p_i = 1$.

$$\therefore \omega_0 : \chi^2 > \chi^2_{\alpha,(k-1)(1-1)}$$

(3) Test for independenceof two attributes

A	B						Total
	B_1	B_2	....	B_j	....	B_l	
A_1	p_{11}	p_{12}	....	p_{1j}	....	p_{1l}	p_{10}
A_2	p_{21}	p_{22}	....	p_{2j}	....	p_{2l}	p_{20}
.	.	.	....	.	....	.	.
.	.	.	....	.	....	.	.
A_i	p_{i1}	p_{i2}		p_{ij}		p_{il}	p_{i0}
.	.	.		.		.	.
.	.	.		.		.	.
A_k	p_{k1}	p_{k2}		p_{kj}		p_{kl}	p_{k0}
Total	p_{01}	p_{02}	....	p_{0j}	....	p_{0l}	1

We are to test
H_0 : A and B are independent, i.e. to test

$$H_0 : \; p_{ij} = p_{i0} x p_{0j} \; \forall (i,j)$$

To do this we draw a sample of size n and suppose the sample observations be classified as shown below:

A	B						Total
	B_1	B_2	....	B_j	....	B_l	
A_1	n_{11}	n_{12}	....	n_{1j}	....	n_{1l}	n_{10}
A_2	n_{21}	n_{22}	....	n_{2j}	....	n_{2l}	n_{20}
.	.	.	....	.	....	.	.
.	.	.	....	.	....	.	.
A_i	n_{i1}	n_{i2}		n_{ij}		n_{il}	n_{i0}
.	.	.		.		.	.
.	.	.		.		.	.
A_k	n_{k1}	n_{k2}		n_{kj}		n_{kl}	n_{k0}
Total	n_{01}	n_{02}	....	n_{0j}	....	n_{0l}	n

$$P(n_{11}, \ldots, n_{kl}) = \frac{n!}{\prod_i \prod_j (n_{ij}!)} \prod_i \prod_j (p_{ij})^{n_{ij}}$$

$$E(n_{ij}) = np_{ij},$$

$$i = 1(1)k, j = 1(1)1.$$

$$\therefore \sum_i \sum_j \frac{\left(n_{ij} - np_{ij}\right)^2}{np_{ij}} \overset{a}{\sim} \chi^2_{k1-1}$$

Under H_0, $\chi^2 = \sum_i \sum_j \frac{\left(n_{ij} - np_{i0}p_{0j}\right)^2}{np_{i0}p_{0j}} \overset{a}{\sim} \chi^2_{k1-1}$

Now, unknown p_{i0} and p_{0j} are estimated by

$\hat{p}_{i0} = \frac{n_{i0}}{n}$ and $\hat{p}_{0j} = \frac{n_{0j}}{n}$

$\therefore$ under H_0, $\chi^2 = \sum_i \sum_j \frac{\left(n_{ij} - \frac{n_{i0}n_{0j}}{n}\right)^2}{\frac{n_{i0}n_{0j}}{n}} \overset{a}{\sim} \chi^2_{(k1-1)-(k+1-2)}$

$$\overset{a}{\sim} \chi^2_{(k-1)(1-1)}$$

i.e., $\chi^2 = n \sum_i \sum_j \frac{n_{ij}^2}{n_{i0}n_{0j}} - n \overset{a}{\sim} \chi^2_{(k-1)(1-1)}$

$$\therefore \omega_0 : \chi^2 > \chi^2_{\alpha,(k-1)(1-1)}.$$

Particular cases: (i) $l = 2$

A	B		Total
	B_1	B_2	
A_1	a_1	b_1	T_1
A_2	a_2	b_2	T_2
.	.	.	.
A_i	a_i	b_i	T_i
.	.	.	.
A_k	a_k	b_k	T_k
Total	T_a	T_b	n

Here,

$$\chi^2 = \sum_1^k \frac{\left(a_i - \frac{T_iT_a}{n}\right)^2}{\frac{T_iT_a}{n}} + \sum_1^k \frac{\left(b_i - \frac{T_iT_b}{n}\right)^2}{\frac{T_iT_b}{n}}$$

Now, $b_i - \frac{T_iT_b}{n} = T_i - a_i - \frac{T_i(n-T_a)}{n}$

$$= T_i - a_i - T_i + \frac{T_iT_a}{n} = -\left(a_i - \frac{T_iT_a}{n}\right)$$

$$\therefore \chi^2 = n\sum_1^k \left(a_i - \frac{T_iT_a}{n}\right)^2 \left(\frac{1}{T_a} + \frac{1}{T_b}\right)\frac{1}{T_i}$$

$$= n\sum_1^k \left(a_i - \frac{T_iT_a}{n}\right)^2 \frac{n}{T_iT_aT_b}$$

$$= \frac{n^2}{T_aT_b}\sum_1^k \left(\frac{a_i^2}{T_i} + \frac{T_iT_a^2}{n^2} - 2\frac{a_iT_a}{n}\right)$$

$$= \frac{n^2}{T_aT_b}\left[\sum_1^k \frac{a_i^2}{T_i} + \frac{T_a^2}{n^2}n - 2\frac{T_a}{n}T_a\right]$$

$$= \frac{n^2}{T_aT_b}\left[\sum_1^k \frac{a_i^2}{T_i} - \frac{T_a^2}{n^2}\right]$$

This formula or its equivalent $\chi^2 = \frac{n^2}{T_aT_b}\left[\sum_1^k \frac{b_i^2}{T_i} - \frac{T_b^2}{n^2}\right]$ will be found more convenient for computational purpose.

$$\omega_0 : \chi^2 > \chi^2_{\alpha,k-1}$$

(ii) $k = 2$, $l = 2$:

A	B		Total
	B_1	B_2	
A_1	a	b	$a + b$
A_2	c	d	$c + d$
Total	$a + c$	$b + d$	$n = a + b + c + d$

Here,

$$\chi^2 = \frac{\left\{a - \frac{(a+b)(a+c)}{n}\right\}^2}{\frac{(a+b)(a+c)}{n}} + \frac{\left\{b - \frac{(a+b)(b+d)}{n}\right\}^2}{\frac{(a+b)(b+d)}{n}} + \frac{\left\{c - \frac{(c+d)(a+c)}{n}\right\}^2}{\frac{(c+d)(a+c)}{n}} + \frac{\left\{d - \frac{(c+d)(b+d)}{n}\right\}^2}{\frac{(c+d)(b+d)}{n}}$$

Now, $a - \frac{(a+b)(a+c)}{n} = \frac{1}{n}[a(a+b+c+d) - (a+b)(a+c)] = \frac{ad-bc}{n}$

Similarly; $b - \frac{(a+b)(b+d)}{n} = -\frac{ad-bc}{n}$; $c - \frac{(c+d)(a+c)}{n} = -\frac{ad-bc}{n}$
and $d - \frac{(b+d)(c+d)}{n} = \frac{ad-bc}{n}$

$$\therefore \chi^2 = \frac{(ad-bc)^2}{n}\left[\frac{1}{(a+b)(a+c)}+\frac{1}{(a+b)(b+d)}+\frac{1}{(c+d)(a+c)}+\frac{1}{(c+d)(b+d)}\right]$$
$$= \frac{(ad-bc)^2}{n}\left[\frac{n}{(a+b)(a+c)(b+d)}+\frac{n}{(a+c)(c+d)(b+d)}\right]$$
$$= \frac{(ad-bc)^2 n}{(a+b)(c+d)(a+c)(b+d)}$$

This turns out to be much easier to apply.

Corrections for continuity

We know that for the validity of the χ^2-approximation it is necessary that the expected frequency in each class should be sufficiently large (say > 4). When expected frequencies are smaller we pool some of the classes in order to satisfy this condition. However, it should be apparent that this procedure should be ruled out in case of 2 × 2 table. For 2 × 2 table the following two methods of correction may be applied.

(I) Yates' correction: Yates has suggested a correction to be applied to the observed frequencies in a 2 × 2 table in case any expected frequency is found to be too small. This is done by increasing or decreasing the frequencies by half $\left(1/2\right)$ in such a way that the marginal totals remain unaltered.

Case 1 Say $ad < bc$

A	*B*		Total
	B_1	B_2	
A_1	$a+\frac{1}{2}$	$b-\frac{1}{2}$	$a+b$
A_2	$c-\frac{1}{2}$	$d+\frac{1}{2}$	$c+d$
Total	$a+c$	$b+d$	$a+b+c+d$

Here, $\left(a+\frac{1}{2}\right)\left(d+\frac{1}{2}\right)-\left(b-\frac{1}{2}\right)\left(c-\frac{1}{2}\right)=(ad-bc)+\frac{n}{2}$
$= -|ad-bc|+\frac{n}{2} = -\left[|ad-bc|-\frac{n}{2}\right]$ (since $ad-bc<0$)

Case 2 If $ad > bc$

A	*B*		Total
	B_1	B_2	
A_1	$a-\frac{1}{2}$	$b+\frac{1}{2}$	$a+b$
A_2	$c+\frac{1}{2}$	$d-\frac{1}{2}$	$c+d$
Total	$a+c$	$b+d$	$a+b+c+d$

Here, $\left(a-\frac{1}{2}\right)\left(d-\frac{1}{2}\right)-\left(b+\frac{1}{2}\right)\left(c+\frac{1}{2}\right)$

$$= (ad - bc) - \frac{n}{2}$$

$$= |ad - bc| - \frac{n}{2}$$

$\therefore$ For both the cases $\chi^2 = \frac{n\left[|ad-bc|-\frac{n}{2}\right]^2}{(a+b)(c+d)(a+c)(b+d)}$.

(ii) **Dandekar's correction**: A slightly different method suggested by V.N. Dandekar involves the calculation of χ_0^2, χ_1^2 and χ_{-1}^2 for the observed 2×2 configuration

where $\chi_0^2 = \frac{n(ad-bc)^2}{(a+b)(c+d)(a+c)(b+d)}$

χ_1^2 = the chi-square obtained by decreasing the smallest frequency by '1' keeping marginal totals fixed and

χ_{-1}^2 = the chi-square obtained by increasing the smallest frequency by '1' keeping the marginal totals fixed.

Then the test statistic is given by

$$\chi^2 = \chi_0^2 - \frac{\chi_0^2 - \chi_{-1}^2}{\chi_1^2 - \chi_{-1}^2}\left(\chi_1^2 - \chi_0^2\right).$$

A.14 Some Convergence Results

Definition 1 A sequence of random variables $\{X_n\}$, $n = 1, 2, \ldots$, is said to be convergent in probability to a random variable X if for any $\in\ > 0$, however small,

$$P\{|X_n - X| < \in\} \to 1 \quad \text{as} \quad n \to \infty$$

and we write it as $X_n \xrightarrow{P} X$. If X is degenerate, i.e. a constant, say c, then this convergence is known as WLLN.

Definition 2 Let $\{X_n\}, n = 1, 2, \ldots$ be a sequence of random variables having distribution functions $\{F_n(x)\}$ and X be a random variable having distribution function$F(x)$. If $F_n(x) \to F(x)$ as $n \to \infty$ at all continuity points of $F(x)$, then we say X_n converges in law to X and we write it as $X_n \xrightarrow{L} X$. i.e., the asymptotic distribution of X_n is nothing but the distribution of X.

Result 1(a): If $X_n \xrightarrow{P} X$ and $g(x)$ be a continuous function for all x, then $g(X_n) \xrightarrow{P} g(X)$.

Result 1(b): If $X_n \xrightarrow{P} C$ and $g(x)$ is continuous in the neighbourhood of C, then $g(X_n) \xrightarrow{P} g(C)$.

Result 2(a):

$$X_n \xrightarrow{P} X \Rightarrow X_n \xrightarrow{L} X$$

$$X_n \xrightarrow{P} C \Leftrightarrow X_n \xrightarrow{L} C$$

Result 2(b): $X_n \xrightarrow{L} X \Rightarrow g(X_n) \xrightarrow{L} g(x)$ if g be a continuous function.

Result 3: Let $\{X_n\}$ and $\{Y_n\}$ be sequences of random variables such that $X_n \xrightarrow{L} X$ and $Y_n \xrightarrow{P} C$, where X is a random variable and C is a constant, then

(a) $X_n + Y_n \xrightarrow{L} X + C$; (b) $X_n Y_n \xrightarrow{L} XC$;

(c) $\frac{X_n}{Y_n} \xrightarrow{L} \frac{X}{C}$, if $C \neq 0$ and

(d) $X_n Y_n \xrightarrow{P} 0$, if $C = 0$.

Theorem 1 *Let* $\{T_n\}$*be a sequence of statistics such that* $\sqrt{n}(T_n - \theta) \xrightarrow{L} X \sim N(0, \sigma^2(\theta))$.*If* $g(\xi)$*be a function admitting* $g'(\xi)$*in the neighbourhood of* θ, *then* $\sqrt{n}(g(T_n) - g(\theta)) \xrightarrow{L} Y \sim N(0, \sigma^2(\theta) g'^2(\theta))$.

Proof By mean value theorem

$g(T_n) = g(\theta) + (T_n - \theta)\{g'(\theta) + \in_n\}\ldots$ (A) where $\in_n \to 0$ as $T_n \to \theta$. Since $\in_n \to 0$ as $T_n \to \theta$, we can determine a $\delta > 0$, for any small positive quantity η, such that $|T_n - \theta| < \eta \Rightarrow |\in_n| < \delta$.

$$\therefore P\{|T_n - \theta| < \eta\} \leq P\{|\in_n| < \delta\} \tag{A.7}$$

i.e., $P\{|\in_n| < \delta\} \geq P\{-\eta < T_n - \theta < \eta\}$

$$= P\{-\sqrt{n}\eta < \sqrt{n}(T_n - \theta) < \sqrt{n}\eta\}$$

$$\to \int_{-\infty}^{\infty} \frac{1}{\sqrt{2\pi}\sigma(\theta)} e^{-\frac{x^2}{2\sigma^2(\theta)}} dx = 1$$

$\therefore P\{|\in_n| < \delta\} \to 1$ as $n \to \infty$

$$\therefore \in_n \xrightarrow{P} 0 \tag{A.8}$$

$$\text{Again, } \sqrt{n}(T_n - \theta) \xrightarrow{L} X \sim N\left(0, \sigma^2(\theta)\right) \tag{A.9}$$

Combining (A.8) and (A.9) and using result 3(d), we can write

$$\sqrt{n}(T_n - \theta) \in_n \xrightarrow{P} 0 \tag{A.10}$$

Again, (A) gives

$$\sqrt{n}(g(T_n) - g(\theta)) - \sqrt{n}(T_n - \theta)g'(\theta) = \sqrt{n}(T_n - \theta) \in_n$$

i.e. $X_n - Y_n = \sqrt{n}(T_n - \theta) \in_n \xrightarrow{P} 0$

where $X_n = \sqrt{n}(g(T_n) - g(\theta))$ and $Y_n = \sqrt{n}(T_n - \theta)g'(\theta)$ i.e. $X_n - Y_n \xrightarrow{P} 0$

(A.11)

$$\text{Also, } Y_n = \sqrt{n}(T_n - \theta)g'(\theta) \xrightarrow{L} Y \sim N\left(0, \sigma^2(\theta)g'^2(\theta)\right) \tag{A.12}$$

Combining (A.11) and (A.12) and using result 3(a),
$Y_n + (X_n - Y_n) \xrightarrow{L} Y + 0$, i.e. $X_n \xrightarrow{L} Y$

i.e., $\sqrt{n}(g(T_n) - g(\theta)) \xrightarrow{L} Y \sim N(0, g'^2(\theta)\sigma^2(\theta))$

i.e., $\sqrt{n}(g(T_n) - g(\theta)) \overset{a}{\sim} N(0, g'^2(\theta)\sigma^2(\theta))$

Note 1 If $T_n \overset{a}{\sim} N\left(0, \frac{\sigma^2(\theta)}{n}\right)$, then $g(T_n) \overset{a}{\sim} N\left(g(\theta), g'^2(\theta)\frac{\sigma^2(\theta)}{n}\right)$ provided $g(\xi)$ be a continuous function in the neighbourhood of θ admitting the1st derivative.

Note 2 $\frac{\sqrt{n}(g(T_n) - g(\theta))}{g'(T_n)} \overset{a}{\sim} N(0, \sigma^2(\theta))$, provided $g'(\xi)$ is continuous.

Proof $\frac{\sqrt{n}(g(T_n) - g(\theta))}{g'(\theta)} \overset{a}{\sim} N(0, \sigma^2(\theta))$

Since $T_n \xrightarrow{P} \theta$ and $g'(\xi)$ is continuous

$$\therefore g'(T_n) \xrightarrow{P} g'(\theta) \Rightarrow \frac{g'(\theta)}{g'(T_n)} \xrightarrow{P} 1$$

$$\therefore \frac{\sqrt{n}(g(T_n) - g(\theta))}{g'(T_n)} = \frac{\sqrt{n}(g(T_n) - g(\theta))}{g'(\theta)} \cdot \frac{g'(\theta)}{g'(T_n)}$$

As first part of the R.H.S converges in law to $X \sim N(0, \sigma^2(\theta))$ and the second part converges in probability to 1,

$\therefore$ their product converges in law to $N(0, \sigma^2(\theta))$.

Note 3 Further if $\sigma(\varsigma)$ is continuous, then

$$\frac{\sqrt{n}(g(T_n) - g(\theta))}{g'(T_n)\sigma(T_n)} \overset{a}{\sim} N(0, 1).$$

Proof $\frac{\sqrt{n}(g(T_n)-g(\theta))}{g'(T_n)\sigma(T_n)} = \frac{\sqrt{n}(g(T_n)-g(\theta))}{g'(T_n)\sigma(\theta)} \frac{\sigma(\theta)}{\sigma(T_n)}$

By note-2, $\frac{\sqrt{n}(g(T_n)-g(\theta))}{g'(T_n)\sigma(\theta)} \overset{a}{\sim} N(0, 1)$

Also, $T_n \xrightarrow{P} \theta$ and $\sigma(\xi)$ is continuous

$$\sigma(T_n) \xrightarrow{P} \sigma(\theta) \Rightarrow \frac{\sigma(\theta)}{\sigma(T_n)} \xrightarrow{P} 1.$$

$$\therefore \frac{\sqrt{n}(g(T_n) - g(\theta))}{g'(T_n)\sigma(T_n)} \xrightarrow{L} N(0, 1)$$

Generalization of theorem 1

Theorem 2

Let $\left\{ \underset{\sim n}{T} = \begin{pmatrix} T_{1n} \\ T_{2n} \\ \cdot \\ \cdot \\ T_{kn} \end{pmatrix} \text{ for } n = 1, 2\ldots \right\}$ be a sequence of statistics such that

$\sqrt{n}\left(\underset{\sim n}{T} - \underset{\sim}{\theta}\right) = \begin{pmatrix} \sqrt{n}(T_{1n} - \theta_1) \\ \sqrt{n}(T_{2n} - \theta_2) \\ \cdot \\ \cdot \\ \sqrt{n}(T_{kn} - \theta_k) \end{pmatrix} \overset{a}{\sim} N_k\left(\underset{\sim}{0}, \sum^{kxk}\left(\underset{\sim}{\theta}\right)\right)$, *where* $\sum\left(\underset{\sim}{\theta}\right) = \left(\sigma_{ij}\left(\underset{\sim}{\theta}\right)\right)$.

Let $g(\ldots)$ be a function of k variables such that it is totally differentiable. Then

$$\sqrt{n}\left(g\left(\underset{\sim n}{T}\right) - g\left(\underset{\sim}{\theta}\right)\right) \xrightarrow{L} X \sim N_1\left(0, V\left(\underset{\sim}{\theta}\right)\right)$$

where $V\left(\underset{\sim}{\theta}\right) = \sum_i^k \sum_j^k \frac{\partial g}{\partial \theta_i} \frac{\partial g}{\partial \theta_j} \sigma_{ij}\left(\underset{\sim}{\theta}\right)_j; \frac{\partial g}{\partial \theta_i} = \left.\frac{\partial g}{\partial T_{in}}\right]_{\underset{\sim n}{T} = \underset{\sim}{\theta}}$

Proof Since g is totally differentiable, so by mean value theorem,

$$g\left(\underset{\sim n}{T}\right) = g\left(\underset{\sim}{\theta}\right) + \sum_{i=1}^{k} (T_{in} - \theta_i)\frac{\partial g}{\partial \theta_i} + \in_n \left\|\underset{\sim n}{T} - \underset{\sim}{\theta}\right\| \tag{A.13}$$

where $\in_n \to 0$ as $T_{in} \to \theta_i \; \forall \, i = 1(1)K$.

$\therefore$ For any given small $\eta > 0$ we can find a $\delta > 0$, however small, such that $|T_{in} - \theta_i| < \eta \Rightarrow |\in_n| < \delta$

$$\Rightarrow P\{|\in_n| < \delta\} \geq P\{|T_{in} - \theta_i| < \eta\} \to 1$$

as $\sqrt{n}(T_{in} - \theta_i) \overset{a}{\sim} N$

$\therefore T_{in} \xrightarrow{P} \theta_i$ and $\in_n \xrightarrow{P} 0$

Again $\sqrt{n}(T_{in} - \theta_i) \overset{a}{\sim} N$

$\therefore \sqrt{n}\left\|\underset{\sim n}{T} - \underset{\sim}{\theta}\right\| = \left\{n \sum_1^k (T_{in} - \theta_i)^2\right\}^{1/2}$ has an asymptotic distribution.

Suppose $\sqrt{n}\left\|\underset{\sim n}{T} - \underset{\sim}{\theta}\right\| \xrightarrow{L} Y$

$$\therefore \sqrt{n}\left\|\underset{\sim n}{T} - \underset{\sim}{\theta}\right\| \cdot \in_n \xrightarrow{P} 0$$

$\therefore$ (A.13) implies $\sqrt{n}\left\{g\left(\underset{\sim n}{T}\right) - g\left(\underset{\sim}{\theta}\right)\right\} - \sqrt{n}\sum_1^k (T_{in} - \theta_i)\frac{\partial g}{\partial \theta_i} = \sqrt{n} \in_n \left\|\underset{\sim n}{T} - \underset{\sim}{\theta}\right\| \xrightarrow{P} 0$

i.e., $Y_n - X_n \xrightarrow{P} 0$

where $Y_n = \sqrt{n}\left\{g\left(\underset{\sim n}{T}\right) - g\left(\underset{\sim}{\theta}\right)\right\}$ and $X_n = \sqrt{n}\sum_1^k (T_{in} - \theta_i)\frac{\partial g}{\partial \theta_i}$

We note that X_n, being linear function of normal variables $\sqrt{n}(T_{in} - \theta_i)$, $i = 1(1)K$, will be asymptotically normal with mean 0 and variance $= \sum_i^k \sum_j^k \frac{\partial g}{\partial \theta_i}\frac{\partial g}{\partial \theta_j}\sigma_{ij}(\theta) = V\left(\underset{\sim}{\theta}\right)$

i.e.,

$$X_n \xrightarrow{L} X \sim N\left(0, V\left(\underset{\sim}{\theta}\right)\right)$$

$$\therefore (Y_n - X_n) + X_n \xrightarrow{L} X \sim N\left(0, V\left(\underset{\sim}{\theta}\right)\right)$$

i.e., $Y_n \xrightarrow{L} X \sim N\left(0, V\left(\underset{\sim}{\theta}\right)\right)$

i.e., $\sqrt{n}\left\{g\left(\underset{\sim n}{T}\right) - g\left(\underset{\sim}{\theta}\right)\right\} \overset{a}{\sim} N\left(0, V\left(\underset{\sim}{\theta}\right)\right)$

A.15 Large Sample Standard Errors of Sample Moments

We have $F(x)$ a continuous c.d.f. We draw a random sample $(x_1, x_2, \ldots, x_n)$ from it. We have

$$\begin{cases} \mu'_r = E(X^r), \mu'_1 = \mu \\ \mu_r = E(X - \mu'_1)^r = E(X - \mu)^r \end{cases}$$

and the sample moments as

$$\begin{cases} m'_r = \frac{1}{n}\sum_1^n x_i^r, m'_1 = \bar{x} \\ m_r^0 = \frac{1}{n}\sum (x_i - \mu)^r \\ m_r = \frac{1}{n}\sum (x_i - \bar{x})^r \end{cases}$$

(i) To find $E(m'_r),\ V(m'_r),\ \mathrm{Cov}(m'_r, m'_s)$

$$E(m'_r) = \frac{1}{n}\sum_1^n E(x_i^r) = \frac{1}{n}\sum_1^n \mu'_r = \mu'_r$$

$$Cov(m'_r, m'_s) = E(m'_r m'_s) - \mu'_r\mu'_s$$

$$= \frac{1}{n^2}E\left\{\left(\sum x_i^r\right)\left(\sum x_i^s\right)\right\} - \mu'_r\mu'_s$$

$$= \frac{1}{n^2}\left[\sum E(x_i^{r+s}) + \sum\sum_{i \neq j} E\left\{\left(x_i^r\right)\left(x_j^s\right)\right\}\right] - \mu'_r\mu'_s$$

$$= \frac{\mu'_{r+s} - \mu'_r\mu'_s}{n}$$

$$\therefore V(m'_r) = \frac{1}{n}\left(\mu'_{2r} - \mu'^2_r\right)$$

$$\Rightarrow \frac{\sqrt{n}\left(m'_r - \mu'_r\right)}{\sqrt{\mu'_{2r} - \mu'^2_r}} \xrightarrow{L} N(0, 1)$$

This fact can be used for testing of hypothesis related to μ'_r.
For $r = 1$,

$$\frac{\sqrt{n}\left(m'_1 - \mu'_1\right)}{\sqrt{\mu'_2 - \mu'^2_1}} = \frac{\sqrt{n}(\bar{x} - \mu)}{\sigma} \xrightarrow{L} N(0, 1).$$

Since the sample s.d $s = \sqrt{\frac{1}{n}\sum_{i=1}^{n}(x_i - \bar{x})^2}$ is consistent estimator of σ, $s \xrightarrow{P} \sigma$, i.e. $\frac{\sigma}{s} \xrightarrow{P} 1$

$$\therefore \frac{\sqrt{n}(\bar{x} - \mu)}{s} = \frac{\sqrt{n}(\bar{x} - \mu)}{\sigma} \cdot \frac{\sigma}{s} \xrightarrow{L} N(0, 1)$$

(ii) To find $E(m_r^0)$, $V(m_r^0)$, $\mathrm{Cov}(m_r^0, m_s^0)$:

$$m_r^0 = \frac{1}{n}\sum_{i=1}^{n}(x_i - \mu)^r; \therefore E(m_r^0) = \mu_r$$

$$E(m_r^0 m_s^0) = \frac{1}{n^2}E\left(\sum_{i=1}^{n}(x_i - \mu)^r\right)\left(\sum_{i=1}^{n}(x_i - \mu)^s\right)$$

$$= \frac{1}{n^2}\left[\sum_{1}^{n}E(x_i - \mu)^{r+s} + \sum\sum_{i \neq j = 1}^{n}E(x_i - \mu)^r E(x_j - \mu)^s\right]$$

$$= \frac{1}{n^2}\left[n\mu_{r+s} + n(n-1)\mu_r\mu_s\right]$$

$$= \frac{1}{n}\left[\mu_{r+s} + (n-1)\mu_r\mu_s\right]$$

$$\therefore \mathrm{Cov}\left(m_r^0, m_s^0\right) = \frac{1}{n}\left[\mu_{r+s} + (n-1)\mu_r\mu_s\right] - \mu_r\mu_s$$

$$= \frac{1}{n}\left[\mu_{r+s} - \mu_r\mu_s\right]$$

$$\therefore V(m_r^0) = \frac{1}{n}\left[\mu_{2r} - \mu_r^2\right]$$

We note that, $m_r^0 = \frac{1}{n}\sum_{i=1}^{n}(x_i - \mu)^r = \frac{1}{n}\sum_i^n Z_i$

where $Z_i = (x_i - \mu)^r, E(Z_i) = \mu_r$ and $V(Z_i) = \mu_{2r} - \mu_r^2$

For $x_1, x_2, \ldots x_n$ i.i.d $\Rightarrow Z_1, Z_2, \ldots Z_n$ are also i.i.d

$$\therefore \frac{\sqrt{n}(\bar{Z} - \mu_r)}{\sqrt{\mu_{2r} - \mu_r^2}} \xrightarrow{L} N(0, 1).$$

That is, $\frac{\sqrt{n}(m_r^0 - \mu_r)}{\sqrt{\mu_{2r} - \mu_r^2}} \overset{a}{\sim} N(0, 1)$

(iii) To find $E(m_r),\ V(m_r),\ \mathrm{Cov}(m_r, m_s)$ **:**

$$m_r = \frac{1}{n}\sum_{i=1}^{n}(x_i - \bar{x})^r = \frac{1}{n}\sum[(x_i-\mu)-(\bar{x}-\mu)]^r$$
$$= \frac{1}{n}\sum\left[(x_i-\mu) - \frac{1}{n}\sum(\bar{x}-\mu)\right]^r$$
$$= \frac{1}{n}\sum[(X_i-\mu) - m_1^0]^r$$
$$= \frac{1}{n}\left[(x_i-\mu)^r - \binom{r}{1}(x_i-\mu)^{r-1}\cdot m_1^0 + \ldots + \sum_1^n(-1)^{r-1}\binom{r}{r-1}(x_i-\mu)m_1^{0^{r-1}} + (-1)^r m_1^{0^r}\right]$$
$$= m_r^0 - \binom{r}{1}m_{r-1}^0 m_1^0 + \cdots + (-1)^r m_1^{0^r}$$
$$= g(m_1^0, m_2^0 \ldots m_r^0) = g\left(\underset{\sim}{m}^0\right)$$

We have observed that $\sqrt{n}\left(m_j^0 - \mu_j\right) \overset{a}{\sim} N\left(0, \mu_{2j} - \mu_j^2\right)\ \forall j = 1(1)r$

$$\therefore \sqrt{n}\left(\underset{\sim}{m}^0 - \underset{\sim}{\mu}\right) = \sqrt{n}\begin{pmatrix} m_1^0 - \mu_1 \\ m_2^0 - \mu_2 \\ \cdot \\ \cdot \\ m_r^0 - \mu_r \end{pmatrix} \overset{a}{\sim} N_r\left(\underset{\sim}{0}, \sum{}^{rxr}\right)$$

where $\sum^{rxr} = \left(\sigma_{ij}\left(\underset{\sim}{\mu}\right)\right)$ and $\sigma_{ij}\left(\underset{\sim}{\mu}\right) = \mathrm{Cov}\left(\sqrt{n}(m_i^0 - \mu_i), \sqrt{n}\left(m_j^0 - \mu_j\right)\right)$

$$= n\mathrm{Cov}\left(m_i^0, m_j^0\right) = (\mu_{i+j} - \mu_i\mu_j)$$

So by Theorem 2,

$$\sqrt{n}\left(g\left(\underset{\sim}{m}^0\right) - g\left(\underset{\sim}{\mu}\right)\right) \overset{a}{\sim} N\left(0, V\left(\underset{\sim}{\mu}\right)\right)$$

where $V\left(\underset{\sim}{\mu}\right) = \sum_{i=1}^r\sum_{j=1}^r\left(\frac{\delta g}{\delta\mu_i}\right)\left(\frac{\delta g}{\delta\mu_j}\right)\sigma_{ij}\left(\underset{\sim}{\mu}\right),\ \frac{\delta g}{\delta\mu_i} = \left(\frac{\delta g}{\delta m_i^0}\right)_{\underset{\sim}{m}^0 = \underset{\sim}{\mu}}$

$$g(\mu_1, \mu_2, \ldots \mu_r) = \mu_r - \binom{r}{1}\mu_{r-1}\mu_1 + \cdots + (-1)^r \mu_1^r = \mu_r$$

$$\frac{\delta g}{\delta \mu_1} = \left(\frac{\delta g}{\delta m_i^0}\right)_{\underset{\sim}{m}^0 = \underset{\sim}{\mu}} = -r\mu_{r-1}$$

$$\frac{\delta g}{\delta \mu_r} = \left(\frac{\delta g}{\delta m_r^0}\right)_{\underset{\sim}{m}^0 = \underset{\sim}{\mu}} = 1 \text{ and } \frac{\delta g}{\delta \mu_i} = 0 \; \forall \, i = 2(1)r - 1$$

$$\therefore V\left(\underset{\sim}{\mu}\right) = \left(\frac{\delta g}{\delta \mu_1}\right)^2 \sigma_{11}\left(\underset{\sim}{\mu}\right) + \left(\frac{\delta g}{\delta \mu_r}\right)^2 \sigma_{rr}\left(\underset{\sim}{\mu}\right) + 2\left(\frac{\delta g}{\delta \mu_1}\right)\left(\frac{\delta g}{\delta \mu_r}\right)\sigma_{1r}\left(\underset{\sim}{\mu}\right)$$

$$= r^2\mu_{r-1}^2\left(\mu_2 - \mu_1^2\right) + \left(\mu_{2r} - \mu_r^2\right) + 2(-r\mu_{r-1})\left(\mu_{r+1} - \mu_1\mu_r\right)$$

$$= r^2\mu_{r-1}^2\mu_2 + \left(\mu_{2r} - \mu_r^2\right) - 2r\mu_{r-1}\mu_{r+1}$$

$$\therefore \sqrt{n}(m_r - \mu_r) \overset{a}{\sim} N\left(0, V\left(\underset{\sim}{\mu}\right)\right)$$

i.e.,

$$m_r \overset{a}{\sim} N\left(\mu_r, \frac{V\left(\underset{\sim}{\mu}\right)}{n}\right)$$

In particular,

for $r = 2,\; m_2 = s^2 \overset{a}{\sim} N\left(\mu_2 = \sigma^2, \frac{\mu_4 - \mu_2^2}{n}\right)$, i.e. $s^2 \overset{a}{\sim} N\left(\sigma^2, \frac{\mu_4 - \sigma^4}{n}\right)$

for $r = 3,\; m_3 \overset{a}{\sim} N\left(\mu_3, \frac{9\mu_2^3 + \mu_6 - \mu_3^2 - 6\mu_2\mu_4}{n}\right)$

for $r = 4,\; m_4 \overset{a}{\sim} N\left(\mu_4, \frac{16\mu_3^2\mu_2 + \mu_8 - \mu_4^2 - 8\mu_3\mu_5}{n}\right)$

Again, if sampling is from normal distribution $N(\mu, \sigma^2)$ then $\mu_3 = \mu_5 = \cdots = 0$ and $\mu_{2r} = (2r-1)(2r-3)\ldots 3.1\;\sigma^{2r}$

i.e.,

$\mu_4 = 3\sigma^4,\; \mu_6 = 15\sigma^6,\; \mu_8 = 105\sigma^8.$

$$\therefore s^2 \overset{a}{\sim} N\left(\sigma^2, \frac{2\sigma^4}{n}\right)$$

$$m_3 \overset{a}{\sim} N\left(0, \frac{6\sigma^6}{n}\right)$$

$$m_4 \overset{a}{\sim} N\left(3\sigma^4, \frac{96\sigma^8}{n}\right).$$

Thus, $\frac{\sqrt{n}\left(s^2-\sigma^2\right)}{\sigma^2} \overset{a}{\sim} N(0,2)$ and as $s^2 \xrightarrow{P} \sigma^2$, $\frac{\sqrt{n}\left(s^2-\sigma^2\right)}{s^2} \overset{a}{\sim} N(0,2)$ and this can be used for testing hypothesis regarding σ^2.

Note For testing $H_0 : \sigma_1 = \sigma_2$

$s_1 \overset{a}{\sim} N\left(\sigma_1, \frac{\sigma_1^2}{2n_1}\right)$ and $s_2 \overset{a}{\sim} N\left(\sigma_2, \frac{\sigma_2^2}{2n_2}\right)$

$$\therefore s_1 - s_2 \overset{a}{\sim} N\left(\sigma_1 - \sigma_2, \frac{\sigma_1^2}{2n_1} + \frac{\sigma_2^2}{2n_2}\right)$$

Under H_0, $\frac{s_1 - s_2}{\sigma\sqrt{\frac{1}{2n_1}+\frac{1}{2n_2}}} \overset{a}{\sim} N(0,1)$ where unknown σ is estimated as

$$\hat{\sigma} = \frac{n_1 s_1 + n_2 s_2}{n_1 + n_2}.$$

(iv) $Cov(m_r, \bar{x}) = Cov\left(m_r, m_1^0 + \mu\right) \left[\bar{x} = \frac{1}{n}\sum_{i=1}^{n}(x_i - \mu) + \mu = m_1^0 + \mu\right]$

$$\begin{aligned} &= \mathrm{Cov}\left(m_r^0, m_1^0\right) - r\mu_{r-1} V\left(m_1^0\right) \\ &= \frac{1}{n}\mu_{r+1} - r\mu_{r-1}\frac{\mu_2}{n} = \frac{1}{n}\left[\mu_{r+1} - r\mu_{r-1}\mu_2\right] \end{aligned}$$

$\mathrm{Cov}(m_2, \bar{x}) \simeq \frac{1}{n}\mu_3 = 0$ if the sampling is from $N(\mu, \sigma^2)$.

Note The exact expression for $\mathrm{Cov}(m_2, \bar{x}) = \frac{n-1}{n^2}\mu_3$.

(v) Large sample distribution of C.V.

$$v = \frac{\sqrt{m_2}}{m_1'} = g\left(m_2, m_1'\right), \quad \text{say}$$

$= g(T_{1n}, T_{2n}) = g\left(\underset{\sim n}{T}\right)$ where $\underset{\sim n}{T} = \begin{pmatrix} T_{1n} \\ T_{2n} \end{pmatrix} = \begin{pmatrix} m_2 \\ m_1' \end{pmatrix}$

Writing

$$\underset{\sim}{\theta} = \begin{pmatrix} \theta_1 \\ \theta_2 \end{pmatrix} = \begin{pmatrix} \mu_2 \\ \mu_1' \end{pmatrix}$$

we observed that $\sqrt{n}\left(\underset{\sim n}{T} - \underset{\sim}{\theta}\right) = \sqrt{n}\begin{pmatrix} m_2 - \mu_2 \\ m_1' - \mu_1' \end{pmatrix} \overset{a}{\sim} N_2(0, \sum)$

where $\sum = \left(\sigma_{ij}\left(\underset{\sim}{\theta}\right)\right) = \begin{pmatrix} \mu_4 - \mu_2^2 & \mu_3 \\ \mu_3 & \mu_2 \end{pmatrix}$

If $g\left(\underset{\sim}{\theta}\right) = g(\mu_2, \mu_1') = \frac{\sqrt{\mu_2}}{\mu_1'} = V$, Population C.V., then by Theorem 2,

$\sqrt{n}\left(g\left(\underset{\sim n}{T}\right) - g\left(\underset{\sim}{\theta}\right)\right) \overset{a}{\sim} N\left(0, V\left(\underset{\sim}{\theta}\right)\right)$, i.e. $\sqrt{n}(v - V) \overset{a}{\sim} N\left(0, V\left(\underset{\sim}{\theta}\right)\right)$

where $V\left(\underset{\sim}{\theta}\right) = \left(\frac{\delta g}{\delta\theta_1}\right)^2 \sigma_{11}\left(\underset{\sim}{\theta}\right) + \left(\frac{\delta g}{\delta\theta_2}\right)^2 \sigma_{22}\left(\underset{\sim}{\theta}\right) + 2\left(\frac{\delta g}{\delta\theta_1}\right)\left(\frac{\delta g}{\delta\theta_2}\right)\sigma_{12}\left(\underset{\sim}{\theta}\right)$

Now, $\frac{\delta g}{\delta \theta_1} = \frac{1}{2\sqrt{\mu_2}\mu_1'}$, $\sigma_{11}\left(\underset{\sim}{\theta}\right) = \mu_4 - \mu_2^2$

$$\frac{\delta g}{\delta \theta_2} = -\frac{\sqrt{\mu_2}}{\mu_1'^2},\ \sigma_{22}\left(\underset{\sim}{\theta}\right) = \mu_2,\ \sigma_{12}\left(\underset{\sim}{\theta}\right) = \mu_3$$

$$V\left(\underset{\sim}{\theta}\right) = \frac{1}{4\mu_2\mu_1'^2}(\mu_4 - \mu_2^2) + \frac{\mu_2}{\mu_1'^4}\mu_2 - \frac{1}{\sqrt{\mu_2}\mu_1'}\frac{\sqrt{\mu_2}}{\mu_1'^2}\mu_3$$

$$= \frac{\mu_4 - \mu_2^2}{4\mu_2\mu_1'^2} + \frac{\mu_2^2}{\mu_1'^4} - \frac{\mu_3}{\mu_1'^3}$$

$$= \left(\frac{\mu_4 - \mu_2^2}{4\mu_2^2} + V^2 - \frac{\mu_3}{\mu_2\mu_1'}\right)V^2$$

If the sampling is from $N(\mu, \sigma^2)$, $\mu_2 = \sigma^2$, $\mu_3 = 0$, $\mu_4 = 3\sigma^4$, then

$$V\left(\underset{\sim}{\theta}\right) = \left(\frac{3\sigma^4 - \sigma^4}{4\sigma^4} + V^2\right)V^2 = \left(\frac{1}{2} + V^2\right)V^2 = \frac{V^2(1 + 2V^2)}{2}$$

Thus $\sqrt{n}(v - V) \overset{a}{\sim} N\left(0, \frac{V^2(1+2V^2)}{2}\right)$.

(vi) Large sample distribution of skewness

Sample skewness = $g_1 = \frac{m_3}{m_2^{3/2}} = g(m_3, m_2) = g\left(\underset{\sim n}{T}\right) = g\begin{pmatrix} T_{1n} \\ T_{2n} \end{pmatrix}$

where $T_{1n} = m_3$ and $T_{2n} = m_2$.

We define, $\underset{\sim}{\theta} = \begin{pmatrix} \theta_1 \\ \theta_2 \end{pmatrix} = \begin{pmatrix} \mu_3 \\ \mu_2 \end{pmatrix} \therefore g\left(\underset{\sim}{\theta}\right) = \frac{\mu_3}{\mu_2^{3/2}} = \gamma_1$

We know, $\sqrt{n}\left(\underset{\sim n}{T} - \underset{\sim}{\theta}\right) = \sqrt{n}\begin{pmatrix} m_3 - \mu_3 \\ m_2 - \mu_2 \end{pmatrix} \overset{a}{\sim} N_2(0, \sum)$

where $\sum^{2\times 2} = \left(\sigma_{ij}\left(\underset{\sim}{\theta}\right)\right) = \begin{pmatrix} \mu_6 - \mu_3^2 + 9\mu_2^3 - 6\mu_4\mu_2 & \mu_5 - 4\mu_2\mu_3 \\ \mu_5 - 4\mu_2\mu_3 & \mu_4 - \mu_2^2 \end{pmatrix}$

$\therefore$ By Theorem 2,

$$\sqrt{n}\left(g\left(\underset{\sim n}{T}\right) - g\left(\underset{\sim}{\theta}\right)\right) \overset{a}{\sim} N\left(0, V\left(\underset{\sim}{\theta}\right)\right)$$

i.e.,

$$\sqrt{n}(g_1 - \gamma_1) \overset{a}{\sim} N\left(0, V\left(\underset{\sim}{\theta}\right)\right)$$

where $V\left(\underset{\sim}{\theta}\right) = \left(\frac{\delta g}{\delta\theta_1}\right)^2 \sigma_{11}\left(\underset{\sim}{\theta}\right) + \left(\frac{\delta g}{\delta\theta_2}\right)^2 \sigma_{22}\left(\underset{\sim}{\theta}\right) + 2\left(\frac{\delta g}{\delta\theta_1}\right)\left(\frac{\delta g}{\delta\theta_2}\right)\sigma_{12}\left(\underset{\sim}{\theta}\right)$

Now, $\frac{\delta g}{\delta\theta_1} = \frac{1}{\mu_2^{3/2}}$; $\frac{\delta g}{\delta\theta_2} = -\frac{3}{2}\frac{\mu_3}{\mu_2^{5/2}}$

$$\therefore V\left(\underset{\sim}{\theta}\right) = \frac{1}{\mu_2^3}(\mu_6 - \mu_3^2 + 9\mu_2^3 - 6\mu_4\mu_2) + \frac{9}{4}\frac{\mu_3^2}{\mu_2^5}(\mu_4 - \mu_2^2) - 3\frac{1}{\mu_2^{3/2}}\frac{\mu_3}{\mu_2^{5/2}}(\mu_5 - 4\mu_2\mu_3)$$

$$= \frac{\mu_6 - \mu_3^2 + 9\mu_2^3 - 6\mu_4\mu_2}{\mu_2^3} + \frac{9}{4}\frac{\mu_3^2(\mu_4 - \mu_2^2)}{\mu_2^5} - \frac{3\mu_3(\mu_5 - 4\mu_2\mu_3)}{\mu_2^4}$$

If the sampling is from $N(\mu, \sigma^2)$ then $\mu_2 = \sigma^2, \mu_3 = \mu_5 = 0, \mu_4 = 3\sigma^4$, $\mu_6 = 15\sigma^6$.

$$\therefore V\left(\underset{\sim}{\theta}\right) = \frac{(15 + 9 - 18)\sigma^6}{\sigma^6} = 6$$

$$\therefore \sqrt{n}(g_1 - \gamma_1) \overset{a}{\sim} N(0, 6)$$

(vii) Large sample distribution of Kurtosis

Sample Kurtosis $= g_2 = \frac{m_4}{m_2^2} - 3 = g(m_4, m_2) = g\left(\underset{\sim n}{T}\right) = g\begin{pmatrix} T_{1n} \\ T_{2n} \end{pmatrix}$

where $T_{1n} = m_4$ and $T_{2n} = m_2$.

Let $\underset{\sim}{\theta} = \begin{pmatrix} \theta_1 \\ \theta_2 \end{pmatrix} = \begin{pmatrix} \mu_4 \\ \mu_2 \end{pmatrix} \therefore g\left(\underset{\sim}{\theta}\right) = \frac{\mu_4}{\mu_2^2} - 3 = \gamma_2$

We know, $\sqrt{n}\left(\underset{\sim n}{T} - \underset{\sim}{\theta}\right) = \sqrt{n}\begin{pmatrix} m_4 - \mu_4 \\ m_2 - \mu_2 \end{pmatrix} \overset{a}{\sim} N_2\left(\underset{\sim}{0}, \Sigma\right)$

where $\Sigma^{2\times 2} = \left(\sigma_{ij}\left(\underset{\sim}{\theta}\right)\right) = \begin{pmatrix} \mu_8 - \mu_4^2 + 16\mu_3^2\mu_2 - 8\mu_3\mu_5 & \mu_6 - \mu_4\mu_2 - 4\mu_3^2 \\ \mu_6 - \mu_4\mu_2 - 4\mu_3^2 & \mu_4 - \mu_2^2 \end{pmatrix}$

$\therefore$ By Theorem 2,

$$\sqrt{n}\left(g\left(\underset{\sim n}{T}\right) - g\left(\underset{\sim}{\theta}\right)\right) \overset{a}{\sim} N\left(0, V\left(\underset{\sim}{\theta}\right)\right)$$

i.e., $\sqrt{n}(g_2 - \gamma_2) \overset{a}{\sim} N\left(0, V\left(\underset{\sim}{\theta}\right)\right)$

where $V\left(\underset{\sim}{\theta}\right) = \left(\frac{\delta g}{\delta\theta_1}\right)^2 \sigma_{11}\left(\underset{\sim}{\theta}\right) + \left(\frac{\delta g}{\delta\theta_2}\right)^2 \sigma_{22}\left(\underset{\sim}{\theta}\right) + 2\left(\frac{\delta g}{\delta\theta_1}\right)\left(\frac{\delta g}{\delta\theta_2}\right)\sigma_{12}\left(\underset{\sim}{\theta}\right)$

Now $\frac{\delta g}{\delta\theta_1} = \frac{1}{\mu_2^2}$ and $\frac{\delta g}{\delta\theta_2} = -\frac{2\mu_4}{\mu_2^3}$

$$V\left(\underset{\sim}{\theta}\right) = \frac{\mu_8 - \mu_4^2 + 16\mu_3^2\mu_2 - 8\mu_3\mu_5}{\mu_2^4} + \frac{4\mu_4^2(\mu_4 - \mu_2^2)}{\mu_2^6} - \frac{4\mu_4(\mu_6 - \mu_4\mu_2 - 4\mu_3^2)}{\mu_2^5}$$

Now, if the sampling is from $N(\mu, \sigma^2)$

$$\mu_2 = \sigma^2,\ \mu_3 = \mu_5 = \mu_7 = 0,\ \mu_4 = 3\sigma^4,\ \mu_6 = 15\sigma^6 \text{ and } \mu_8 = 105\sigma^8$$

$$\therefore V\left(\underset{\sim}{\theta}\right) = 96 + 4.9(3-1) - 4.3(15-3) = 24$$

$$\therefore \sqrt{n}(g_2 - \gamma_2) \overset{a}{\sim} N(0, 24)$$

(viii) Large sample distribution of bivariate moments

Let $F(x, y)$ be c.d.f from which a random sample$(x_1, y_1), (x_2, y_2), \ldots (x_n, y_n)$ is drawn.

We define, $m'_{rs} = \frac{1}{n}\sum x_i^r y_i^s$; $\mu'_{rs} = E(X^r Y^s)$

$$m'_{10} = \frac{1}{n}\sum x_i = \bar{x};\ \mu'_{10} = E(X) = \mu_x$$

$$m'_{01} = \frac{1}{n}\sum y_i = \bar{y};\ \mu'_{01} = E(Y) = \mu_y$$

$$m^0_{rs} = \frac{1}{n}\sum_1^n (x_i - \mu'_{10})^r (y_i - \mu'_{01})^s = \frac{1}{n}\sum_1^n (x_i - \mu_x)^r (y_i - \mu_y)^s$$

$$m_{rs} = \frac{1}{n}\sum_1^n (x_i - \bar{x})^r (y_i - \bar{y})^s = \frac{1}{n}\sum_1^n (x_i - m'_{10})^r (y_i - m'_{01})^s$$

$$\mu_{rs} = E(X - \mu_x)^r (Y - \mu_y)^s = E(X - \mu'_{10})^r (Y - \mu'_{01})^s$$

$$E(m'_{rs}) = \frac{1}{n}\sum_1^n E(x_i^r y_i^s) = \frac{1}{n}\sum \mu'_{rs} = \mu'_{rs}$$

$$E(m'_{rs} m'_{uv}) = \frac{1}{n^2} E\left\{\left(\sum x_i^r y_i^s\right)\left(\sum x_i^u y_i^v\right)\right\}$$

$$= \frac{1}{n^2} E\left\{\sum_1^n x_i^{r+u} y_i^{s+v} + \sum\sum_{i \neq j = 1}^n x_i^r y_i^s x_j^u y_j^v\right\}$$

$$= \frac{1}{n^2}\left[n\mu'_{r+u,s+v} + n(n-1)\mu'_{rs}\mu'_{uv}\right]$$

$$= \frac{\mu'_{r+u,s+v} + (n-1)\mu'_{rs}\mu'_{uv}}{n}$$

$$\therefore \text{Cov}\left(m'_{rs}, m'_{uv}\right) = \frac{1}{n}\left(\mu'_{r+u,s+v} + (n-1)\mu'_{rs}\mu'_{uv}\right) - \mu'_{rs}\mu'_{uv}$$

$$= \frac{1}{n}\left[\mu'_{r+u,s+v} - \mu'_{rs}\mu'_{uv}\right]$$

$$\therefore V\left(m'_{rs}\right) = \frac{1}{n}\left(\mu'_{2r,2s} - \mu'^{2}_{rs}\right)$$

$$E\left(m^0_{rs}\right) = \frac{1}{n}\sum E\left(x_i - \mu'_{10}\right)^r\left(y_i - \mu'_{01}\right)^s = \mu_{rs}$$

$$E\left(m^0_{rs}m^0_{uv}\right) = \frac{1}{n^2}E\left(\sum\left(x_i - \mu'_{10}\right)^r\left(y_i - \mu'_{01}\right)^s\right)\left(\sum\left(x_i - \mu'_{10}\right)^u\left(y_i - \mu'_{01}\right)^v\right)$$

$$= \frac{1}{n^2}\left[n\mu_{r+u,s+v} + n(n-1)\mu_{rs}\mu_{uv}\right]$$

$$= \frac{1}{n}\left[\mu_{r+u,s+v} + (n-1)\mu_{rs}\mu_{uv}\right]$$

$$\therefore \text{Cov}\left(m^0_{rs}, m^0_{uv}\right) = \frac{1}{n}\left[\mu_{r+u,s+v} - \mu_{rs}\mu_{uv}\right]$$

$$\therefore V\left(m^0_{rs}\right) = \frac{1}{n}\left(\mu_{2r,2s} - \mu^2_{rs}\right)$$

$$m_{rs} = \frac{1}{n}\sum_1^n\left(x_i - \bar{x}\right)^r\left(y_i - \bar{y}\right)^s$$

$$= \frac{1}{n}\sum_1^n\left\{\left(x_i - \mu'_{10}\right) - \left(\bar{x} - \mu'_{10}\right)\right\}^r\left\{\left(y_i - \mu'_{01}\right) - \left(\bar{y} - \mu'_{01}\right)\right\}^s$$

Since $\bar{x} - \mu'_{10} = \frac{1}{n}\sum_1^n\left(x_i - \mu'_{10}\right) = m^0_{10}$ and $\bar{y} - \mu'_{01} = \frac{1}{n}\sum_1^n\left(y_i - \mu'_{01}\right) = m^0_{01}$

$$\therefore m_{rs} = \frac{1}{n}\sum_1^n\left\{\left(x_i - \mu'_{10}\right) - m^0_{10}\right\}^r\left\{\left(y_i - \mu'_{01}\right) - m^0_{01}\right\}^s$$

$$= \frac{1}{n}\sum_1^n\left\{\left(x_i - \mu'_{10}\right)^r - \binom{r}{1}\left(x_i - \mu'_{10}\right)^{r-1}m^0_{10} + \cdots + (-1)^r m^{0^r}_{10}\right\}$$

$$\left\{\left(y_i - \mu'_{01}\right)^s - \binom{s}{1}\left(y_i - \mu'_{01}\right)^{s-1}m^0_{01} + \ldots + (-1)^s m^{0^s}_{01}\right\}$$

$$= \frac{1}{n}\sum_1^n\left\{\left(x_i - \mu'_{10}\right)^r\left(y_i - \mu'_{01}\right)^s - \binom{r}{1}\left(x_i - \mu'_{10}\right)^{r-1}\left(y_i - \mu'_{01}\right)^s m^0_{10} - \binom{s}{1}\left(x_i - \mu'_{10}\right)^r\left(y_i - \mu'_{01}\right)^{s-1}m^0_{01}\right.$$

$$\left. + \binom{r}{1}\binom{s}{1}\left(x_i - \mu'_{10}\right)^{r-1}\left(y_i - \mu'_{01}\right)^{s-1}m^0_{10}m^0_{01}\cdots + (-1)^{r+s}\left(m^0_{10}\right)^r\left(m^0_{01}\right)^s\right\}$$

$$= m^0_{rs} - \binom{r}{1}m^0_{r-1,s}m^0_{10} - \binom{s}{1}m^0_{r,s-1}m^0_{01} + \binom{r}{1}\binom{s}{1}m^0_{r-1,s-1}m^0_{10}m^0_{01} + \cdots + (-1)^{r+s}\left(m^0_{10}\right)^r\left(m^0_{01}\right)^s$$

$$= g\left(m^0_{ij}; i = 0(1)r, j = 0(1)s, (i,j) \neq (0,0)\right)$$

$$\therefore m_{rs} = g\left(\underset{\sim}{m}^0\right),$$

, say where $\underset{\sim}{m}^0 = \begin{pmatrix} m_{10}^0 \\ m_{01}^0 \\ \cdot \\ \cdot \\ m_{rs}^0 \end{pmatrix}^{\{(r+1)(s+1)-1\}X1}$

Using the expansion in Taylor's series

$$m_{rs} = g\left(m_{ij}^0; i = 0(1)r, j = 0(1)s, (i,j) \neq (0,0)\right)$$

$$= g(\mu_{ij}, i = 0(1)r, j = 0(1)s, (i,j) \neq (0,0)) + \sum_{\substack{i=0 \\ (i,j)\neq(0,0)}}^{r}\sum_{j=0}^{s}\left(m_{ij}^0 - \mu_{ij}\right)\left(\frac{\delta g}{\delta m_{ij}^0}\right)_{\underset{\sim}{m}^0=\underset{\sim}{\mu}} + \cdots$$

where $\underset{\sim}{\mu} = (\mu_{10}, \mu_{01}, \cdots, \mu_{rs})^1$

$$= \mu_{rs} + \sum_{\substack{i \\ (i,j)\neq(0,0)}}\sum_{j}\left(m_{ij}^0 - \mu_{ij}\right)\left(\frac{\partial g}{\partial m_{ij}^0}\right)_{\underset{\sim}{m}^0=\underset{\sim}{\mu}} \quad (\text{as } \mu_{01} = \mu_{10} = 0)$$

Now $\left(\frac{\partial g}{\partial m_{10}^0}\right)_{\underset{\sim}{m}^0=\underset{\sim}{\mu}} = -r\mu_{r-1,s}$

$$\left(\frac{\partial g}{\partial m_{01}^0}\right)_{\underset{\sim}{m}^0=\underset{\sim}{\mu}} = -s\mu_{r,s-1}$$

$$\left(\frac{\partial g}{\partial m_{rs}^0}\right)_{\underset{\sim}{m}^0=\underset{\sim}{\mu}} = 1 \text{ and } \left(\frac{\partial g}{\partial m_{ij}^0}\right)_{\underset{\sim}{m}^0=\underset{\sim}{\mu}} = 0 \forall i = 0(1)r, j = 0(1)s$$

$(i,j) = (0,0), (r,s), (0,1), (1,0)$.

$\therefore m_{rs} = \mu_{rs} + \left(m_{10}^0 - \mu_{10}\right)\left(-r\mu_{r-1,s}\right) + \left(m_{01}^0 - \mu_{01}\right)\left(-s\mu_{r,s-1}\right) + \left(m_{rs}^0 - \mu_{rs}\right)1$

$\therefore m_{rs} = m_{rs}^0 - r\mu_{r-1,s}m_{10}^0 - s\mu_{r,s-1}m_{01}^0$

$\therefore E(m_{rs}) = E\left(m_{rs}^0\right) - r\mu_{r-1,s}E\left(m_{10}^0\right) - s\mu_{r,s-1}E\left(m_{01}^0\right)$

$= \mu_{rs}$

$$
\begin{aligned}
&\mathrm{Cov}(m_{rs}, m_{uv}) = \mathrm{Cov}\{(m_{rs}^0 - r\mu_{r-1,s}m_{10}^0 - s\mu_{r,s-1}m_{01}^0), (m_{uv}^0 - u\mu_{u-1,v}m_{10}^0 - v\mu_{u,v-1}m_{01}^0)\} \\
&= \mathrm{Cov}(m_{rs}^0, m_{uv}^0) - u\mu_{u-1,v}\mathrm{Cov}(m_{rs}^0, m_{10}^0) - v\mu_{u,v-1}\mathrm{Cov}(m_{rs}^0, m_{01}^0) - r\mu_{r-1,s}\mathrm{Cov}(m_{10}^0, m_{uv}^0) \\
&+ ru\mu_{r-1,s}\mu_{u-1,v}V(m_{10}^0) + rv\mu_{r-1,s}\mu_{u,v-1}\mathrm{Cov}(m_{10}^0, m_{01}^0) - s\mu_{r,s-1}\mathrm{Cov}(m_{01}^0, m_{uv}^0) \\
&+ us\mu_{r,s-1}\mu_{u-1,v}\mathrm{Cov}(m_{01}^0, m_{10}^0) + sv\mu_{r,s-1}\mu_{u,v-1}V(m_{01}^0) \\
&= \frac{1}{n}\left[\begin{array}{l} \mu_{r+u,s+v} - \mu_{rs}\mu_{uv} - u\mu_{u-1,v}\mu_{r+1,s} - v\mu_{u,v-1}\mu_{r,s+1} - r\mu_{r-1,s}\mu_{u+1,v} + ru\mu_{r-1,s}\mu_{u-1,v}\mu_{20} + rv\mu_{r-1,s}\mu_{u,v-1}\mu_{11} \\ - s\mu_{r,s-1}\mu_{u,v+1} + us\mu_{r,s-1}\mu_{u-1,v}\mu_{11} + sv\mu_{r,s-1}\mu_{u,v-1}\mu_{02} \end{array}\right] \\
&\therefore V(m_{rs}) = \frac{1}{n}\left[\mu_{2r,2s} - \mu_{rs}^2 + r^2\mu_{r-1,s}^2\mu_{20} + s^2\mu_{r,s-1}^2\mu_{02} - 2r\mu_{r-1,s}\mu_{r+1,s} - 2s\mu_{r,s-1}\mu_{r,s+1} + 2rs\mu_{r-1,s}\mu_{r,s-1}\mu_{11}\right] \\
&\therefore V(m_{20}) = \frac{1}{n}\left[\mu_{40} - \mu_{20}^2\right], \mathrm{Cov}(m_{20}, m_{02}) = \frac{1}{n}[\mu_{22} - \mu_{20}\mu_{02}] \\
&V(m_{02}) = \frac{1}{n}\left[\mu_{04} - \mu_{02}^2\right], \mathrm{Cov}(m_{20}, m_{11}) = \frac{1}{n}[\mu_{31} - \mu_{20}\mu_{11}] \\
&V(m_{11}) = \frac{1}{n}\left[\mu_{22} - \mu_{11}^2\right], \mathrm{Cov}(m_{02}, m_{11}) = \frac{1}{n}[\mu_{13} - \mu_{02}\mu_{11}]
\end{aligned}
$$

Sample correlation $r = \frac{m_{11}}{\sqrt{m_{20}m_{02}}} = g\left(\underset{\sim}{m}\right) = g(Tn)$, say

where $\underset{\sim}{m} = (m_{20}, m_{02}, m_{11})'$ and $\underset{\sim}{T_n} = (T_{1n}, T_{2n}, T_{3n})' = (m_{20}, m_{02}, m_{11})'$

$$\therefore \sqrt{n}\left(\underset{\sim}{T_n} - \underset{\sim}{\theta}\right) \overset{a}{\sim} N_3\left(\underset{\sim}{0}, \sum\nolimits^{3\times 3}\right)$$

i.e., $\therefore \sqrt{n}\left(\underset{\sim}{m} - \underset{\sim}{\mu}\right) \overset{a}{\sim} N_3\left(\underset{\sim}{0}, \sum\right)$ where $\underset{\sim}{\theta} = \begin{pmatrix}\theta_1\\ \theta_2\\ \theta_3\end{pmatrix} = \begin{pmatrix}\mu_{20}\\ \mu_{02}\\ \mu_{11}\end{pmatrix} = \underset{\sim}{\mu}$

and $\sum = ((\sigma_{ij}(\theta)) = \begin{pmatrix}\mu_{40} - \mu_{20}^2 & \mu_{22} - \mu_{20}\mu_{02} & \mu_{31} - \mu_{20}\mu_{11}\\ & \mu_{04} - \mu_{02}^2 & \mu_{13} - \mu_{02}\mu_{11}\\ & & \mu_{22} - \mu_{11}^2\end{pmatrix}$

$$\rho = \frac{\mu_{11}}{\sqrt{\mu_{20}\mu_{02}}} = g\left(\underset{\sim}{\mu}\right) = g\left(\underset{\sim}{\theta}\right)$$

$$\sqrt{n}\left(g\left(\underset{\sim n}{T}\right) - g\left(\underset{\sim}{\theta}\right)\right) \overset{a}{\sim} N\left(0, V\left(\underset{\sim}{\theta}\right)\right)$$

i.e., $\sqrt{n}(r - \rho) \overset{a}{\sim} N\left(0, V\left(\underset{\sim}{\theta}\right)\right)$

where $V\left(\underset{\sim}{\theta}\right) = \sum_{i=1}^{3}\sum_{j=1}^{3}\left(\frac{\partial g}{\partial \theta_i}\right)\left(\frac{\partial g}{\partial \theta_j}\right)\sigma_{ij}\left(\underset{\sim}{\theta}\right)$

and $\left(\frac{\partial g}{\partial \theta_i}\right) = \left(\frac{\partial g}{\partial T_{in}}\right)_{\underset{\sim n}{T} = \underset{\sim}{\theta}}$

$$\text{i.e.}\, V\left(\underset{\sim}{\theta}\right) = \left(\frac{\partial g}{\partial \theta_1}\right)^2 \sigma_{11}\left(\underset{\sim}{\theta}\right) + \left(\frac{\partial g}{\partial \theta_2}\right)^2 \sigma_{22}\left(\underset{\sim}{\theta}\right) + \left(\frac{\partial g}{\partial \theta_3}\right)^2 \sigma_{33}\left(\underset{\sim}{\theta}\right) + 2\left(\frac{\partial g}{\partial \theta_1}\right)\left(\frac{\partial g}{\partial \theta_2}\right)\sigma_{12}\left(\underset{\sim}{\theta}\right)$$

$$+2\left(\frac{\partial g}{\partial \theta_1}\right)\left(\frac{\partial g}{\partial \theta_3}\right)\sigma_{13}\left(\underset{\sim}{\theta}\right) + 2\left(\frac{\partial g}{\partial \theta_2}\right)\left(\frac{\partial g}{\partial \theta_3}\right)\sigma_{23}\left(\underset{\sim}{\theta}\right)$$

$$= \rho^2\left[\frac{\mu_{22}}{\mu_{11}^2} + \frac{1}{4}\left(\frac{\mu_{40}}{\mu_{20}^2} + \frac{\mu_{04}}{\mu_{02}^2} + 2\frac{\mu_{22}}{\mu_{20}\mu_{02}}\right) - \left(\frac{\mu_{31}}{\mu_{11}\mu_{20}} + \frac{\mu_{13}}{\mu_{11}\mu_{02}}\right)\right]$$

If the sampling is from $N_2\left(\mu_1, \mu_2, \sigma_1^2, \sigma_2^2, \rho\right)$ then

$$\mu_{40} = 3\sigma_1^4, \mu_{04} = 3\sigma_2^4, \mu_{11} = \rho\sigma_1\sigma_2, \mu_{22} = \sigma_1^2\sigma_2^2(1+2\rho^2)$$
$$\mu_{13} = 3\rho\sigma_1\sigma_2^3, \mu_{31} = 3\rho\sigma_1^3\sigma_2, \mu_{20} = \sigma_1^2, \mu_{02} = \sigma_2^2$$

Using these values in the expression of $V\left(\underset{\sim}{\theta}\right)$, we get

$$V\left(\underset{\sim}{\theta}\right) = \left(1-\rho^2\right)^2$$
$$\therefore \sqrt{n}(r-\rho) \overset{a}{\sim} N\left(0, \left(1-\rho^2\right)^2\right)$$

i.e., $r \overset{a}{\sim} N\left(\rho, \frac{(1-\rho^2)^2}{n}\right)$

This result can be used for testing hypothesis regarding ρ.

(i) $H_0 : \rho = \rho_0$; under $H_0 : \tau = \frac{\sqrt{n}(r-\rho_0)}{1-\rho_0^2} \overset{a}{\sim} N(0,1)$

(ii) $H_0 : \rho_1 = \rho_2 (= \rho, \text{say}); r_1 \overset{a}{\sim} N\left(\rho_1, \frac{(1-\rho_1^2)^2}{n_1}\right); r_2 \overset{a}{\sim} N\left(\rho_2, \frac{(1-\rho_2^2)^2}{n_2}\right)$

$$\therefore r_1 - r_2 \overset{a}{\sim} N\left(\rho_1 - \rho_2, \frac{\left(1-\rho_1^2\right)^2}{n_1} + \frac{\left(1-\rho_2^2\right)^2}{n_2}\right)$$

Under $H_0, \tau = \frac{r_1 - r_2}{(1-\rho^2)\sqrt{\left(\frac{1}{n_1}+\frac{1}{n_2}\right)}} \overset{a}{\sim} N(0,1)$

If ρ is unknown then it is estimated by $\hat{\rho} = \frac{n_1 r_1 + n_2 r_2}{n_1 + n_2}$

If ρ is known, then the efficiency of the test will be good enough, but if it is unknown then the efficiency will be diminished. We can use the estimate of ρ only when the sample sizes are very very large. Otherwise, we transform the statistic so that its distribution is independent of ρ.

A.16 Transformation of Statistics

If a sequence of statistics $\{T_n\}$ for estimating θ are such that $\sqrt{n}(T_n - \theta) \overset{a}{\sim} N(0, \sigma^2(\theta))$, then for large samples the normal distribution can be used for testing hypothesis regarding θ if $\sigma^2(\theta)$ is independent of θ. Otherwise, it may be necessary to transform the statistic T_n such that the new statistic $g(T_n)$ has an asymptotic variance independent of θ. This is known as *transformation of statistics*. Another important advantage of such transformation is that in many cases the distribution of $g(T_n)$ tends more rapidly to normality than T_n itself, so that large sample tests can be made even for moderately large sample sizes. Also, in analysis of variance, where the assumption of homoscedasticity is made, such transformation of statistics may be useful.

A general formula We know that, if $\{T_n\}$ is a sequence of statistics $\sqrt{n}(T_n - \theta) \overset{a}{\sim} N(0, \sigma^2(\theta))$, then $\sqrt{n}(g(T_n) - g(\theta)) \overset{a}{\sim} N(0, g'^2(\theta)\sigma^2(\theta))$ provided $g(\cdot)$ is a function admitting 1st derivative and $g'(\theta) \neq 0$.

By equating the standard deviation $g'(\theta)\sigma(\theta)$ to a constant c, we get the differentiated equation

$$\mathrm{d}g(\theta) = \frac{c}{\sigma(\theta)}\mathrm{d}\theta$$

Solving this equation we get, $g(\theta) = \int \frac{c}{\sigma(\theta)}\mathrm{d}\theta + k$, where k is the constant of integration. Using this formula and suitably choosing c and k we can obtain a number of transformations of statistics of different important cases.

I. $\sin^{-1}$ transformationof the square root of the binomial proportion

We know $\sqrt{n}(p - P) \overset{a}{\sim} N(0, P(1 - P) = \sigma^2(P))$. We like to have a function $g(\cdot)$ such that $\sqrt{n}(g(p) - g(P)) \overset{a}{\sim} N(0, c^2)$ where c is independent of P.

From the differentiated equation, we have

$$\begin{aligned} g(P) &= \int \frac{c}{\sigma(P)} d(P) + k \\ &= c\int \frac{1}{\sqrt{P(1-P)}} d(P) + k = c.2\theta + k \\ &= c.2\sin^{-1}\sqrt{P} + k \qquad \left[\text{where } \sin^2\theta = P\right] \end{aligned}$$

Now selecting $c = \frac{1}{2}$ and $k = 0$, we have $g(P) = \sin^{-1}\sqrt{P}$

$\therefore g(p) = \sin^{-1}\sqrt{P}$ and $\sqrt{n}(\sin^{-1}\sqrt{p} - \sin^{-1}\sqrt{P}) \overset{a}{\sim} N(0, c^2 = \frac{1}{4})$
i.e.,

$$\left(\sin^{-1}\sqrt{p}\right) \overset{a}{\sim} N\left(\sin^{-1}\sqrt{P}, \frac{1}{4n}\right)$$

This fact can be used for testing hypothesis regarding P.

Note Ascomble (1948) has shown that a slightly better transformation assuming more stability in variance is $\sin^{-1}\sqrt{\frac{p+\frac{3}{8n}}{1+\frac{3}{4n}}}$ which has asymptotic variance $\frac{1}{4n+2}$.

Uses: (i) $H_0 : P = P_0$

Under $H_0,\ \tau = \left(\sin^{-1}\sqrt{p} - \sin^{-1}\sqrt{P_0}\right)2\sqrt{n} \overset{a}{\sim} N(0, 1)$

$w_0 : |\tau| > \tau_{\alpha/2}$ where $H_1 : P \neq P_0$.

Interval estimate of P

$$P_r\left[-\tau_{\alpha/2} \leq 2\sqrt{n}\left(\sin^{-1}\sqrt{p} - \sin^{-1}\sqrt{P}\right) \leq \tau_{\alpha/2}\right] = 1 - \alpha$$

i.e., $P_r\left[\sin^2\left(\sin^{-1}\sqrt{p} - \frac{\tau_{\alpha/2}}{2\sqrt{n}}\right) \leq P \leq \sin^2\left(\sin^{-1}\sqrt{p} + \frac{\tau_{\alpha/2}}{2\sqrt{n}}\right)\right] = 1 - \alpha$

(ii) $H_0 : P_1 = P_2 (=P)$ **say**

$$\sin^{-1}\sqrt{p_1} \overset{a}{\sim} N\left(\sin^{-1}\sqrt{P_1}, \frac{1}{4n_1}\right)$$
$$\sin^{-1}\sqrt{p_2} \overset{a}{\sim} N\left(\sin^{-1}\sqrt{P_2}, \frac{1}{4n_2}\right)$$
$$\therefore \left(\sin^{-1}\sqrt{p_1} - \sin^{-1}\sqrt{p_2}\right) \overset{a}{\sim} N\left(\sin^{-1}\sqrt{P_1} - \sin^{-1}\sqrt{P_2}, \frac{1}{4n_1} + \frac{1}{4n_2}\right)$$

Under H_0,

$$\tau = \frac{\left(\sin^{-1}\sqrt{p_1} - \sin^{-1}\sqrt{p_2}\right)}{\sqrt{\frac{1}{4n_1} + \frac{1}{4n_2}}} \overset{a}{\sim} N(0, 1)$$

$\therefore w_0 : |\tau| > \tau_{\alpha/2}$ if $H_1 : P_1 \neq P_2$.

If H_0 is accepted then to find the confidence interval for P:

$$\widehat{\sin}^{-1}\sqrt{P} = \frac{4n_1 \times \sin^{-1}\sqrt{p_1} + 4n_2 \sin^{-1}\sqrt{p_2}}{4n_1 + 4n_2} = \frac{n_1 \sin^{-1}\sqrt{p_1} + n_2 \sin^{-1}\sqrt{p_2}}{n_1 + n_2}$$

$$E\left(\widehat{\sin}^{-1}\sqrt{P}\right) = \frac{n_1 \sin^{-1}\sqrt{P_1} + n_2 \sin^{-1}\sqrt{P_2}}{n_1 + n_2} = \sin^{-1}\sqrt{P}\ [As P_1 = P_2 = P]$$

$$V\left(\widehat{\sin}^{-1}\sqrt{P}\right) = \frac{n_1^2 \times \frac{1}{4n_1} + n_2^2 \times \frac{1}{4n_2}}{(n_1+n_2)^2} = \frac{1}{4(n_1+n_2)}$$

$$\therefore \widehat{\sin}^{-1}\sqrt{P} \overset{a}{\sim} N\left(\sin^{-1}\sqrt{P}, \frac{1}{4(n_1+n_2)}\right)$$

$$P_r\left[-\tau_{\alpha/2} \le \left(\widehat{\sin}^{-1}\sqrt{P} - \sin^{-1}\sqrt{P}\right)2\sqrt{(n_1+n_2)} \le \tau_{\alpha/2}\right] = 1-\alpha$$

$$\Rightarrow P_r\left[\sin^2\left(\widehat{\sin}^{-1}\sqrt{P} - \frac{\tau_{\alpha/2}}{2\sqrt{(n_1+n_2)}}\right) \le P \le \sin^2\left(\widehat{\sin}^{-1}\sqrt{P} + \frac{\tau_{\alpha/2}}{2\sqrt{(n_1+n_2)}}\right)\right] = 1-\alpha.$$

If H_0 is rejected, then to find the confidence interval for the difference $(P_1 - P_2)$: Since $\sin^{-1}\sqrt{p_1} \overset{a}{\sim} N\left(\sin^{-1}\sqrt{P_1}, \frac{1}{4n_1}\right)$

$$\therefore P_r\left[\sin^2\left(\sin^{-1}\sqrt{p_1} - \frac{\tau_{\alpha/2}}{2\sqrt{n_1}}\right) \le P_1 \le \sin^2\left(\sin^{-1}\sqrt{p_1} + \frac{\tau_{\alpha/2}}{2\sqrt{n_1}}\right)\right] = 1-\alpha$$

i.e., $P(A) = 1-\alpha$ where $A = \{L_1 \le P_1 \le U_1\}$ having $L_1 = \sin^2(\sin^{-1}\sqrt{p_1} - \frac{\tau_{\alpha/2}}{2\sqrt{n_1}})$

$$U_1 = \sin^2\left(\sin^{-1}\sqrt{p_1} + \frac{\tau_{\alpha/2}}{2\sqrt{n_1}}\right)$$

Similarly, $\sin^{-1}\sqrt{p_2} \overset{a}{\sim} N\left(\sin^{-1}\sqrt{P_2}, \frac{1}{4n_2}\right)$ and $P_r\{L_2 \le P_2 \le U_2\} = 1-\alpha$ where

$$L_2 = \sin^2\left(\sin^{-1}\sqrt{p_2} - \frac{\tau_{\alpha/2}}{2\sqrt{n_2}}\right)$$
$$U_2 = \sin^2\left(\sin^{-1}\sqrt{p_2} + \frac{\tau_{\alpha/2}}{2\sqrt{n_2}}\right)$$

i.e., $P(B) = 1-\alpha$ where $B = \{L_2 \le P_2 \le U_2\}$
As $P(AB) \ge P(A) + P(B) - 1$

$$\therefore P_r\{L_1 \le P_1 \le U_1, L_2 \le P_2 \le U_2\} \ge (1-\alpha) + (1-\alpha) - 1$$
$$\therefore P_r\{L_1 - U_2 \le P_1 - P_2 \le U_1 - L_2\} \ge (1-2\alpha).$$

(iii) $H_0 : P_1 = P_2 = \cdots = P_k (= P)$ say

$$\sin^{-1}\sqrt{p_i} \overset{a}{\sim} N\left(\sin^{-1}\sqrt{P_i}, \frac{1}{4n_i}\right), i = 1(1)k$$

$\therefore$ under H_0, $\sum_{i=1}^{k}\left(\sin^{-1}\sqrt{p_i} - \sin^{-1}\sqrt{P}\right)^2 4n_i \sim \chi_k^2$
$\widehat{\sin}^{-1}\sqrt{P} = \frac{\sum n_i \sin^{-1}\sqrt{p_i}}{\sum n_i}$ and thus $\chi^2 = \sum_{i=1}^{k}\left(\sin^{-1}\sqrt{p_i} - \widehat{\sin}^{-1}\sqrt{P}\right)^2 4n_i \sim \chi_{x-1}^2$

If H_0 is accepted, then to find the interval estimate of P:

$$E\left(\widehat{\sin}^{-1}\sqrt{P}\right) = \frac{\sum n_i \sin^{-1}\sqrt{P_i}}{\sum n_i} = \frac{\sum n_i \sin^{-1}\sqrt{P}}{\sum n_i} = \sin^{-1}\sqrt{P} \because [P_1 = P_2 = \cdots = P_k = P]$$

$$V\left(\widehat{\sin}^{-1}\sqrt{P}\right) = \frac{\sum n_i^2 \times \frac{1}{4n_i}}{\left(\sum n_i\right)^2} = \frac{1}{4\left(\sum n_i\right)}$$

$$\therefore \widehat{\sin}^{-1}\sqrt{P} \overset{a}{\sim} N\left(\sin^{-1}\sqrt{P}, \frac{1}{4\left(\sum n_i\right)}\right)$$

$$P_r\left[\sin^2\left(\widehat{\sin}^{-1}\sqrt{P} - \frac{\tau_{\alpha/2}}{2\sqrt{\sum n_i}}\right) \le P \le \sin^2\left(\widehat{\sin}^{-1}\sqrt{P} + \frac{\tau_{\alpha/2}}{2\sqrt{\sum n_i}}\right)\right] = 1 - \alpha$$

II Square root transformation of Poisson variate

If $X \sim P(\lambda)$, then $E(X) = V(X) = \lambda$

We know, $(X - \lambda) \overset{a}{\sim} N(0, \lambda = \sigma^2(\lambda))$. We would like to have a function $g(.)$ such that $g(X) - g(\lambda) \overset{a}{\sim} N(0, c^2)$ where c^2 is independent of λ. $g(\lambda) = c\int \frac{d\lambda}{\sigma(\lambda)} + k = c\int \frac{d\lambda}{\sqrt{\lambda}} + k = c2\sqrt{\lambda} + k$.

Taking $k = 0$ and $c = 1/2$, $g(\lambda) = \sqrt{\lambda}$

$\therefore g(X) = \sqrt{X}$ and $c^2 = \frac{1}{4}$; $\therefore \left(\sqrt{X} - \sqrt{\lambda}\right) \overset{a}{\sim} N\left(0, \frac{1}{4}\right)$

i.e., $\sqrt{X} \overset{a}{\sim} N\left(\sqrt{\lambda}, \frac{1}{4}\right)$.

Uses: (i) $H_0 : \lambda = \lambda_0$

Under H_0, $\tau = 2\left(\sqrt{X} - \sqrt{\lambda_0}\right) \overset{a}{\sim} N(0, 1)$

$w_0 : |\tau| > \tau_{\alpha/2}$ where $H_1 : \lambda \neq \lambda_0$

Interval estimate of λ:

$$P\left[-\tau_{\alpha/2} \le 2\left(\sqrt{X} - \sqrt{\lambda}\right) \le \tau_{\alpha/2}\right] = 1 - \alpha$$

$$\therefore P\left[\left(\sqrt{X} - \frac{1}{2}\tau_{\alpha/2}\right)^2 \le \lambda \le \left(\sqrt{X} + \frac{1}{2}\tau_{\alpha/2}\right)^2\right] = 1 - \alpha$$

(ii) $H_0 : \lambda_1 = \lambda_2 (= \lambda)$,**Say**

$$\sqrt{X_1} \overset{a}{\sim} N\left(\sqrt{\lambda_1}, \frac{1}{4}\right), \qquad \sqrt{X_2} \overset{a}{\sim} N\left(\sqrt{\lambda_2}, \frac{1}{4}\right)$$

$$\therefore \left(\sqrt{X_1} - \sqrt{X_2}\right) \overset{a}{\sim} N\left(\sqrt{\lambda_1} - \sqrt{\lambda_2}, \frac{1}{2}\right)$$

$\therefore$ Under H_0, $\tau = \left(\sqrt{X_1} - \sqrt{X_2}\right)2 \overset{a}{\sim} N(0,1)$
$w_0 : |\tau| > \tau_{\alpha/2}$ if $H_1 : \lambda_1 \neq \lambda_2$.
If H_0 is accepted, then to find the confidence interval for λ:

$$\widehat{\sqrt{\lambda}} = \frac{4 \times \sqrt{X_1} + 4 \times \sqrt{X_2}}{4+4} = \frac{\sqrt{X_1} + \sqrt{X_2}}{2}$$

$$E\left(\widehat{\sqrt{\lambda}}\right) = \frac{\sqrt{\lambda} + \sqrt{\lambda}}{2} = \sqrt{\lambda} \quad \left[\because \sqrt{\lambda_1} = \sqrt{\lambda_2} = \sqrt{\lambda}\right]$$

$$V\left(\widehat{\sqrt{\lambda}}\right) = \frac{\frac{1}{4} + \frac{1}{4}}{4} = \frac{1}{8}$$

So $\widehat{\sqrt{\lambda}} \overset{a}{\sim} N\left(\sqrt{\lambda}, \frac{1}{8}\right)$

$$\therefore \text{Probability}\left[-\tau_{\alpha/2} \leq \left(\widehat{\sqrt{\lambda}} - \sqrt{\lambda}\right)\sqrt{8} \leq \tau_{\alpha/2}\right] = 1 - \alpha$$

$$\Rightarrow \text{Probability}\left[\left(\widehat{\sqrt{\lambda}} - \frac{\tau_{\alpha/2}}{\sqrt{8}}\right)^2 \leq \lambda \leq \left(\widehat{\sqrt{\lambda}} + \frac{\tau_{\alpha/2}}{\sqrt{8}}\right)^2\right] = 1 - \alpha$$

If H_0 is rejected, then to find the confidence interval for the difference $(\lambda_1 - \lambda_2)$:
Since $\sqrt{X_1} \overset{a}{\sim} N\left(\sqrt{\lambda_1}, \frac{1}{4}\right)$

$$\Rightarrow \text{Probability}\left[\left(\sqrt{X_1} - \frac{\tau_{\alpha/2}}{2}\right)^2 \leq \lambda_1 \leq \left(\sqrt{X_1} + \frac{\tau_{\alpha/2}}{2}\right)^2\right] = 1 - \alpha$$

i.e. $P(A) = 1 - \alpha$ where $A = \{L_1 \leq \lambda_1 \leq U_1\}$ where $L_1 = \left(\sqrt{X_1} - \frac{\tau_{\alpha/2}}{2}\right)^2$ and $U_1 = \left(\sqrt{X_1} + \frac{\tau_{\alpha/2}}{2}\right)^2$
Similarly, $\sqrt{X_2} \overset{a}{\sim} N\left(\sqrt{\lambda_2}, \frac{1}{4}\right)$

$$\therefore \text{Probability}\left[\left(\sqrt{X_2} - \frac{\tau_{\alpha/2}}{2}\right)^2 \leq \lambda_2 \leq \left(\sqrt{X_2} + \frac{\tau_{\alpha/2}}{2}\right)^2\right] = 1 - \alpha$$

i.e. $P(B) = 1 - \alpha$ where $B = \{L_2 \leq \lambda_2 \leq U_2\}$ having $L_2 = \left(\sqrt{X_2} - \frac{\tau_{\alpha/2}}{2}\right)^2$, $U_2 = \left(\sqrt{X_2} + \frac{\tau_{\alpha/2}}{2}\right)^2$

As, $P(AB) \geq P(A) + P(B) - 1$

$$\Rightarrow \text{Probability}\{L_1 \leq \lambda_1 \leq U_1, L_2 \leq \lambda_2 \leq U_2\} \geq (1-\alpha) + (1-\alpha) - 1$$
$$\Rightarrow \text{Probability}\{L_1 - U_2 \leq \lambda_1 - \lambda_2 \leq U_1 - L_2\} \geq 1 - 2\alpha$$

(iii) $H_0 : \lambda_1 = \lambda_2 = \cdots = \lambda_k (= \lambda)$ **say**

$$\sqrt{X_i} \overset{a}{\sim} N\left(\sqrt{\lambda_i}, \frac{1}{4}\right), i = 1(1)k$$

$\therefore$ under H_0, $\sum_{i=1}^{k} \left(\sqrt{X_i} - \sqrt{\lambda_i}\right)^2 \cdot 4 \sim \chi_k^2$
$\hat{\sqrt{\lambda}} = \frac{\sum \sqrt{X_i}}{k}$ and then

$$\chi^2 = \sum_{i=1}^{k} \left(\sqrt{X_i} - \hat{\sqrt{\lambda}}\right)^2 \cdot 4 \sim \chi_{k-1}^2$$
$$w_0 : \chi^2 > \chi_{\alpha,k-1}^2.$$

If H_0 is accepted, then to find the interval estimate of λ: $E\left(\hat{\sqrt{\lambda}}\right) = \frac{\sum \sqrt{\lambda_i}}{k} = \frac{\sum \sqrt{\lambda}}{k} = \sqrt{\lambda}$ $[As \lambda_1 = \lambda_2 = \cdots = \lambda_k = \lambda]$

$$V\left(\widehat{\sqrt{\lambda}}\right) = \frac{\sum V(\sqrt{X_i})}{k^2} = \frac{1}{4k}$$
$$\therefore \widehat{\sqrt{\lambda}} \overset{a}{\sim} N\left(\sqrt{\lambda}, \frac{1}{4k}\right)$$
$$\therefore \tau = \left(\widehat{\sqrt{\lambda}} - \sqrt{\lambda}\right)\sqrt{4k} \sim N(0,1)$$
$$\therefore \text{Probability}\left[-\tau_{\alpha/2} \leq \left(\widehat{\sqrt{\lambda}} - \sqrt{\lambda}\right)2\sqrt{k} \leq \tau_{\alpha/2}\right] = 1 - \alpha$$
$$\Rightarrow \text{Probability}\left[\left(\widehat{\sqrt{\lambda}} - \frac{\tau_{\alpha/2}}{2\sqrt{k}}\right)^2 \leq \lambda \leq \left(\widehat{\sqrt{\lambda}} + \frac{\tau_{\alpha/2}}{2\sqrt{k}}\right)^2\right] = 1 - \alpha$$

Note It can be shown that

$$E\left(\sqrt{X}\right) = \sqrt{\lambda} + 0\left(\frac{1}{\sqrt{\lambda}}\right)$$
$$V\left(\sqrt{X}\right) = \frac{1}{4} + 0\left(\frac{1}{\lambda}\right)$$

whereas $E\left(\sqrt{X + 3/8}\right) = \sqrt{\lambda + 3/8} + 0\left(\frac{1}{\sqrt{\lambda}}\right)$ and $V\left(\sqrt{X + 3/8}\right) = \frac{1}{4} + 0\left(\frac{1}{\lambda^2}\right)$.

Comparing $V(\sqrt{X})$ and $V\left(\sqrt{X+{}^3/_8}\right)$ we observe that $\sqrt{X+{}^3/_8}$ is better transformation than $\sqrt{X}$.

III Logarithmic transformation of sample variance for $N(\mu, \sigma^2)$

$$s^2 = \frac{1}{n-1}\sum (x_i - \bar{x})^2$$

$E(s^2) = \sigma^2$ and $V(s^2) \simeq \frac{2\sigma^4}{n}$
Also $E(S^2) \to \sigma^2$ and $V(S^2) \simeq \frac{2\sigma^4}{n}$ for $S^2 = \frac{\sum (x_i - \bar{x})^2}{n}$

$$\therefore s^2 \overset{a}{\sim} N\left(\sigma^2, \frac{2\sigma^4}{n}\right)$$

We like to get a function $g(\cdot)$ such that $g(s^2) \overset{a}{\sim} N(g(\sigma^2), c^2)$ where c^2 is independent of σ^2.

$$g(\sigma^2) = \int \frac{c}{\sqrt{\frac{2\sigma^4}{n}}} d\sigma^2 = c\sqrt{\frac{n}{2}}\int \frac{d\sigma^2}{\sigma^2}$$
$$= c\sqrt{\frac{n}{2}}\log_e \sigma^2 + k$$

Choosing $k = 0$ and $c = \sqrt{\frac{2}{n}}$. We get $g(\sigma^2) = \log_e \sigma^2$

$$\therefore g(s^2) = \log_e s^2 \overset{a}{\sim} N\left(\log_e \sigma^2, \frac{2}{n}\right)$$

Uses: (i) $H_0 : \sigma^2 = \sigma_0^2$
Under H_0, $\tau = \sqrt{\frac{n}{2}}(\log s^2 - \log \sigma_0^2) \sim N(0, 1)$
$w_0 : |\tau| > \tau_{\alpha/2}$ if $H_1 : \sigma^2 \neq \sigma_0^2$.
Interval estimate of σ^2 is given as

$$\text{Probability}\left[-\tau_{\alpha/2} \leq \sqrt{\frac{n}{2}}(\log s^2 - \log \sigma^2) \leq \tau_{\alpha/2}\right] = 1 - \alpha$$

i.e., $\text{Probability}\left[e^{\log s^2 - \sqrt{\frac{2}{n}}\tau_{\alpha/2}} \leq \sigma^2 \leq e^{\log s^2 + \sqrt{\frac{2}{n}}\tau_{\alpha/2}}\right] = 1 - \alpha.$

(ii) $H_0 : \sigma_1^2 = \sigma_2^2 (=\sigma^2)$ **say**
Under $H_0 : \tau = \frac{\log s_1^2 - \log s_2^2}{\sqrt{\frac{2}{n_1} + \frac{2}{n_2}}} \overset{a}{\sim} N(0, 1)$
$w_0 : |\tau| \geq \tau_{\alpha/2}$ if $H_1 : \sigma_1^2 \neq \sigma_2^2$.

If H_0 is accepted, thus the interval estimate of the common variance σ^2 can be obtained by the

$\widehat{\log \sigma^2}$ where $\widehat{\log \sigma^2} = \dfrac{\frac{n_1}{2}\log s_1^2 + \frac{n_2}{2}\log s_2^2}{\frac{n_1}{2} + \frac{n_2}{2}} = \dfrac{n_1 \log s_1^2 + n_2 \log s_2^2}{n_1 + n_2}$.

$E\left(\widehat{\log \sigma^2}\right) = \log \sigma^2$ and $V\left(\widehat{\log \sigma^2}\right) = \frac{2}{n_1 + n_2}$

$$\widehat{\log \sigma} \overset{a}{\sim} N\left(\log \sigma^2, \frac{2}{n_1 + n_2}\right)$$

$$\therefore \text{Probability}\left[e^{\widehat{\log \sigma^2} - \sqrt{\frac{2}{n_1+n_2}}\tau_{\alpha/2}} \le \sigma^2 \le e^{\widehat{\log \sigma^2} + \sqrt{\frac{2}{n_1+n_2}}\tau_{\alpha/2}}\right] = 1 - \alpha.$$

If H_0 is rejected, then the confidence interval for $\left(\sigma_1^2 - \sigma_2^2\right)$ can be obtained in the following way:

$$\text{Probability}\left[e^{\log s_1^2 - \sqrt{\frac{2}{n_1}}\tau_{\alpha/2}} \le \sigma_1^2 \le e^{\log s_1^2 + \sqrt{\frac{2}{n_1}}\tau_{\alpha/2}}\right] = 1 - \alpha$$

i.e., $P(A) = 1 - \alpha$ where $A = \{L_1 \le \sigma_1^2 \le U_1\}$ having $L_1 = e^{\log s_1^2 - \sqrt{\frac{2}{n_1}}\tau_{\alpha/2}}$

$$U_1 = e^{\log s_1^2 + \sqrt{\frac{2}{n_1}}\tau_{\alpha/2}}$$

Also, Probability $\left[e^{\log s_2^2 - \sqrt{\frac{2}{n_2}}\tau_{\alpha/2}} \le \sigma_2^2 \le e^{\log s_2^2 + \sqrt{\frac{2}{n_2}}\tau_{\alpha/2}}\right] = 1 - \alpha$

i.e., $P(B) = 1 - \alpha$ where $B = \{L_2 \le \sigma_2^2 \le U_2\}$

As $P(AB) \ge P(A) + P(B) - 1$

$$\therefore \text{Probability}\{L_1 \le \sigma_1^2 \le U_1, L_2 \le \sigma_2^2 \le U_2\} \ge (1-\alpha) + (1-\alpha) - 1$$

Or Probability$\{L_1 - U_2 \le \sigma_1^2 - \sigma_2^2 \le U_1 - L_2\} \ge 1 - 2\alpha$

(iii) $H_0 : \sigma_1^2 = \sigma_2^2 = \cdots = \sigma_k^2 (= \sigma^2)$**say**

$$\log_e s_i^2 \overset{a}{\sim} = N\left(\log_e \sigma_i^2, \frac{2}{n_i}\right)$$

$\therefore$ under H_0, $\sum_{i=1}^k \left(\log_e s_i^2 - \widehat{\log \sigma^2}\right)^2 \frac{n_i}{2} \overset{a}{\sim} \chi^2_{k-1}$

where $\widehat{\log_e \sigma^2} = \dfrac{\sum n_i \log_e s_i^2}{\sum n_i}$;

$$\therefore w_0 : \chi^2 > \chi^2_{\alpha, k-1}$$

If H_0 is accepted, then the interval estimate of σ^2 can be obtained as follows:

$$\widehat{\log_e \sigma^2} \overset{a}{\sim} N\left(\log_e \sigma^2, \frac{2}{\sum n_i}\right)$$

$$\therefore \text{Probability}\left[-\tau_{\alpha/2} \le \frac{\widehat{\log_e \sigma^2} - \log_e \sigma^2}{\sqrt{\frac{2}{\sum n_i}}} \le \tau_{\alpha/2}\right] = 1 - \alpha$$

$$\text{So, Probability}\left[e^{\widehat{\log_e \sigma^2} - \sqrt{\frac{2}{\sum n_i}}\tau_{\alpha/2}} \le \sigma^2 \le e^{\widehat{\log_e \sigma^2} + \sqrt{\frac{2}{\sum n_i}}\tau_{\alpha/2}}\right] = 1 - \alpha.$$

IV Logarithmic transformation of sample s.d.

$$s \overset{a}{\sim} N\left(\sigma, \frac{\sigma^2}{2n}\right)$$

We like to get a $g(\cdot)$ such that $g(s) \overset{a}{\sim} N(g(\sigma), c^2)$ where c^2 is independent of σ.

$g(\sigma) = \int \frac{c}{\sigma/\sqrt{2n}} d\sigma = \sqrt{2n}c \log_e \sigma + k$. Choosing $c = \frac{1}{\sqrt{2n}}$ and $k = 0$. We have $g(\sigma) = \log_e \sigma$

$\therefore g(s) = \log_e s \overset{a}{\sim} N\left(\log_e \sigma, \frac{1}{2n}\right)$.

We may use this result for testing hypothesis related to σ.

V Z-transformation of sample correlation coefficient from $N_2\left(\mu_1, \mu_2, \sigma_1^2, \sigma_2^2, \rho\right)$:

$E(r) \sim \rho$ and $V(r) \sim \frac{\left(1-\rho^2\right)^2}{n}$

$$\Rightarrow r \overset{a}{\sim} N\left(\rho, \frac{\left(1-\rho^2\right)^2}{n}\right).$$

We like to get a function $g(\cdot)$ such that $g(r)$ is asymptotically normal with variance independent of ρ.

$$\therefore g(\rho) = \sqrt{n}\int \frac{c}{1-\rho^2} dp = \sqrt{n}c\frac{1}{2}\log_e \frac{1+\rho}{1-\rho} + k$$

We choose $c = \frac{1}{\sqrt{n}}$ and $k = 0$ and then

$$\therefore g(\rho) = \frac{1}{2}\log_e \frac{1+\rho}{1-\rho} = \tan h^{-1}\rho = \xi, \quad \text{(say)}$$

$$\therefore g(r) = \frac{1}{2}\log_e \frac{1+r}{1-r} = \tan h^{-1} r = Z, \quad \text{(say)}$$

$$\therefore Z = g(r) \overset{a}{\sim} N\left(\xi, \frac{1}{n}\right).$$

Note Putting $Z - \xi = y$, the distribution of y may be derived using the distribution of r. The first four moments were found by Fisher and later they were revised by Gayen (1951).

In fact $E(Z) = \xi + \frac{\rho}{2(n-1)} + 0\left(\frac{1}{n^2}\right)$

$$\mu_2(Z) = \frac{1}{n-1} + \frac{4-\rho^2}{2(n-1)^2} + 0\left(\frac{1}{n^3}\right)$$

Now, $\frac{1}{n-3} = \frac{1}{(n-1)\left(\frac{n-3}{n-1}\right)} = \frac{1}{(n-1)\left(1-\frac{2}{n-1}\right)} = \frac{1}{n-1}\left(1-\frac{2}{n-1}\right)^{-1}$

$$= \frac{1}{n-1}\left[1 + \frac{2}{n-1} + \frac{4}{(n-1)^2} + 0\left(\frac{1}{n^3}\right)\right]$$

$$= \frac{1}{n-1} + \frac{2}{(n-1)^2} + 0\left(\frac{1}{n^3}\right)$$

Again, $\mu_2(Z) = \frac{1}{n-1} + \frac{2}{(n-1)^2} - \frac{\rho^2}{2(n-1)^2} + 0\left(\frac{1}{n^3}\right)$

$$= \frac{1}{n-3} - \frac{\rho^2}{2(n-1)^2} + 0\left(\frac{1}{n^3}\right)$$

$$\therefore \mu_2(Z) \simeq \frac{1}{n-3}$$

In fact, $V(Z) \simeq \frac{1}{n}$ for large n
$\simeq \frac{1}{n-3}$ for moderately large n.

$\therefore$ For moderately large n,

$$Z = \tan\text{h}^{-1} r = \frac{1}{2}\log_e \frac{1+r}{1-r} \overset{a}{\sim} N\left(\xi, \frac{1}{n-3}\right)$$

where $\xi = \tan\text{h}^{-1}\rho = \frac{1}{2}\log_e \frac{1+\rho}{1-\rho}$.

Uses: (i) $H_0 : \rho = \rho_0$ against $H_1 : \rho \neq \rho_0$
$\Leftrightarrow H_0 : \xi = \xi_0$ against $H_1 : \xi \neq \xi_0$ where $\xi_0 = \frac{1}{2}\log_e \frac{1+\rho_0}{1-\rho_0}$
$\therefore$ Under H_0, $\tau = (Z - \xi_0)\sqrt{n-3} \overset{a}{\sim} N(0, 1)$

$$w_0 : |\tau| \geq \tau_{\alpha/2}$$

Also, the $100(1-\alpha)\%$ confidence interval for ρ is given as

$$\text{Probability}\left[-\tau_{\alpha/2} \le \sqrt{n-3}(Z-\xi) \le \tau_{\alpha/2}\right] = 1-\alpha$$

$$\text{Probability}\left[Z - \frac{\tau_{\alpha/2}}{\sqrt{n-3}} \le \xi \le Z + \frac{\tau_{\alpha/2}}{\sqrt{n-3}}\right] = 1-\alpha$$

$$\therefore \text{Probability}\left[e^{2\left(Z-\frac{\tau_{\alpha/2}}{\sqrt{n-3}}\right)} \le \frac{1+\rho}{1-\rho} \le e^{2\left(Z+\frac{\tau_{\alpha/2}}{\sqrt{n-3}}\right)}\right] = 1-\alpha$$

$$\text{i.e., Probability}\left[\frac{e^{2\left(Z-\frac{\tau_{\alpha/2}}{\sqrt{n-3}}\right)}-1}{e^{2\left(Z-\frac{\tau_{\alpha/2}}{\sqrt{n-3}}\right)}+1} \le \rho \le \frac{e^{2\left(Z+\frac{\tau_{\alpha/2}}{\sqrt{n-3}}\right)}-1}{e^{2\left(Z+\frac{\tau_{\alpha/2}}{\sqrt{n-3}}\right)}+1}\right] = 1-\alpha$$

(ii) $H_0 : \rho_1 = \rho_2 (= \rho)$, **say**

$$\Leftrightarrow H_0 : \xi_1 = \xi_2 (= \xi) \quad \text{say}$$

$$Z_1 = \tanh^{-1} r_1 \overset{a}{\sim} N\left(\xi_1, \frac{1}{n_1-3}\right)$$

$$Z_2 = \tanh^{-1} r_2 \overset{a}{\sim} N\left(\xi_2, \frac{1}{n_2-3}\right)$$

$$\therefore (Z_1 - Z_2) \overset{a}{\sim} N\left(\xi_1 - \xi_2, \frac{1}{n_1-3} + \frac{1}{n_2-3}\right)$$

Under H_0, $\tau = \frac{Z_1 - Z_1}{\sqrt{\frac{1}{n_1-3}+\frac{1}{n_2-3}}} \overset{a}{\sim} N(0,1)$, $\therefore w_0 : |\tau| \ge \tau_{\alpha/2}$ if $H_1 : \rho_1 \ne \rho_2$

If H_0 is accepted $100(1-\alpha)\%$confidence interval for ξ is given as

$$\hat{Z} = \frac{(n_1-3)Z_1 + (n_2-3)Z_2}{(n_1-3)+(n_2-3)} = \frac{(n_1-3)Z_1 + (n_2-3)Z_2}{n_1+n_2-6}$$

$$E(\hat{Z}) = \xi = \frac{1}{2}\log_e \frac{1+\rho}{1-\rho}$$

$$V(\hat{Z}) = \frac{1}{n_1+n_2-6}$$

$$\therefore \text{Probability}\left[\hat{Z} - \tau_{\alpha/2}\Big/\sqrt{n_1+n_2-6} \le \frac{1}{2}\log_e \frac{1+\rho}{1-\rho} \le \hat{Z} + \tau_{\alpha/2}\Big/\sqrt{n_1+n_2-6}\right] = 1-\alpha.$$

We can get $100(1-\alpha)\%$ confidence interval from this.

If H_0 is rejected, then $100(1-2\alpha)\%$ confidence interval can be obtained as follows:

$$\text{Probability}\left[\frac{e^{2\left(Z_1-\frac{\tau_{\alpha/2}}{\sqrt{n_1-3}}\right)}-1}{e^{2\left(Z_1-\frac{\tau_{\alpha/2}}{\sqrt{n_1-3}}\right)}+1} \le \rho_1 \le \frac{e^{2\left(Z_1+\frac{\tau_{\alpha/2}}{\sqrt{n_1-3}}\right)}-1}{e^{2\left(Z_1+\frac{\tau_{\alpha/2}}{\sqrt{n_1-3}}\right)}+1}\right] = 1-\alpha$$

Or, $P(A) = 1-\alpha$ where $A = \{L_1 \le \rho_1 \le U_1\}$ having $L_1 = \frac{e^{2\left(Z_1-\frac{\tau_{\alpha/2}}{\sqrt{n_1-3}}\right)}-1}{e^{2\left(Z_1-\frac{\tau_{\alpha/2}}{\sqrt{n_1-3}}\right)}+1}$

$$U_1 = \frac{e^{2\left(Z_1+\frac{\tau_{\alpha/2}}{\sqrt{n_2-3}}\right)}-1}{e^{2\left(Z_1+\frac{\tau_{\alpha/2}}{\sqrt{n_2-3}}\right)}+1}$$

Similarly we get $P(B) = 1-\alpha$ where $B = \{L_2 \le \rho_2 \le U_2\}$ and

$L_2 = \frac{e^{2\left(Z_2-\frac{\tau_{\alpha/2}}{\sqrt{n_2-3}}\right)}-1}{e^{2\left(Z_2-\frac{\tau_{\alpha/2}}{\sqrt{n_2-3}}\right)}+1}$ and $U_2 = \frac{e^{2\left(Z_2+\frac{\tau_{\alpha/2}}{\sqrt{n_2-3}}\right)}-1}{e^{2\left(Z_2+\frac{\tau_{\alpha/2}}{\sqrt{n_2-3}}\right)}+1}$

As $P(AB) \ge P(A) + P(B) - 1$

$$\therefore \text{Probability}\{L_1 \le \rho_1 \le U_1, L_2 \le \rho_2 \le U_2\} \ge (1-\alpha) + (1-\alpha) - 1$$
$$\therefore \text{Probability}\{L_1 - U_2 \le \rho_1 - \rho_2 \le U_1 - L_2\} \ge (1-2\alpha).$$

(iii) $H_0 : \rho_1 = \rho_2 = \cdots = \rho_k (=\rho)$

$$\Leftrightarrow H_0 : \xi_1 = \xi_2 = \cdots = \xi_k (=\xi)$$
$$Z_i = \frac{1}{2}\log_e \frac{1+r_i}{1-r_i} \overset{a}{\sim} N\left(\xi_i, \frac{1}{n_i-3}\right)$$

Under $H_0, \chi^2 = \sum_1^k (n_i-3)\left(Z_i - \hat{\xi}\right)^2 \overset{a}{\sim} \chi^2_{k-1}$ where $\hat{\xi} = \frac{\sum (n_i-3)Z_i}{\sum (n_i-3)}$

$$w_0 : \chi^2 > \chi^2_{\alpha,k-1}$$

If H_0 is accepted, then $100(1-\alpha)\%$confidence interval for ξ (Subsequently for ρ) can be obtained as follows:

$$E\left(\hat{\xi}\right) = \xi,\; V\left(\hat{\xi}\right) = \frac{1}{\sum n_i - 3k}$$
$$\therefore \text{Probability}\left[-\tau_{\alpha/2} \le \left(\sum n_i - 3k\right)\left(\hat{\xi} - \xi\right) \le \tau_{\alpha/2}\right] = 1-\alpha$$

This will provide us for interval estimate of ξ and thus for ρ.

References

Agresti, A.: Categorical Data Analysis. Wiley, New York (1990)

Aigner D.J.: Basic Econometrics, Prentice-Hall (1971)

Aitken, M., Anderson, D., Francis, B., Hinde, J.: Statistical Modelling in GLIM. Clarendon Press, Oxford (1989)

Akahira, M., Takeuchi, K.: Asymptotic Efficiency of Statistical Estimators. Springer-Verlag, New York (1981)

Allen, R.G.D.: Statistics for Economics. Hutchinson Universal Library (1951)

Amari, S.-I., Barndorff-Nielsen, O.E., Kass, R.E., Lauritzen, S.L., Rao, C.R.: Differential geometry and statistical inference. Institute of Mathematical Statistics, Hayward (1987)

Anderson, T.W.: An Introduction to multivariate analysis. Wiley, New York (1958)

Anderson, T.W.: Introduction to Multivariate Statistical Analysis, 2nd edn. Wiley, New York (1984)

Arnold, S.F.: The Theory of Linear Models and Multivariate Analysis. Wiley, New York (1981)

Arnold, S.F.: Sufficiency and invariance. Statist. Prob. Lett. **3**, 275–279 (1985)

Ash, R.: Real Analysis and Probability. Academic Press, New York (1972)

Bahadur, R.R.: Some Limit Theorems in Statistics. SIAM, Philadelphia (1971)

Bar-Lev, S.K., Enis, P.: On the classical choice of variance stabilizing transformations and an application for a Poisson variate. Biometrika **75**, 803–804 (1988)

Barlow, R., Proschan, F.: Statistical Theory of Life Testing. Holt, Rinehart and Winston, New York (1975)

Barnard, G.A.: Pivotal Inference and the Bayesian Controversy (with discussion). In: Bernardo, J. M., DeGroot, M.H., Lindley, D.V., Smith, A.F.M. (eds.) Bayesian Statistics. University Press, Valencia (1980)

Barnard, G.A.: Pivotal inference. In: Johnson, N.L., Kota, S., Reade, C. (eds.) Encyclopedia Statistical Sciences. Wiley, New York (1985)

Barndorff-Nielsen, O.: Information and Exponential Families in Statistical Theory. Wiley, New York (1978)

Barndorff-Nielsen, O.: Conditionality resolutions. Biometrika **67**, 293–310 (1980)

Barndorff-Nielsen, O.: On a formula for the distribution of the maximum likelihood estimator. Biometrika **70**, 343–365 (1983)

Barndorff-Nielsen, O.: Parametric Statistical Models and Likelihood. Lecture Notes in Statistics 50. Springer, New York (1988)

Barndorff-Nielsen, O., Blaesild, P.: Global maxima, and likelihood in linear models. Research Rept. 57. Department of Theoretical Statistics, University of Aarhus (1980)

Barndorff-Nielsen, O., Cox, D.R.: Inference and Asymptotics. Chapman & Hall (1994)

Barr, D.R., Zehna, P.W.: Probabilit y: Modeling Uncertainty. Addison-Wesley. Reading (1983)

Barnett, V.: Comparitive Statistical Inference, 2nd edn. Wiley, New York (1989)

Barnett, V., Lewis, T.: Outliers in Statistics. John Wiley (1978)

P.K. Sahu et al., *Estimation and Inferential Statistics*,
DOI 10.1007/978-81-322-2514-0

Barnett, V.D.: Evaluation of the maximum likelihood estimator where the likelihood equation has multiple roots. Biometrika **53**, 151–166 (1966)

Barron, A.R.: Uniformly powerful goodness of fit test. Ann. Statist. **17**, 107–124 (1982)

Basawa, I.V., Prakasa Rao, B.L.S.: Statistical Inference in Stochastic Processes. Academic Press, London (1980)

Basu, D.: A note on the theory of unbiased estimation. Ann. Math. Statist. **26**, 345-348. Reprinted as Chapter XX of Statistical Information and Likelihood: A Collection of Critical Essays. Springer-Verlag, New York (1955a)

Basu, D.: On statistics independent of a complete sufficient statistic. Sankhya **15**, 377-380. Reprinted as Chapter XXII of Statistical Information and Likelihood: A Collection of Critical Essays. Springer-Verlag, New York (1955b)

Basu, D.: The concept of asymptotic efficiency. Sankhya **17**, 193–196. Reprinted as Chapter XXI of Statistical Information and Likelihood: A Collection of Critical Essays. Springer-Verlag, New York (1956)

Basu, D.: Statistical Information and Likelihood: A Collection of Critical Essays (J.K. Ghosh, ed.). Springer-Verlag, New York (1988)

Bayes, T.: An essay toward solving a problem in the doctrine of chances. Phil. Trans. Roy. Soc. **153**, 370–418 (1763). Reprinted in (1958) Biometrika **45**, 293-315

Berger, J.: Selecting a minimax estimator of a multivariate normal mean. Ann. Statist. **10**, 81–92 (1982)

Berger, J.0.: The Robust Bayesian Viewpoint (with discussion). Robustness of Bayesian Analysis (J. Kadane, ed.), 63–144. North-Holland. Amsterdam (1984)

Berger, J.0.: Statistical Decision Theory and Bayesian Analysis, 2nd edn. Springer-Verlag, New York (1985)

Berger, J.O.: Estimation in continuous exponential families: Bayesian estimation subject to risk restrictions. In: Gupta, S.S., Berger, J.O. (eds.) Statistical Decision Theory III. Academic Press, New York (1982b)

Berger, J.O.: Statistical Decision Theory and Bayesian Analysis, 2nd edn. Springer-Verlag, New York (1985)

Berger, J.O., Bernardo, J.M. On the development of reference priors. In: Berger, J.O., Bernardo, J. M. (eds.) Bayesian Statist. 4. Clarendon Press, London (1992a)

Berger, J.O., Bernardo, J.M.: Ordered group reference priors with application to multinomial probabilities. Biometrika **79**, 25–37 (1992b)

Berger, J.O., Wolpert, R.W.: The Likelihood Principle, 2nd edn. Institute of Mathematical Statistics, Hayward, CA (1988)

Bernardo, J.M., Smith, A.F.M.: Bayesian Theory. Wiley, New York (1994)

Berndt, E.R.: The practice of Econometrics: Classic and Contemporary. Addison and Wesley (1991)

Bhattacharya, G.K., Johnson, R.A.: Statistical Concepts and Methods. John Wiley (1977)

Bhatttachayra, R., Denker, M.: Asymptotic Statistics. Birkhauser-Verlag, Basel (1990)

Bickel, P.J.: Minimax estimation of the mean of a normal distribution subject to doing well at a point. In: Rizvi, M.H., Rustagi, J.S., Siegmund, D., (eds.) Recent Advances in Statistics: Papers in Honor of Herman Chernoff on his Sixtieth Birthday. Academic Press, New York (1983)

Bickel, P.J., Klaassen, P., Ritov, C.A.J., Wellner, J.: Efficient and Adaptive Estimation for Semiparametric Models. Johns Hopkins University Press, Baltimore (1993)

Billingsley, P.: Probability and Measure, 3rd edn. Wiley, New York (1995)

Blackwell, D., Girshick, M.A.: Theory of Games and Statistical Decision. John Wiley and Sons, New York (1954)

Blackwell, D., Girshick, M.A.: Theory of Games and Statistical Decisions. Wiley, New York (1954)

Blyth, C.R.: Maximum probability estimation in small samples. In: Bickel, P.J., Doksum, K.A., Hodges, J.L., Jr., (eds.) Festschrift for Erich Lehmann. Wadsworth and Brooks/Cole. Pacific Grove, CA (1982)

Bock, M.E.: Employing vague inequality information in the estimation of normal mean vectors (Estimators that shrink toward closed convex polyhedra). In: Gupta, S.S., Berger, J.O. (eds.). Statistical Decision Theory III. Academic Press, New York (1982)

Bock, M.E.: Shrinkage estimators: Pseudo-Bayes estimators for normal mean vectors. In: Gupta, S.S., Berger, J.O. (eds.) Statistical Decision Theory IV. Springer-Verlag, New York (1988)

Bradley, R.A., Gart, J.J.: The asymptotic properties of ML estimators when sampling for associated populations. Biometrika **49**, 205–214 (1962)

Brandwein, A.C., Strawderman, W.E.: Minimax estimation of location parameters for spherically symmetric unimodal distributions under quadratic loss. Ann. Statist. **6**, 377–416 (1978)

Bridge, J.I.: Applied Econometrics. North Holland, Amsterdam (1971)

Brockwell, P.J., Davis, R.A.: Time Series: Theory and Methods. Springer-Verlag, New York (1987)

Brown, D., Rothery, P.: Models in Biology: Mathematics, Statistics and Computing. Wiley, New York (1993)

Brown, L.D.: Fundamentals of Statistical Exponential Families with Applications in Statistical Decision Theory. Institute of Mathematical Statistics Lecture Notes–Monograph Series. Hayward, CA: IMS (1986)

Brown, L.D.: Fundamentals of Statistical Exponential Families. Institute of Mathematical Statistics, Hayward, CA (1986)

Brown, L.D.: Commentary on paper [19]. Kiefer Collected Papers, Supple-mentary Volume. Springer-Verlag, New York (1986)

Brown, L.D.: Minimaxity, more or less. In: Gupta, S.S., Berger, J.O. (eds.) Statistical Decision Theory and Related Topics V. Springer-Verlag, New York (1994)

Brown, L.D., Hwang, J.T.: A unified admissibility proof. In: Gupta, S.S., Berger, J.O. (eds.) Statistical Decision Theory III. Academic Press, New York (1982)

Bucklew, J.A.: Large Deviation Techniques in Decision, Simulation and Estimation (1990)

Burdick, R.K., Graybill, F.A.: Confidence Intervals on Variance Components. Marcel Dekker, New York (1992)

Carlin, B.P., Louis, T.A.: Bayes and Empirical Bayes Methods for Data Analysis. Chapman & Hall, London (1996)

Carroll, R.J., Ruppert, D., Stefanski, L.: Measurment Error in Nonlinear Models. Chapman & Hall, London (1995)

Carroll, R.J., and Ruppert, D.: Transformation and Weighting in Regression. Chapman and Hall, London (1988)

Carroll, R.J., Ruppert, D., Stefanski, L.A.: Measurement Error in Non-linear Models. Chapman and Hall, London (1995)

Casella, G., Berger, R.L.: Statistical Inference.: Wadsworth/Brooks Cole. Pacific Grove, CA (1990)

Cassel, C., Sa¨rndal, C., Wretman, J.H.: Foundations of Inference in Survey Sampling. Wiley, New York (1977)

CBBella., G., Robert, C.P.: Rao-Blackwellisation of Sampling Schemes. Biometrika **83**, 81–94 (1996)

Chatterji, S., Price, B.: Regression Analysis by Example. John Wiley (1991)

Chatterji, S.D.: A remark on the Crame´r-Rao inequality. In: Kallianpur, G., Krishnaiah, P.R., Ghosh, J.K. (eds.) Statistics and Probability: Essays in Honor of C. R. Rao. North Holland, New York (1982)

Chaudhuri, A., Mukerjee, R.: Randomized Response: Theory and Techniques. Marcel Dekker, New York (1988)

Chikka.ra, R.S., Folks, J.L.: The Inverse Gaussian Distribution: Theory, Methodolog y, and Applications.: Marcel Dekker. New York (1989)

Chow, G.C.: Test of equality between sets of coefficient in two linear regressions. Econometrica **28**(3), 591–605 (1960)
Chow, G.C.: EconometricMethods. McGraw-Hill, New York (1983)
Christensen, R.: Plane Answers to Complex Questions: The Theory of Linear Models, 2nd edn. Springer-Verlag, New York (1987)
Christensen, R.: Log-linear Models. Springer-Verlag, New York (1990)
Christensen, R.: Plane Answers to Complex Questions. The Theory of Linear Models, 2nd edn. Springer-Verlag, New York (1996)
Christopher, A.H.: Interpreting and using regression. Sage Publication (1982)
Chung, K.L.: A Course in Probability Theory. Academic Press, New York (1974)
Chung, K.L.: A Course in Probability Theory, 2nd edn. Academic Press, New York (1974)
Chung, K.L.: A Course in Probability Theory, Harcourt. Brace & World, New York (1968)
Cleveland, W.S.: The Elements of Graphing Data. Wadsworth. Monterey (1985)
Clevensen, M.L., Zidek, J.: Simultaneous estimation of the mean of independent Poisson laws. J. Amer. Statist. Assoc. **70**, 698–705 (1975)
Clopper, C.J., Pearson, E.S.: The Use of Confidence or Fiducial Limits Illustrated in the Case of the Binomial. Biometrika **26**, 404–413 (1934)
Cochran, W.G.: Sampling technique. Wiley Eastern Limited, New Delhi (1985)
Cochran, W.G.: Sampling Techniques, 3rd edn. Wiley, New York (1977)
Cox, D.R.: The Analysis of Binary Data. Methuen, London (1970)
Cox, D.R.: Partial likelihood. Biometrika **62**, 269–276 (1975)
Cox, D.R., Oakes, D.O.: Analysis of Survival Data. Chapman & Hall, London (1984)
Cox, D.R., Hinkley, D.V.: Theoretical Statistics. Chapman and Hall, London (1974)
Crame′r, H.: Mathematical Methods of Statistics. Princeton Univer-sity Press, Princeton (1946a)
Crow, E.L., Shimizu, K.: Lognormal Distributions: Theory and Practice. Marcel Dekker, New York (1988)
Crowder, M.J., Sweeting, T.: Bayesian inference for a bivariate binomial distribution. Biometrika **76**, 599–603 (1989)
Croxton, F.E., Cowden, D.J.: Applied General Statistics. Prentice-Hall (1964)
Daniels, H.E.: Exact saddlepoint approximations. Biometrika **67**, 59–63 (1980)
DasGupta, A.: Bayes minimax estimation in multiparameter families when the parameter space is restricted to a bounded convex set. Sankhya **47**, 326–332 (1985)
DasGupta, A.: An examination of Bayesian methods and inference: In search of the truth. Technical Report, Department of Statistics, Purdue University (1994)
DasGupta, A., Rubin, H.: Bayesian estimation subject to minimaxity of the mean of a multivariate normal distribution in the case of a common unknown variance. In: Gupta, S.S., Berger, J.O. (eds.) Statistical Decision Theory and Related Topics IV. Springer-Verlag, New York (1988)
Datta, G.S., Ghosh, J.K.: On priors providing frequentist validity for Bayesian inference. Biometrika **82**, 37–46 (1995)
Dean, A., Voss, D.: Design and Analysis of Experiments.: Springer- Verlag, New York (1999)
deFinetti, B.: Probability, Induction, and Statistics. Wiley, New York (1972)
DeGroot, M.: Optimal Statistical Decisions. McGraw-Hill, New York (1970)
DeGroot, M.H.: Probability and Statistics, 2nd edn. Addison-Wesley, New York (1986)
Raj, D., Chandhok, P.: Samlpe Survey Theory. Narosa Publishing House, New Delhi (1999)
Devroye, L.: Non-Uniform Random Variate Generation. Springer-Verlag, New York (1985)
Devroye, L., Gyoerfi, L.: Nonparametric Density Estimation: The L1 View. Wiley, New York (1985)
Diaconis, P.: Theories of data analysis, from magical thinking through classical statistics. In: Hoaglin, F. Mosteller, J (eds.) Exploring Data Tables, Trends and Shapes (1985)
Diaconis, P.: Group Representations in Probability and Statistics. Institute of Mathematical Statistics, Hayward (1988)
Dobson, A.J.: An Introduction to Generalized Linear Models. Chapman & Hall, London (1990)
Draper, N.R., Smith, H.: Applied Regression Analysis, 3rd edn. Wiley, New York (1998)

Draper, N.R., Smith, H.: Applied Regression Analysis. John Wiley and Sons, New York (1981)
Dudley, R.M.: Real Analysis and Probability. Wadsworth and Brooks/Cole, Pacific Grove, CA (1989)
Durbin, J.: Estimation of parameters in time series regression model. J. R. Statis. Soc.-Ser-B, **22**, 139–153 (1960)
Dutta, M.: Econometric Methods. South Western Publishing Company, Cincinnati (1975)
Edwards, A.W.F.: Likelihood. Johns Hopkins University Press, Baltimore (1992)
Efron, B., Hinkley, D.: Assessing the accuracy of the maximum likelihood estimator: Observed vs. expected Fisher information. Biometrica **65**, 457–481 (1978)
Efron, B., Morris, C.: Empirical Bayes on vector observations-An extension of Stein's method. Biometrika **59**, 335–347 (1972)
Efron, B., Tibshirani, R.J.: An Introduction to the Bootstrap. Chapman and Hall, London (1993)
Everitt, B.S.: The Analysis of Contingency Tables, 2nd edn. Chap-man & Hall, London (1992)
Everitt, B.S.: The Analysis of Contingency Tables. John Wiley (1977)
Everitt, B.S., Hand, D.J.: Finite Mixture Distributions. Chapman & Hall, London (1981)
Ezekiel, M., Fox, K.A.: Methods of Correlation and Regression Analysis. John Wiley (1959)
Faith, R.E.: Minimax Bayes point and set estimators of a multivariate normal mean. Ph.D. thesis, Department of Statistics, University of Michigan (1976)
Feller, W.: An Introduction to Probability Theory and Its Applications, vol. 1, 3rd edn. Wiley, New York (1968)
Feller, W.: An Introduction to Probability Theory and Its Applications, vol. II. Wiley, New York (1971)
Feller, W.: An Introduction to Probability Theory and Its Applications, vol II, 2nd edn. John Wiley, New York (1971)
Ferguson, T.S.: Mathematical Statistics: A Decision Theoretic Approach. Academic Press, New York (1967)
Ferguson, T.S.: A Course in Large Sample Theory. Chapman and Hall, London (1996)
Ferguson, T.S.: Mathematical Statistics. Academic Press, New York (1967)
Field, C.A., Ronchetti, E.: Small Sample Asymptotics. Institute of Mathematical Statistics. Hayward, CA (1990)
Finney, D.J.: Probit Analysis. Cambridge University Press, New York (1971)
Fisher, R.A.: Statistical Methods and Scientific Inference, 2nd edn. Hafner, New York. Reprinted (1990). Oxford University Press, Oxford (1959)
Fisz, M.: Probability Theory and Mathematical Statistics, 3rd edn. John Wiley (1963)
Fleming, T.R., Harrington, D.P.: Counting Processes and Survival Analysis. Wiley, New York (1991)
Fox, K.: Intermediate Economic Statistics. Wiley (1968)
Fraser, D.A.S.: The Structure of Inference. Wiley, New York (1968)
Fraser, D.A.S.: Inference and Linear Models. McGraw-Hill, New York (1979)
Fraser, D.A.S.: Nonparametric Methods in Statistics. John Wiley, New York (1965)
Freedman, D., Pisani, R., Purves, R., Adhikari, A.: Statistics, 2nd edn. Norton, New York (1991)
Freund, J.E.: Mathematical Statistics. Prentice-Hall of India (1992)
Fuller, W.A.: Measurement Error Models. Wiley, New York (1987)
Gelman, A., Carlin, J., Stern, H., Rubin, D.B.: Bayesian Data Analysis. Chapman & Hall, London (1995)
Ghosh, J.K., Mukerjee, R.: Non-informative priors (with discussion). In: Bernardo, J.M., Berger, J. O., Dawid, A.P., Smith, A.F.M. (eds.) Bayesian Statistics IV. Oxford University Press, Oxford (1992)
Ghosh, J.K., Subramanyam, K.: Second order efficiency of maximum likelihood estimators. Sankhya A **36**, 325–358 (1974)
Ghosh, M., Meeden, G.: Admissibility of the MLE of the normal integer mean. Wiley, New York (1978)
Gibbons, J.D.: Nonparametric Inference. McGraw-Hill, New York (1971)

Gibbons, J.D., Chakrabarty, S.: Nonparametric Methods for Quantitative Analysis. American Sciences Press (1985)
Gilks, W.R., Richardson, S., Spiegelhalter, D.J. (eds.): Markov Chain Monte Carlo in Practice. Chapman & Hall, London (1996)
Girshick, M.A., Savage, L.J.: Bayes and minimax estimates for quadratic loss functions. University of California Press (1951)
Glejser, H.: A new test for heteroscedasticity, J. Am. Stat. Assoc. *64* 316–323 (1969)
Gnedenko, B.V.: The Theory of Probabilit y. MIR Publishers, Moscow (1978)
Godambe, V.P.: Estimating Functions. Clarendon Press, UK (1991)
Goldberg, S.: Probability, an Introduction. Prentice-Hall (1960)
Goldberger, A.S.: Econometric Theory. John Wiley and Sons, New York (1964)
Goldfield, S.M., Quandt, R.E.: Nonlinear methods in Econometrics. North Holland Publishing Company, Amsterdam (1972)
Goon, A.M., Gupta, M.K., Dasgupta, B.: Fundamentals of Statistics, vol. 1. World Press. Kolkata (1998)
Goon, A.M., Gupta, M.K., Dasgupta, B.: Fundamentals of Statistics, vol. 2. World Press. Kolkata, India (1998)
Goon, A.M., Gupta, M.K., Dasgupta, B.: Outline of Statistics, vol. 1. World Press. Kolkata (1998)
Goon, A.M., Gupta, M.K., Dasgupta, B.: Outline of Statistics, vol. 2. World Press. Kolkata (1998)
Granger, C.W.J., Mowbold, P.: R^2 and the transformation of regression variables. J. Econ. **4** 205–210 (1976)
Granger, C.W.J.: Investigating Causal Relations by Econometric Models and Cross- spectral Methods. Econometrica, 424–438 (1969)
Graybill, F.A.: Introduction to Linear Statistical Models, vol. 1. Mc-Graw Hill Inc., New York (1961)
Gujarati, D.N.: Basic Econometrics. McGraw-Hill, Inc., Singapore (1995)
Gupta, S.C., Kapoor, V.K.: Fundamentals of Mathematical Statistics. Sultan Chand and Sons. New Delhi (2002)
Haberman, S.J.: The Analysis of Frequency Data. University of Chicago Press. Chicago (1974)
Hall, P.: Pseudo-likelihood theory for empirical likelihood. Ann. Statist. **18**, 121–140 (1990)
Hall, P.: The Bootstrap and Edgeworth Expansion. Springer-Verlag, New York (1992)
Halmos, P.R.: Measure Theory. Van Nostrand, New York (1950)
Hampel, F.R., Ronchetti, E.M., Rousseeuw, P.J., Stahel, W.A.: Robust Statistics: The Approach Based on Influence Functions. Wiley, New York (1986)
Hardy, G.H., Littlewood, J.E., Polya, G.: Inequalities, 2nd edn. Cambridge University Press, London (1952)
Hedayat, A.S., Sinha, B.K.: Design and Inference in Finite Population Sampling. Wiley, New York (1991)
Helms, L.: Introduction to Potential Theory. Wiley, New York (1969)
Hinkley, D.V., Reid, N., Snell, L.: Statistical Theory and Modelling. In honor of Sir David Cox. Chapman & Hall, London (1991)
Hobert, J.: Occurrences and consequences of nonpositive Markov chains in Gibbs sampling. Ph.D. Thesis, Biometrics Unit, Cornell University (1994)
Hogg, R.V., Craig, A.T.: Introduction to Mathematical Statistics. Amerind (1972)
Hollander, M., Wolfe, D.A..: Nonparametric Statistical Methods. John Wiley (1973)
Hsu, J.C.: Multiple Comparisons: Theory and Methods. Chapman and Hall, London (1996)
Huber, P.J.: Robust Statistics. Wiley, New York (1981)
Hudson, H.M.: Empirical Bayes estimation. Technical Report No. 58, Department of Statistics, Stanford University ((1974))
Ibragimov, I.A., Has'minskii, R.Z.: Statistical Estimation: Asymptotic Theory. Springer-Verlag, New York (1981)

James, W., Stein, C.: Estimation with Quadratic Loss. In: Proceedings of the Fourth Berkele y Symposium on Mathematical Statistics and Probability 1, pp. 361–380. University of California Press, Berkeley (1961)

Johnson, N.L., Kotz, S., Kemp, A.W.: Univariate Discrete Distributions, 2nd edn. Wiley, New York (1992)

Johnson, N.L., Kotz, S.: Distributions in Statistics (4 vols.). Wiley, New York (1969–1972)

Johnson, N.L., Kotz, S., Balakrishnan, N.: Continuous Univariate Distri- butions, vol 1, 2nd edn. Wiley, New York (1994)

Johnson, N.L., Kotz. S., Balakrishnan, N.: Continuous Univariate Distributions, vol. 2, 2d edn. Wiley, New York (1995)

Johnston, J.: Econometric Methods, 3rd edn. Mc-Grawl-Hill Book Company (1985)

Kagan, A.M., Linnik, YuV, Rao, C.R.: Characterization Problems in Mathe- matical Statistics. Wiley, New York (1973)

Kalbfleisch, J.D., Prentice, R.L.: The Statistical Analysis of Failure Time Data. Wiley, New York (1980)

Kane, E.J.: Econmic Statistics and Econometrics. Harper International (1968)

Kapoor, J.N., Saxena, H.C.: Mathematical Statistics. S Chand and Co (Pvt) Ltd, New Delhi (1973)

Kelker, D.: Distribution Theory of Spherical Distributions and a Location-Scale Parameter Generalization. Sankhya. Ser. A **32**, 419–430 (1970)

Kempthorne, P.: Dominating inadmissible procedures using compromise decision theory. In: Gupta, S.S., Berger, J.O. (eds.) Statistical Decision Theory IV. Springer-Verlag, New York (1988a)

Kendall, M.G., Stuart, A.: The Advance Theory of Statistics vol. 3, 2nd edn. Charles Griffin and Company Limited, London (1968)

Kendall, M., Stuart, A.: The Advance Theory of Statistics, vol. 2. Charles Griffin and Co. Ltd., London (1973)

Kendall, M., Stuart, A.: The Advance Theory of Statistics. vol 1. Charles Griffin and Co. Ltd., London (1977)

Kendall, M.G.: Rank Correlation Methods, 3rd edn. Griffin, London (1962)

Kendall, M., Stuart, A.: The Advanced Theory of Statistics, Volume II: Inference and Relationship, 4th edn. Macmillan, New York (1979)

Kiefer, J.: Multivariate optimality results. In: Krishnaiah, P. (ed.) Multivariate Analysis. Academic Press, New York (1966)

Kirk, R.E.: Experimental Design: Procedures for the Behavioral Sciences, 2nd edn. Brooks/Cole, Pacific Grove (1982)

Klien, L.R., Shinkai, Y.: An Econometric Model of Japan, 1930-1959. International Economic Review **4**, 1–28 (1963)

Klien, L.R.: An Introduction to Econometrics. Prentice-Hall (1962)

Kmenta, J.: Elements of Econometrics, 2nd edn. Macmillan, New York (1986)

Kolmogorov, A.N., Fomin, S.V.: Elements of the Theory of Functions and Functional Analysis, vol. 2. Graylock Press, Albany, New York (1961)

Koroljuk, V.S., Borovskich, YuV: Theory of U-Statistics. Kluwer Academic Publishers, Boston (1994)

Koutsoyiannis, A.: Theory of Econometrics. Macmillan Press Ltd., London (1977)

Kraft, C.H., Van Eeden, C.: A Nonparametric Introduction to Statistics. Mac-millan, New York (1968)

Kramer, J.S.: The logit Model for Economists. Edward Arnold publishers, London (1991)

Kuehl, R.O.: Design of Experiments: Statistical Principles of Research Design and Analysis, 2nd edn. Pacific Grove, Duxbury (2000)

Lane, D.A.: Fisher, Jeffreys, and the nature of probability. In: Fienberg, S.E., Hinkley, D.V. (eds.) R.A. Fisher: An Appreciation. Lecture Notes in Statistics 1. Springer-Verlag, New York (1980)

Lange, N., Billard, L., Conquest, L., Ryan, L., Brillinger, D., Greenhouse, J. (eds.): Case Studies in Biometry. Wiley-Interscience, New York (1994)

Le Cam, L.: Maximum Likelihood: An Introduction. Lecture Notes in Statistics No. 18. University of Maryland, College Park, Md (1979)

Le Cam, L.: Asymptotic Methods in Statistical Decision Theory. Springer-Verlag, New York (1986)

Le Cam, L., Yang, G.L.: Asymptotics in Statistics: Some Basic Concepts. Springer-Verlag, New York (1990)

Lehmann, E.L.: Testing Statistical Hypotheses, 2nd edn. Wiley, New York (1986)

Lehmann, E.L.: Introduction to Large-Sample Theory. Springer-Verlag, New York (1999)

Lehmann, E.L.: Testing Statistical Hypotheses, Second Edition (TSH2). Springer-Verlag, New York (1986)

Lehmann, E.L.: Elements of Large-Sample Theory. Springer-Verlag, New York (1999)

Lehmann, E.L.: Testing Statistical Hypotheses. John Wiley, New York (1959)

Lehmann, E.L., Scholz, F.W.: Ancillarity. In: Ghosh, M., Pathak, P.K. (eds.) Current Issues in Statistical Inference: Essays in Honor of D. Basu. Institute of Mathematical Statistics, Hayward (1992)

Lehmann, E.L., Casella, G.: Theory of Point Estimation, 2nd edn. Springer-Verlag, New York (1998)

LePage, R., Billard, L.: Exploring the Limits of Bootstrap. Wiley, New York (1992)

Leser, C.: Econometric Techniques and Problemss. Griffin (1966)

Letac, G., Mora, M.: Natural real exponential families with cubic variance functions. Ann. Statist. **18**, 1–37 (1990)

Lindgren, B.W.: Statistical Theory, 2nd edn. The Macmillan Company, New York (1968)

Lindley, D.V.: The Bayesian analysis of contingency tables. Ann. Math. Statist. **35**, 1622–1643 (1964)

Lindley, D.V.: Introduction to Probability and Statistics. Cambridge University Press, Cambridge (1965)

Lindley, D.V.: Introduction to Probability and Statistics from a Bayesian Viewpoint. Part 2. Inference. Cambridge University Press, Cambridge (1965)

Little, R.J.A., Rubin, D.B.: Statistical Analysis with Missing Data. Wiley, New York (1987)

Liu, C., Rubin, D.B.: The ECME algorithm: A simple extension of EM and ECM with faster monotone convergence. Biometrika **81**, 633–648 (1994)

Loeve, M.: Probability Theory, 3rd edn. Van Nostrand, Princeton (1963)

Luenberger, D.G.: Optimization by Vector Space Methods. Wiley, New York (1969)

Lukacs, E.: Characteristic Functions, 2nd edn. Hafner, New York (1970)

Lukacs, E.: Probability and Mathematical Statistics. Academic Press, New York (1972)

Madala: Limited Dependent and Qualitative Variables in Econometrics. Cambridge University Press, New York (1983)

Madnani, J.M.K.: Introduction to Econometrics: Principles and Applications, 4th edn. Oxford and 1BH publishing Co. Pvt. Ltd (1988)

Maritz, J.S., Lwin, T.: Empirical Bayes Methods, 2nd edn. Chapman & Hall, London (1989)

Marshall, A., Olkin, I.: Inequalities—Theory of Majorization and its Applications. Academic Press. New York (1979)

McCullagh, P.: Quasi-likelihood and estimating functions. In: Hinkley, D., Reid, N., Snell, L. (eds.) Statistical Theory and Modelling: In Honor of Sir David Cox. Chapman & Hall, London (1991)

McCullagh, P., Nelder, J.A.: Generalized Linear Models, 2nd edn. Chapman & Hall, London (1989)

McLa.chlan, G., Krishnan, T.: The EM Algorithm and Extensions. Wiley, New York (1997)

McLachlan, G.: Recent Advances in Finite Mixture Models. Wiley, New York (1997)

McLachlan, G., Basford, K.: Mixture Models: Inference and Applications to Clustering. Marcel Dekker, New York (1988)

McLachlan, G., Krishnan, T.: The EM Algorithm and Extensions. Wiley, New York (1997)
McPherson, G.: Statistics in Scientific Investigation. Springer-Verlag, New York (1990)
Meng, X.-L., Rubin, D.B.: Maximum likelihood estimation via the ECM algo-rithm: A general framework. Biometrika **80**, 267–278 (1993)
Meyn, S., Tweedie, R.: Markov Chains and Stochastic Stability. Springer-Verlag, New York (1993)
Miller, R.G.: Simultaneous Statistical Inference, 2nd edn. Springer-Verlag, New York (1981)
Montgomery, D., Elizabeth, P.: Introduction to Linear Regression Analysis. John Wiley & Sons (1982)
Mood, A.M., Graybill, F.A., Boes, D.C.: Introduction to the Theory of Statistics. McGraw-Hill (1974)
Murray, M.K., Rice, J.W.: Differential Geometry and Statistics. Chap-man & Hall, London (1993)
Neter, J., Wasserman, W., Whitmore, G.A.: Applied Statistics. Allyn & Bacon, Boston (1993)
Novick, M.R., Jackson, P.H.: Statistical Methods for Educational and Psycho-logical Research. McGraw-Hill, New York (1974)
Oakes, D.: Life-table analysis. Statistical Theory and Modelling, in Honor of Sir David Cox, FRS. Chapman & Hall, London (1991)
Olkin, I., Selliah, J.B.: Estimating covariances in a multivariate distribution. In: Gupta, S.S., Moore, D.S. (eds) Statistical Decision Theory and Related Topics II. Academic Press, New York (1977)
Owen, A.: Empirical likelihood ratio confidence intervals for a single functional. Biometrika **75**, 237–249 (1988)
Panse, V.G., Sukhatme, P.V.: Statistical methods for agricultural workers. Indian Council of Agricultural Research, New Delhi (1989)
Park, R.E.: Estimation with heteroscedastic error terms. Econometrica. **34**(4), 888 (1966)
Parzen, E.: Modern Probability Theory and Its Applications. Wiley Eastern (1972)
Pfanzagl, J.: Parametric Statistical Theory. DeGruyter, New York (1994)
Raifa, H., Schlaifer, R.: Applied Statistical Decision Theory. Published by Division of Research, Harvard Business School, Harvard University, Boston (1961)
Rao, C.R.: Simultaneous estimation of parameters—A compound decision problem. In: Gupta, S. S., Moore, D.S. (eds.) Decision Theory and Related Topics. Academic Press, New York (1977)
Rao, C.R.: Linear Statistical Inference and Its Applications. John Wiley, New York (1965)
Rao, C.R., Kleffe, J.: Estimation of variance components and applications. North Holland/Elsevier, Amsterdam (1988)
Ripley, B.D.: Stochastic Simulation. Wiley, New York (1987)
Robbins, H.: Asymptotically subminimax solutions of compound statistical decision problems. In: Proceedings Second Berkeley Symposium Mathematics Statistics Probability. University of California Press, Berkeley (1951)
Robert, C., Casella, G.: Improved confidence statements for the usual multivariate normal confidence set. In: Gupta, S.S., Berger, J.O. (eds.) Statistical Decision Theory V. Springer-Verlag, New York (1994)
Robert, C., Casella, G.: Monte Carlo Statistical Methods. Springer-Verlag, New York (1998)
Robert, C.P.: The Bayesian Choice. Springer-Verlag, New York (1994)
Rohatgi, V.K.: Statistical Inference. Wiley, New York (1984)
Romano, J.P., Siegel, A.F.: Counter examples in Probability and Statistics. Wadsworth and Brooks/Cole, Pacific Grove (1986)
Rosenblatt, M.: Markov Processes. Structure and Asymptotic Behavior. Springer-Verlag, New York (1971)
Ross, S.M.: A First Course in Probability Theory, 3rd edn. Macmillan, New York (1988)
Ross, S.: Introduction to Probability Models, 3rd edn. Academic Press, New York (1985)
Rothenberg, T.J.: The Bayesian approach and alternatives in econometrics. In: Fienberg, S., Zellner, A. (eds.) Stud- ies in Bayesian Econometrics and Statistics, vol. 1. North-Holland, Amsterdam (1977)

Rousseeuw, P.J., Leroy, A.M.: Robust Regression and Outlier Detection. Wiley, New York (1987)
Royall, R.M.: Statistical Evidence: A Likelihood Paradigm. Chapman and Hall, London (1997)
Rubin, D.B.: Using the SIR Algorithm to Simulate Posterior Distributions. In: Bernardo, J.M., DeGroot, M.H., Lindley, D.V., Smith, A.F.M. (eds.) Bayesian Statistics, pp. 395–402. Oxford University Press, Cambridge (1988)
Rudin, W.: Principles of Real Anal ysis. McGraw-Hill, New York (1976)
Sahu, P.K.: Agriculture and Applied Statistics-I.2nd Reprint. Kalyani Publishers, New Delhi, India (2013)
Sahu, P.K., Das, A.K.: Agriculture and Applied Statistics-II, 2nd edn. Kalyani Publishers, New Delhi, India (2014)
Sahu, P.K.: Research Methodology-A Guide for Researchers in Agricultural Science. Springer, Social science and other related fields (2013)
Sa¨rndal, C-E., Swenson, B., and retman, J.: Model Assisted Survey Sampling. Springer-Verlag, New York (1992)
Savage, L.J.: The Foundations of Statistics. Wiley, Rev. ed., Dover Publications, New York (1954, 1972)
Savage, L.J.: On rereading R. A. Fisher (with discussion). Ann. Statist. **4**, 441–500 (1976)
Schafer, J.L.: Analysis of Incomplete Multivariate Data. Chapman and Hall, London (1997)
Scheffe, H.: The Analysis of Variance. John Wiley and Sons, New York (1959)
Schervish, M.J.: Theory of Statistics. Springer-Verlag, New York (1995)
Scholz, F.W.: Maximum likelihood estimation. In: Kotz, S., Johnson, N.L., Read, C.B. (eds.) Encyclopedia of Statistical Sciences **5**. Wiley, New York (1985)
Searle, S.R.: Linear Models. Wiley, New York (1971)
Searle, S.R.: Matrix Algebra Useful for Statistics. Wiley, New York (1982)
Searle, S.R.: Linear Models for Unbalanced Data. Wiley, New York (1987)
Searle, S.R., Casella, G., McCulloch, C.E.: Variance Components. Wiley, New York (1992)
Seber, G.A.F.: Linear Regression Analysis. Wiley, New York (1977)
Seber, G.A.F., Wild, C.J.: Nonlinear Regression. John Wiley (1989)
Seshadri, V.: The Inverse Gaussian Distribution. A Case Stud y in Exponential Families. Clarendon Press, New York (1993)
Shao, J.: Mathematical Statistics. Springer-Verlag, New York (1999)
Shao, J., Tu, D.: The Jackknife and the Bootstrap. Springer- Verlag, New York (1995)
Siegel, S.: Nonparametric Statistics for the Behavioral Sciences. McGraw-Hill (1956)
Silverman, B.W.: Density Estimation for Statistic and Data Analysis. Chap-man & Hall, London (1986)
Daroga, S., Chaudhary, F.S.: Theory and Analysis of Sample Survey Designs. Wiley Eastern Limited. New Delhi (1989)
Singh, R.K., Chaudhary, B.D.: Biometrical methods in quantitative genetic analysis. Kalyani Publishers. Ludhiana (1995)
Snedecor, G.W., Cochran, W.G.: Statistical Methods, 8th edn. Iowa. State University Press, Ames (1989)
Snedecor, G.W., Cochran, W.G.: Statistical Methods. Iowa State University Press (1967)
Spiegel, M.R.: Theory and Problems of Statistics. McGraw-Hill Book Co., Singapore (1988)
Staudte, R.G., Sheather, S.J.: Robust Estimation and Testing. Wiley, New York (1990)
Stein, C.: Efficient nonparametric testing and estimation. In: Proceedings Third Berkeley Symposium Mathematics Statististics Probability 1. University of California Press (1956a)
Stein, C.: Inadmissibility of the usual estimator for the mean of a multivariate distribution. In: Proceedings Third Berkeley Symposium Mathematics Statististics Probability 1. University of California Press (1956b)
Stigler, S.: The History of Statistics: The Measurement of Uncertainty before 1900. Harvard University Press, Cambridge (1986)
Stuart, A., Ord, J.K.: Kendall' s Advanced Theory of Statistics, vol. I, 5th edn. Oxford University Press, New York (1987)

Stuart, A., Ord, J.K.:Kendall's Advanced Theory of Statistics, Volume I: Distribution Theory, 5th edn. Oxford University Press, New York (1987)
Stuart, A., Ord, J.K.: Kendall' s Advanced Theory of Statistics, vol. II, 5th edn. Oxford University Press, New York (1991)
Stuart, A., Ord, J.K., Arnold, S.: Advanced Theory of Statistics, Volume 2A: Classical Inference and the Linear Model, 6th edn. Oxford University Press, London (1999)
Susarla, V.: Empirical Bayes theory. In: Kotz, S., Johnson, N.L., Read, C.B. (eds.) Encyclopedia of Statistical Sciences **2**. Wiley, New York (1982)
Tanner, M.A.: Tools for Statistical Inference: Observed Data and Data Augmentation Methods, 3rd edn. Springer-Verlag, New York (1996)
The Selected Papers of E. S. Pearson. Cambridge University Press, New York (1966)
Theil, H.: On the Relationships Involving Qualitative Variables. American J. Sociol. **76**, 103–154 (1970)
Theil, H.: Principles of Econometrics. North Holland (1972)
Theil, H.: Introduction to Econometrics. Prentice-Hall (1978)
Thompson, W.A. Jr.: Applied Probability, Holt, Rinehart and Winston. New York (1969)
Tintner, G.: Econometrics. John Wiley and Sons, New York (1965)
Tukey, J.W.: A survey of sampling from contaminated distributions. In: Olkin, I. (ed.) Contributions to Probability and Statistics. Stanford University Press. Stanford (1960)
Unni, K.: The theory of estimation in algebraic and analytical exponential families with applications to variance components models. PhD. Thesis, Indian Statistical Institute, Calcutta, India ((1978))
Wald, A.: Statistical Decision Functions. Wiley, New York (1950)
Walker, H.M., Lev, J.: Statistical Inference. Oxford & IBH (1965)
Wand, M.P., Jones, M.C.: Kernel Smoothing. Chapman & Hall, London (1995)
Wasserman, L.: Recent methodological advances in robust Bayesian inference (with discussion). In: Bernardo, J.M, Berger, J.O., David, A.P. (eds.) Bayesian Statistics 4 (1990)
Weiss, L., Wolfowitz, J.: Maximum Probability Estimators and Related Topics. Springer-Verlag, New York (1974)
White, H.: A heterosedasticity consistent covariance matrix estimator and direct test of heterosedasticity. Econometrica **48** 817–898 (1980)
Wilks, S.S.: Mathematical Statistics. John Wiley, New York (1962)
Williams, E.J.: Regression Analysis. Wiley, New York (1959)
Wu, C.F.J.: On the convergence of the EM algorithm. Ann. Statist. **11**, 95–103 (1983)
Yamada, S. and Morimoto, H. (1992). Sufficiency. In: Ghosh, M., Pathak, P.K. (eds.) Current Issues in Statistical Inference: Essays in Honor of D. Basu. Institute of Mathematical Statistics, Hayward, CA
Yamane, T.: Statistics. Harper International (1970)
Yule, G.U., Kendell, M.G.: Introduction to the Theory of Statistics (Introduction). Charles Griffin, London (1950)
Zacks, S.: The Theory of Statistical Inference. John Wiley, New York (1971)
Zellner, A.: An Introduction to Bayesian Inference in Econometrics. Wiley, New York (1971)

Stuart, A., Ord, J.K.: Kendall's Advanced Theory of Statistics, [illegible] Distribution Theory, 5th edn. Oxford University Press, [illegible]
Stuart, A., Ord, J.K.: Kendall's Advanced Theory of Statistics, [illegible] Hafner, New York [illegible]
Stuart, A., [illegible] Arnold, S.: Advanced Theory of Statistics, Volume 2A: Classical Inference and the Linear Model, 6th edn. Oxford University Press, London (1999)
Susarla, V.: [illegible] theory. In: Kotz, S., Johnson, N.L., Read, C.B. (eds.) Encyclopedia of Statistical Sciences, [illegible] Wiley, New York (1985)
Tanner, M.A.: Tools for Statistical Inference: Observed Data and Data Augmentation Methods, [illegible] Springer-Verlag, New York (1996)
Thisted, R.A.: [illegible] Cambridge University Press, New York (1988)
[illegible] Quality [illegible] Journal of Quality Technology [illegible] 103–124 (1971)
[illegible] Smith, Elder (1902)
[illegible] Prentice-Hall (1958)
Thompson, [illegible] Sampling [illegible] Wiley, New York (1992)
[illegible] Wiley and Sons, New York (1996)
[illegible] sampling from populations [illegible]
[illegible] Statistics [illegible]
[illegible] estimation [illegible] mixture [illegible] models. PhD [illegible] Institute [illegible]
[illegible] Wiley, New York (1976)
[illegible]
[illegible] Sampling [illegible] Computing [illegible]
[illegible] Statistical [illegible]
[illegible] Vol. 3 [illegible] (1994)
[illegible] Springer-Verlag, New York [illegible]
[illegible] consistent [illegible] and [illegible] Test [illegible] 81 (1998) [illegible]
Wilks, [illegible] John Wiley, New York (1962)
[illegible] Wiley, New York [illegible]
[illegible]
Yamada, [illegible] (1992) [illegible]
[illegible] Statistical Inference [illegible] Mathematics [illegible]
[illegible]
[illegible] Introduction to the Theory of [illegible] Institute, [illegible]
[illegible] Statistical Inference [illegible] Wiley, New York (1971)
Zellner, A.: An Introduction to Bayesian Inference in Econometrics. Wiley, New York (1971)

Index

P.K. Sahu et al., *Estimation and Inferential Statistics*,
DOI 10.1007/978-81-322-2514-0

Printed in the United States
By Bookmasters